Comprehensive

Coronary

Care

Second Edition

KT-386-797

Comprehensive Coronary Care

Second Edition

Nigel I Jowett

MD, MRCP, MB, BS, MRCS, LRCP
Director of Clinical Medicine and Consultant Physician
Pembrokeshire Health Trust

and

David R Thompson

BSc, MA, PhD, RN, FRCN
Professor of Nursing Studies
University of Hull

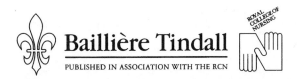

Baillière Tindall
PUBLISHED IN ASSOCIATION WITH THE RCN

Baillière Tindall   24–28 Oval Road
London NW1 7DX

The Curtis Center
Independence Square West
Philadelphia, PA 19106-3399, USA

Harcourt Brace & Company
55 Horner Avenue
Toronto, Ontario M8Z 4X6, Canada

Harcourt Brace & Company, Australia
30–52 Smidmore Street
Marrickville
NSW 2204, Australia

Harcourt Brace & Company, Japan
Ichibancho Central Building
22-1 Ichibancho
Chiyoda-ku, Tokyo 102, Japan

© 1996 Baillière Tindall

This book is printed on acid-free paper

All rights reserved. No part of this publication may be reproduced, stored in a retrieval system or transmitted, in any form or by any other means, electronic, mechanical, photocopying or otherwise, without the prior permission of Baillière Tindall, 24–28 Oval Road, London NW1 7DX

First printed 1995 by Scutari Press

A catalogue record for this book is available from the British Library

ISBN 1-873853-21-2

Printed and bound in Great Britain by WBC Book Manufacturers Ltd, Bridgend, Mid Glamorgan

Contents

Contents

Acknowledgements

We would like to thank all those readers who have been kind enough to contact us with both praise and constructive criticism of the first edition. We invite current readers to do the same. We have hopefully addressed the errors and omissions of our first attempt, and would specifically like to thank doctors Roger Hall, Liam Penny, Mike Wort and Ian Martin and nurses Tom Quinn and Rose Webster for their contributions. Special and very grateful thanks to Sheena Jowett for typing the manuscript, and to Val Creese for generally co-ordinating things.

NIJ
DRT

Preface

There can be few areas of medicine in which clinical practice has changed so radically over the last 5 years as acute cardiac care. The publication of the first edition of our book, in 1989, coincided with that of several major cardiological trials and was only able to give a glimpse of what was to come. Nowadays, the modern management of patients with acute myocardial infarction requires more than diamorphine and a defibrillator, and we can now deliver optimal coronary care, based almost entirely on the results of good clinical trials. The benefits of thrombolysis, aspirin, beta-blockers and ACE-inhibitors are now clear, and nitrates, magnesium, antidysrhythmic agents and calcium-channel blockers have been shown to have no place in the routine management of acute myocardial infarction. The concept of triage has brought cardiac nurses back into the front line, to minimise the 'door-to-needle' time for thrombolysis, and the new, simplified resuscitation guidelines have underscored the value of a practised coronary care team in providing rapid life support and defibrillation.

In July 1992, the British government set out its health strategy in a White Paper, *The Health of the Nation*. Coronary heart disease was chosen as a key area for investment and intervention for the reduction of cardiac morbidity and mortality. The role of acute coronary care has never been stronger, and we hope this book continues to provide a useful guide for all who practise this exciting discipline.

Nigel I Jowett
David R Thompson

Note: Throughout this book the authors have avoided the use of 'him/her', 'he/she' etc. and have opted for the male pronoun when refering to the patient and the female pronoun for the nurse, whenever possible, to make for ease of reading.

Preface to the First Edition

The role of coronary care has changed markedly since its inception in the early 1960s, and it now has an extended importance for patients with other manifestations of coronary artery disease, and for those with critical cardiac dysfunction who require intensive care and cardiovascular monitoring. This book is intended as an up-to-date guide to this current practice of 'cardiac intensive care', and to provide a basis for further exploration of the subject. Because we believe that such practice is not the sole domain of either nursing or medical staff we have tried to utilise an integrated approach, suitable for all those concerned in patient management on the coronary care unit. Some of our material extends outside the traditional boundaries of coronary care, but we think it important that it is appreciated how the patients come to be there, and what may happen to them after they leave.

Whilst we hope that nurses never lose sight of their primary caring role, in reality much of their work in the area of coronary care involves a high degree of medical and technical expertise, and our book reflects this. We have assumed that nurse-readers have a basic understanding of primary nursing, the nursing process, nursing theories and conceptual models, and only salient features are mentioned in the text.

Nigel I Jowett
David R Thompson

1

Introduction to Coronary Care

Coronary heart disease is the major cause of morbidity and mortality in all Western industrialised countries (Figure 1.1). In the UK, there is a death due to coronary heart disease in a person under the age of 65 years every 16 minutes, and one in five men will have a heart attack before retirement. In women, it is the second major cause of death, cancer being the first. Overall, coronary heart disease was responsible for 26% of all deaths in England in 1991, with even higher rates in the rest of the UK. Although coronary mortality continues to decline in the West, it is still depriving the economy of people in their most productive years and many young families of their parents (Office of Health Economics, 1990). Coronary heart disease events account for 2.5% of the total NHS expenditure; approximately 30% of acute medical beds are occupied by patients with coronary heart disease, and there are about

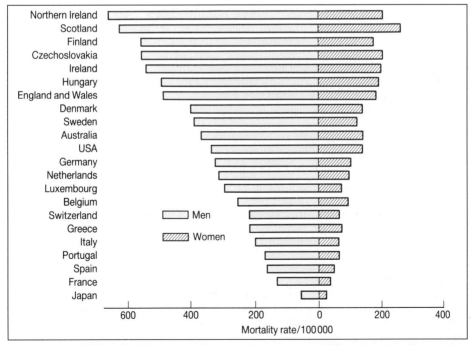

Fig. 1.1 Coronary heart disease mortality rates in 1988 for men and women aged 35–74 years. Data from *WHO Statistics Annual* (1988). Geneva: WHO.

115 000 hospital discharges annually in England and Wales with the diagnosis of coronary heart disease, placing an enormous drain on health-care budgets (Mann and Marmot, 1987). In addition, the economic cost in terms of lost industrial production time and sickness benefit payments is enormous; there were 35 million lost working days in 1990. Thus, it can be seen that coronary heart disease has a major impact, in both human and economic terms.

Over the past 10 years, there have been considerable advances in the medical management of coronary heart disease, many of which have resulted from applying the findings of huge clinical trials involving many thousands of patients with acute myocardial infarction. It was the Clinical Trial Service Unit in Oxford which started the trend for 'mega-trials', from the first International Study of Infarct Survival (ISIS-1) in 1988, with over 16 000 patients studied, to the recently-reported results of the largest ever randomised trial, ISIS-4, which recruited a huge total of 58 000 patients (ISIS-4, 1995). Whilst ISIS-1 studied the acute administration of beta-blockers following myocardial infarction (mortality reduced by 15 per cent), ISIS-2 (1988), ISIS-3 (1992) and ISIS-4 have investigated the role of various thrombolytic agents with other drugs (such as heparin, magnesium, aspirin, nitrates and ACE-inhibitors) in the management of acute myocardial infarction (Table 1.1). There have been several other similar randomised trials, all including over one thousand patients and demonstrating that fibrinolytic therapy can reduce mortality in acute myocardial infarction, a conclusion that has had probably the biggest impact on current cardiological practice in the last decade (Ridker et al, 1993). The overview of these trials by the Fibrinolytic Therapy Trialists' Collaborative Group (1994) has indicated that fibrinolytic therapy is, in fact, beneficial in a much wider group of patients than currently receive it routinely, offering this life-saving treatment to an even greater number of patients.

The World Health Organization (1979) has outlined the concept of 'comprehensive coronary care' as a systematic approach to the control of heart

Table 1.1 Summary results of the 'mega-trials'

ASPIRIN for ALL suspected acute myocardial infarction or unstable angina (+ LONG-TERM aspirin after hospital)
Benefit: 20–30 lives/1000 (+ definite EXTRA from LONG TERM)

FIBRINOLYTICS for patients with bundle branch block or ST elevation who are within 0–12 hours of pain onset
Benefit: 30 lives/1000 in these patients (or more, with EARLIER treatment)

BETA-BLOCKERS, STARTED EARLY with iv dose (except in shock or persistent hypotension) and continued LONG TERM
Benefit: about 5 lives/1000 in first month (+ definite EXTRA from LONG TERM)

ACE-INHIBITORS, STARTED EARLY (except in shock or persistent hypotension) and continued LONG TERM, especially if failure threatens
Benefit: about 5 lives/1000 in first month (perhaps 10 lives/1000 in high-risk groups + EXTRA from LONG TERM in those with left ventricular dysfunction)

NB Heparin, magnesium, nitrates: little or no net benefit (and little difference in net clinical benefit between different antiplatelet agents, or between different fibrinolytic agents).

disease throughout the whole of its natural history. For the management of acute myocardial infarction, this will include:

- Primary and secondary prevention
- Prehospital coronary care
- Acute and intermediate coronary care
- Rehabilitation

PRIMARY AND SECONDARY PREVENTION

Coronary heart disease may present as congestive heart failure, conduction defects, dysrhythmias, angina pectoris or myocardial infarction. Most cases of unexpected death are also attributable to coronary heart disease. The detection of coronary atherosclerosis is often delayed, because the extent of coronary atheroma may be masked by collateral coronary circulation; coronary insufficiency only becomes obvious when there is disequilibrium between the demand for oxygen by the myocardium and the coronary blood supply. The estimated prevalence of coronary heart disease in asymptomatic, middle-aged men is 4%, and their typical course is shown in Figure 1.2. Often, by the time that the clinical signs and symptoms of coronary heart disease have developed, atherosclerosis is found to be in an advanced stage, with stenosed arteries lined by calcified and necrotic atheromatous

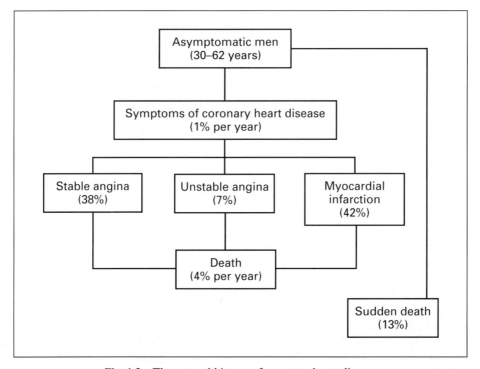

Fig. 1.2   The natural history of coronary heart disease

plaques. Therapy at this stage would seem nothing more than palliative and provides good reason for particular emphasis on preventative measures.

Primary prevention of coronary heart disease aims either to prevent the first heart attack or to delay the appearance of other symptoms related to myocardial ischaemia, such as dysrhythmias, heart failure and angina. Secondary prevention includes any treatment that reduces the risk of death or a second heart attack in a patient who has already suffered a myocardial infarction. The two modes of prevention will not necessarily be the same, since the underlying pathological processes and relative risks are not the same. The benefits of therapy will not necessarily be the same, either.

Many different factors may lead to damage of the coronary vasculature to produce the same final result – accumulation of atheroma and coronary heart disease. Attention is usually focused on certain factors that have been implicated in the accelerated development of coronary heart disease (British Cardiac Society Working Group on Coronary Prevention, 1987). These include hypertension, hyperlipidaemia, diabetes mellitus, cigarette smoking, obesity, physical inactivity and stress. However, these disorders alone are not implicated in all cases of coronary heart disease, and there may, additionally, be an inherited risk. The presence of early coronary heart disease in a first-degree relative is very common in young patients who present with myocardial infarction and, as such, represents a strong risk factor. This, of course, may simply reflect the similarity of a shared environment and life-style, but it is likely that there is a significant genetic predisposition (Jowett, 1984).

In July 1992, the Department of Health set out its health strategy in a White Paper *The Health of the Nation* (Secretary of State for Health, 1992). As a major cause of premature death, coronary heart disease (along with stroke) was chosen as a key area for investment and intervention. The stated aim is to reduce coronary heart disease in people aged under 65 by 40% by the year 2000, and in those over 65 by 30%. These targets are neither unrealistic nor particularly ambitious, and they have already been achieved by Australia and the USA in the decade 1978–1988 (Stamler, 1985). In fact, coronary heart disease mortality in the West has been falling steadily since the decade 1970–1980. Explanations of why the mortality rate is falling have pointed to a combination of factors, rather than a single cause, and it may be attributed to the combined effects of prevention and medical treatments (Gillum et al, 1984; Goldman and Cook, 1984; Kannel and Thom, 1984).

The marked fall in mortality amongst younger patient groups is consistent with a primary prevention effect (Figure 1.3). In those countries with the fastest falling coronary mortality rate, there has been a general change in life-style, with a reduction in the smoking rate and ingestion of saturated fats and an increase in levels of physical activity (especially jogging). This has been seen particularly in Wales, where there may be additional benefits from the prevention project 'Heartbeat Wales' (Osmond and Barker, 1991). In England, the large and comprehensive coronary prevention programme 'Look After Your Heart' (LAYH) was launched in April 1987 by the Department of Health and has published its prevention strategy for reducing deaths by 25% by the year 2000 (Department of Health, 1990). Indeed, if the present rate of decline in the mortality from coronary heart disease

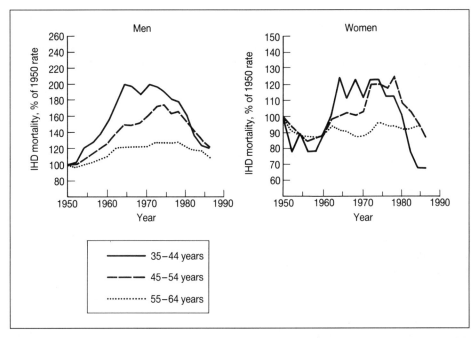

Fig. 1.3 Deaths from coronary heart disease (IHD) in England and Wales compared with rates in 1950–1951. Data from *Office of Population Censuses and Surveys Mortality Statistics 1950–90*. London: HMSO.

continues, we may hope to see it disappear as the major cause of death in people under 70 years within the next 20 years (Mulcahy et al, 1993).

Improved medical management of coronary heart disease has been responsible for a large and continuing reduction in coronary mortality (Beaglehole, 1986). The accomplishments of coronary care units, where the detection and treatment of potentially fatal dysrhythmias following myocardial infarction are of major importance, have been emphasised. The incidence of ventricular fibrillation is about 5% of admissions to coronary care, of which over 90% are now usually reversed. Strategies to limit infarct size are now having a major impact on the falling cardiovascular mortality, with the introduction of new drugs (such as the ACE-inhibitors and thrombolytic agents) plus the revival of some old ones (e.g. aspirin). The contribution of improved surgical techniques (bypass surgery and coronary angioplasty) is acting significantly to enhance the prognosis. Finally, prehospital resuscitation and therapeutic intervention are playing an increasing role in patient management with a superior outcome.

PREHOSPITAL CORONARY CARE

'Sudden death' is a term used to describe an event that affects a group of people who at one moment appear fit and well and then suddenly collapse, to die in less than an hour (and often immediately). Some of these will have experienced chest pain or dyspnoea in the preceding few days, and most will have a previous history of cardiovascular disease. The chances of survival are directly related to the speed with which resuscitative· measures can be instituted. The event is presumably caused by a ventricular dysrhythmia (ventricular tachycardia or fibrillation), but whether this is triggered by coronary emboli, coronary thrombosis or biochemical abnormalities is unknown.

Two-thirds of the deaths associated with myocardial infarction occur outside hospital, mostly within 2 hours of the onset of symptoms. Since these are mainly due to ventricular fibrillation, urgent resuscitative measures and defibrillation are required. If the recognition and prompt treatment of cardiac arrest were more widely appreciated by the general public, many more lives could be saved. In Seattle, USA, up to half the general population are fully trained in bystander-initiated resuscitation. Such a programme of public education has resulted in a doubling of survival rates, from 21 to 43%, following witnessed cardiac arrest, and of those resuscitated, half leave hospital (Thompson et al, 1979). Wider availability of automatic, semi-automatic or transtelephonic defibrillators could further increase the likelihood of survival from out-of-hospital cardiac arrest (Dickey and Adgey, 1992).

With the recognition that the provision of early and skilled intervention is of major importance, prehospital care has taken on a more important role in recent years. Coronary ambulances, as described by Pantridge and Geddes (1967), have been further developed, with specialist medical, nursing or paramedical staff employed as mobile emergency units, giving appreciable benefits (Lewis et al, 1993). Initially, the idea was to get a defibrillator to the patient and then to relieve pain and stabilise rhythm before travel to hospital (Mathewson et al, 1985). Now, these mobile units have a potentially critical role in the administration of thrombolytic agents. Acute coronary thrombosis often leads rapidly to myocardial necrosis, leaving little time for therapeutic intervention. The position is better if a collateral coronary blood circulation has developed, or if coronary occlusion evolves gradually (stuttering ischaemia), but myocardial necrosis will still take place if adequate perfusion is not restored. The prognosis of the survivor of a heart attack is mainly dependent on the quantity of myocardium destroyed; infarcted tissue cannot be repaired, and damage will affect the heart's function as an efficient pump. The resultant cardiac failure and dysrhythmias caused by areas of necrosis and regional anoxia are, then, the main treatable areas that will influence outcome.

Since most cases of coronary thrombosis occur at home, there is a real opportunity for general practitioners to be very much in the forefront of prehospital myocardial salvage (Colquhoun, 1993). Currently, only about 16% of patients in the UK receive thrombolytic therapy within 2 hours of the onset of chest pain (J S Birkhead, personal communication). Patients treated by mobile coronary ambulances receive thrombolysis up to 1 hour before those who are taken to hospital (EMIP, 1988), and where general practitioners offer a first response service, the 'call-to-needle' time may be as little as 43 minutes (GREAT study group, 1992). Prehospital thrombolysis could become widespread in the UK, with sufficient organisation and training, especially in rural areas where the journey may be prolonged or treatment within hospital may be delayed (Rawles, 1992). The potential benefits of prehospital coronary care for patients with acute myocardial infarction are great (Waine et al, 1993). Unfortunately, even the simplest interventions of prehospital opiate and aspirin administration to patients with suspected myocardial infarction are seldom undertaken (Wyllie and Dunn, 1994; Moher and Johnson, 1994), so that much training is needed (Rawles, 1992).

It is important to appreciate that intensive cardiac care facilities will not reduce mortality in patients who delay a call for help (Table 1.2). It is not known why patients who call their general practitioner do so much later than those who call the emergency services or make their own way to hospital. The perception of severity of symptoms is identical in these patient groups, but those who call their general practitioner take twice as long to reach hospital. Whilst improvement of within-hospital delay can be achieved within a short time scale, improvement in out-of-hospital delays will require long-term patient education, especially of patients at high risk of or with known coronary heart disease.

Table 1.2   Time between onset of coronary symptoms and call for medical help in 200 patients admitted to coronary care*, with and without previous myocardial infarction (MI)

Time (hr)	Previous MI	No previous MI
<0.5	28	20
0.5–1	18	15
1–3	42	27
3–24	5	9
>24	7	29
Total	100	100

*Leicester General Hospital

An analysis of the records of out-of-hospital cardiac deaths found that 91% of people were dead before a call for help was made (Fitzpatrick et al, 1992) and only 16% of witnesses attempted resuscitation. It appears that although the public in general understand the value of bystander resuscitation, they have not taken the steps to acquire the necessary skills. Worse still, for those who know what to do, the effectiveness of their resuscitative attempts is doubtful (Wiseman et al, 1989). Success will only be likely if there has been a prompt call for help, efficient bystander cardiopulmonary resuscitation, fast response times from emergency teams and rapid admission to hospital.

Guidelines for the early management of patients with myocardial infarction have been issued by a British Heart Foundation Working Group (Weston et al, 1994) and are summarised in Table 1.3.

ACUTE AND INTERMEDIATE CORONARY CARE

The first priority within hospital is to identify patients with acute ischaemic myocardial syndromes (e.g. unstable angina or acute myocardial infarction) who need immediate attention for haemodynamic stabilisation, relief of pain, early

Table 1.3 Principles of early management of myocardial infarction

1. The overall goal is to reduce mortality and morbidity of heart attack. A means to this end is to reduce the time interval from the onset of symptoms to the provision of resuscitation skills, adequate analgesia, adequate assessment and accurate diagnosis and, where appropriate, early thrombolytic treatment.

2. Patients with obvious acute myocardial infarction should expect to receive thrombolytic treatment (in the absence of contraindications) within 90 minutes of alerting the medical or paramedical service (the 'call-to-needle' time).

3. The above could be achieved through a variety of options, depending on local circumstances. In general, a prompt integrated response by general practitioners, ambulance services and hospital staff is required. Patients with coronary disease, and their relatives, must be provided with guidelines on when to summon help.

Responsibilities of general practitioners
● General practitioners need to develop practice policies for responding rapidly to patients with chest pain. This will involve educating ancillary practice staff. Patients deemed to be at high risk of acute myocardial infarction and their close associates should be informed of the practice policy.

● Where possible, general practitioners should arrange to rendezvous with an emergency ambulance at the patient's home, providing the patient does not suffer additional delay.

● General practitioners must be prepared to give oxygen, aspirin and nitrates.

● Adequate analgesia is essential. The analgesic of choice is intravenous diamorphine with an antiemetic.

● Other drugs that should be available include adrenaline, atropine, lignocaine, frusemide and naloxone.

● General practitioners starting thrombolytic treatment outside hospital need to be fully aware of the indications, contraindications and side-effects of such treatment and should have a defibrillator available. They should confirm the diagnosis by a 12-lead electrocardiogram.

Responsibilities of ambulance services
● Ambulance services should continue to improve training for control staff (ambulance despatchers) and improve prioritisation of emergency and urgent calls using 'criteria-based response'.

● All patients with chest pain require an emergency response, with a vehicle containing a defibrillator and staff trained in its use.

● By 1996, all emergency ambulances must be staffed by at least one paramedic fully capable of advanced cardiac life support.

● Once an ambulance has been despatched, the patient's general practitioner should (when feasible) be informed; this is particularly important in areas where general practitioners are responsible for initiating thrombolytic treatment.

● Cardiac monitoring must be instituted as soon as possible.

● Protocols should be developed to allow the appropriate administration of oxygen, nitrates and aspirin.

● Direct communication between the ambulance and the admitting hospital department should be developed.

Responsibilities of hospitals
● Admitting hospitals should streamline their admissions policies by developing 'fast tracking' of patients with obvious myocardial infarction.

● If direct admission to a coronary care unit is not possible, thrombolytic treatment should be started in the accident and emergency department.

● Senior hospital staff have a responsibility to educate undergraduates, junior staff, general practitioners and ambulance staff and to provide audit data of delays in treatment.

Responsibilities of health authorities
● Regional, district and family health service authorities need to formulate and monitor appropriate local protocols to achieve a 90 minute call-to-needle time.

assessment and administration of thrombolytic agents and, finally, aggressive treatment of any complications. Whether the patient is received in the accident and emergency department or (preferably) directly by the coronary care unit, a system of triage must exist to ensure that the appropriate cases get urgent treatment at the earliest opportunity (Burns et al, 1989).

Triage or 'fast-track' systems allow patients to be selected for treatment by the coronary care team, and routine evaluation by the hospital's admitting medical team or casualty staff is bypassed. Immediately on arrival at hospital, the presentation should be recognised as an acute cardiac problem. It should take no more than a few minutes to confirm or reject the diagnosis of acute myocardial infarction, obtain a 12-lead electrocardiogram and ensure that there are no contraindications to thrombolysis. Patients may then be classified as:

- *Fast track*: myocardial infarction, qualifying ECG (ST elevation or bundle branch block) and no contraindications for thrombolysis
- *Slow track*: probable myocardial infarction, with dubious ECG changes or relative contraindications to thrombolysis
- *No track*: myocardial infarction unlikely or thrombolysis is contraindicated

'Fast-track' patients should be able to receive thrombolytic treatment within 15 minutes of admission. For this and other effective interventions to be implemented, a specialist unit is required, where trained staff are available immediately and where patients at risk can be monitored under constant supervision. It was for a similar reason that the concept of coronary care units emerged. Before these units existed, treatment of acute myocardial infarction was directed towards the healing of the infarct and the prevention of cardiac rupture. Hospital mortality in most hospitals was around 25–30%. However, with the recognition of the importance of rhythm monitoring and prompt defibrillation, the management of coronary patients was revolutionised (Julian, 1961).

The first purpose-built coronary care unit was opened on 20 May 1962 by Hughes Day in Kansas City, and others, in Toronto, Sydney and Philadelphia, quickly followed (Day, 1972). From then on, medical and public demand led to the development of many similar units, so that by the early 1970s, most large hospitals had facilities for monitoring the acute coronary patient, either as part of a general ward or on a separate intensive care unit.

Coronary care units essentially exist for three purposes:

1. To provide a separate area within the hospital for the care and monitoring of patients with acute myocardial infarction and other acute cardiac conditions.

2. To provide care by nurses and physicians with specialist training.

3. To provide an environment for rapid and effective resuscitation.

Roughly half of the patients admitted to coronary care have a complicated clinical course, and their problems mostly occur soon after admission. In general, patients with larger myocardial infarcts have more complications and a poorer prognosis; much depends upon how much functional myocardium is preserved. Intervention to salvage ischaemic myocardium has become a major goal in the modern management of myocardial infarction, with special attention paid to relieving coronary obstruction and acutely improving myocardial perfusion, by coronary thrombolysis or percutaneous coronary angioplasty. Whilst the early success of coronary care units was due to better recognition and treatment of dysrhythmias, effective myocardial salvage, improved haemodynamic monitoring methods and effective pharmaceutical agents for the treatment of heart failure have now led to a further reduction in peri-infarction mortality. In fact, coronary care units have now extended their role to the management of cardiac problems not specifically due to acute myocardial infarction. These include congestive heart failure, dysrhythmias, crescendo angina and cardiogenic shock, so perhaps the term 'cardiac care unit' is more appropriate (Julian, 1987).

Staffing

The staffing and organisation of the coronary care unit is of great importance. The style of management will vary from unit to unit, but it is probably important that decisions are democratic, rather than autocratic. This is more likely to encourage individual initiative and help to reduce stress levels in staff members on the unit, which would otherwise be transmitted to the patient (Henderson, 1980). The unit is usually under the direction of a physician responsible for administration, but it is desirable that selection and training of staff, unit policy and therapy are subject to discussion by all staff on the unit.

In the UK and Scandinavia, intensive care units have principally become part of the department of anaesthesia. Elsewhere in Europe, anaesthetists are in charge of surgical intensive care, and the department of internal medicine runs the medical intensive care units. Coronary care units have become entirely separate areas, usually managed by physicians and/or cardiologists. Despite all the advances with machinery, recording equipment and other useful technology on coronary care units, the most important resource remains their staff. Both the equipment and the staff must work smoothly, reliably and efficiently at all times. There is usually a high workload, with many responsibilities and emotional demands, and although many people relish this atmosphere, others may find it overpowering. Ashworth has made reference to the classification of staff (and patients) as 'drains or radiators' (Ashworth, 1986). The former group leave one drained and exhausted after an encounter, whilst the 'radiators' radiate warmth and other good qualities, leaving one feeling better. Coronary care units need to develop a functional maturity, where each member is a radiator of professional competence and support. Although there will be times when, under pressure, we all become 'drains', interprofessional teamwork requires everybody involved to make a valued contribution from their personal resources towards efficient patient care.

Patients are usually investigated and treated by two groups of doctors: the junior house physicians and the supervising consultants. Whilst the consultant staff direct the management of the patients, it is the junior medical staff who are responsible for the day-to-day care of the patients on the unit. Since patients on these units require constant supervision, it is usually not possible for this to be undertaken on a 24-hour basis by medical staff. Accordingly, the responsibility has fallen to the nursing staff, and this has caused a major change in the role of nursing. Because of the increased duties and responsibility assumed by intensive care nurses, the traditional doctor–nurse relationship has been altered, which often proves awkward to the uninitiated (Jowett, 1986). The nursing staff have a vital role in the smooth running of coronary care units and, in some units, are almost entirely responsible for the care of patients. In the team approach, the nurse has emerged as the key to successful patient management.

Coronary care and the cardiac nurse specialist

Since the introduction of coronary care units, the role of the nurse has not been able to remain static. The nursing profession has continually had to redefine its function, to keep pace with advances in medical treatment and technology, rather than remain in the sphere of traditional nursing. Coronary care units have a small, well-defined technician requirement for specific activities (e.g. echocardiographers and ECG technicians), although their role tends to be less well defined than in other high-technology areas, such as renal units or intensive care units (Ball and Stock, 1993). Nurses and technicians have horizontally-integrated roles, and whilst the two groups cannot substitute for one another, teamwork can enhance quality and efficiency. The concept of intensive cardiac nursing is based on a team approach, with the nurse, technician and attending physician sharing the responsibility for patient care. It is, perhaps, more important for nurses to concentrate primarily on nursing matters, rather than becoming too engrossed in medical and technical areas.

Cardiac care by the nurse requires that he or she be skilled at:

- Giving complete nursing care to the patient and family under his or her care
- Collecting and recording clinical data and taking prompt and appropriate action when necessary
- Communicating with the patient, relatives, colleagues and co-professionals

The nurse needs to be competent in assessing the various needs of the patient and his family, to ensure the provision of physical comfort and emotional support (Thompson, 1990). The illness itself, hospitalisation and therapy present their own problems, to say nothing of the effect of the alien and technical atmosphere of an intensive care unit, which frequently frightens trained medical and nursing staff on their first visit, let alone patients and their relatives. Good cardiac care nursing is based upon general nursing principles of maintaining as near normal a life-style as possible and helping the patient to perform daily activities. It is only in addition to this that the nurse needs to be skilled in technological advances, although experience in advanced cardiac life support and defibrillation is obviously indispensable.

Until recently, nurses have tended to rely on others for guidance and direction, rather than assuming the role of decision-maker. The ability to make decisions quickly has become essential within coronary care and can only come with expertise and knowledge (Webster and Thompson, 1992). As professionals, nurses have a responsibility to themselves, as well as to their patients and colleagues, for continuing education. This includes frequent updating by reading relevant literature and keeping informed of professional issues and clinical practice. The recent reforms in nurse education will ensure that this is an obligatory and not an optional part of patient care. Already, the medical profession is under pressure to take compulsory, rather than optional, study leave to keep updated. Research and its clinical application is also a normal part of medical training but a relatively new concept in coronary care nursing. It should not be seen to be the sole domain of the medical staff.

Design and organisation of the coronary care unit

The design and layout of the unit has to be a compromise between desirability and practicality. For psychological reasons, patients may be better accommodated in individual rooms, so that they are unaware of other patients' problems and are protected from the high drama of cardiac arrests. However, although this design may allow privacy and promote rest, it makes no allowance for direct vision of the patient by the staff. This arrangement may often lead to a feeling of isolation in the patients and fear about not being discovered were they to collapse. Constant visual observation is a prime consideration in acute coronary care and, apart from its main role of spotting early signs of distress, may contribute towards the patients' overall feeling of well-being.

It should be possible to move patients around without transfer between beds or trollies, which causes a great deal of physical effort, especially if the patient is over-weight or arthritic. It may also involve involuntary use of the Valsalva manoeuvre, producing potentially adverse vagal stimulation. Doors should, therefore, be wide enough to permit the passage of beds in and out of the unit. Patient bed areas must be large enough to accommodate staff and equipment and probably no smaller than $10\,m^2$. Each bed should have piped oxygen and suction and must be of suitable design for manoeuvring in case of cardiac arrest. The bed-head must be easily removable, and the base must be rigid (or easily made so with an 'arrest board'). Equipment should be located on the walls and fixed securely. There should be sufficient natural (and artificial) light, with window views to the outside world, so that the patient does not become unduly disorientated. The ability to see a clock is particularly helpful in this respect. Noise insulation and air-conditioning are important for comfort and to promote rest. A separate procedure room away from the main unit is desirable for elective cardioversion and temporary pacing. Provision should be made for interviewing relatives in private and should be additional to a normal visitors' waiting room. Staff coffee and rest rooms are useful for periods of relaxation. A lecture room could also be included in coronary care unit design, equipped with projection facilities and audiovisual aids, for continuing medical education and rehabilitation group meetings.

Intermediate coronary care

In-hospital mortality following myocardial infarction treated by thrombolysis is currently about 8% in men and 14% in women, ranging from about 4% in those under 55 years of age to 25% in patients over 75 years. Without thrombolysis, an excess mortality up to 20% may be expected. Since the risk of primary ventricular fibrillation is highest in the first 36 hours, there is little need for uncomplicated cases of myocardial infarction to remain on the coronary care unit for longer than 48 hours. However, patients may remain at risk of delayed complications for up to 10 days, and these late complications may be responsible for about one-third of in-

Table 1.4 Typical physical activity plan following acute myocardial infarction

Time	Activity
Day 1	Bed-chair rest
Day 2	Sit out of bed or chair; discharge from CCU
Day 3	Walk around ward and to toilet
Day 4	Try stairs
Day 5–7	Discharge home
Day 7–14	Exercise within home and garden
Day 14–28	Gradual increased walking outside home
	Enrol in rehabilitation programme
Day 28–35	Exercise stress test*
Week 4–6	Outpatient review
	Return to work
	Recommence driving (in line with DVLA regulations)

*Predischarge exercise stress testing may be preferable if resources allow

hospital deaths (Graboys, 1975). The provision of intermediate ('step-down') coronary care wards might reduce this excess mortality. Most cardiac units have a policy for encouraging the patient quickly back to normal activity (Table 1.4), and this could take place on step-down units, where the use of telemetry to monitor cardiac rhythm, in the presence of immediate and practised resuscitation facilities, may be of advantage (Kuchar et al, 1987). An additional benefit may be that early rehabilitation and education can take place with all the patients together, as a form of group therapy, perhaps with their husband or wife being present.

REHABILITATION (see Chapter 12)

A heart attack is usually a devastating experience for most patients, particularly for those who have never been ill before and have always considered themselves to be fit. Whilst most make a good cardiological recovery, some degree of chronic invalidism is common, often affecting their vocation, hobbies, social life and sexual activity. For example, only 50–70% of patients return to work following their heart attack, but only in a minority of cases are there genuine medical reasons for the non-return to their former occupation (Monpere et al, 1988). There seems to be no doubt that the quality of life may be improved for cardiac patients by the relief of stress and anxiety and other measures to prevent cardiac neurosis (Horgan et al, 1992). The value of rehabilitation programmes in terms of improving prognosis, however, still needs investigation (Chua and Lipkin 1993).

Whilst the role of cardiac rehabilitation after myocardial infarction and cardiac surgery is generally established, rehabilitation may also be beneficial for patients with angina who have not had a myocardial infarct, patients with class II/III heart failure or following the implantation of physiological pacemakers. Care should be directed not only towards physical problems, but also towards the patient's psychosocial well-being, with an optimistic but realistic approach. Early ambulation following acute myocardial infarction and early discharge from hospital should be encouraged for low-risk patients. This will prevent the complications caused by enforced bed-rest, particularly thromboembolic disorders, and will additionally reduce depression and physical weakness. Entry into a cardiac rehabilitation programme is desirable to restore patients to their optimal physical, psychosocial, emotional and vocational status. Those who benefit most are those with multiple risk factors or low exercise capacity and those who are finding psychological difficulty in coping with their illness. Unfortunately, these services are poorly developed in the UK, with less than half the health districts having established programmes.

Cardiac rehabilitation programmes differ in organisation, but most comprise sections on exercise and relaxation, with discussion and education. Whilst the programme needs to be multidisciplinary, a nurse or physiotherapist usually co-ordinates activities. Cardiac nurses can play a significant role in family education and physical rehabilitation of the patient, and their input is increasing in counselling sessions, exercise programmes and relaxation classes (Thompson, 1994). Free discussion is to be encouraged at all times, with particular advice on diet, smoking, exercise, work and sexual activity. Videotapes and pamphlets may be useful in this context, with rehabilitation tailored to individual patient needs.

The average general practice has approximately 10–12 cases of myocardial infarction per annum. This is too small a number upon which an individual practice can run an effective rehabilitation programme. Active participation in rehabilitation by the cardiac team in the community is probably what is needed, and, perhaps in the coming years, nurses will not view themselves as exclusively hospital based within the isolation of the coronary care unit. There may be a role for the coronary care nurse as a specialist in both the hospital and the community (Webster and Thompson, 1992).

References

Ashworth P (1986) Doctors, nurses and others in ICU – 'drains' or 'radiators'. *Intensive Care Nursing,* 1: 165–167.

Ball J and Stock J (1993) *Nurses and Technicians in High Technology Areas.* IMS Report No. 240. Brighton: Institute of Manpower Studies, University of Sussex.

Beaglehole R (1986) Medical management and the decline in mortality from coronary heart disease. *British Medical Journal,* 292: 33–35.

British Cardiac Society Working Group on Coronary Prevention (1987) Conclusions and recommendations. *British Heart Journal,* 57: 188–189.

Burns J M A, Hogg K J, Rae A P, Hillis W S and Dunn F G (1989) Impact of a policy of direct admissions to a coronary care unit on use of thrombolytic treatment. *British Heart Journal,* 61: 322–325.

Chua T P and Lipkin D P (1993) Cardiac rehabilitation. *British Medical Journal,* 306: 731–732.

Colquhoun M C (1993) General practitioners and the treatment of myocardial infarction: the place of thrombolytic treatment. *British Heart Journal,* 70: 215–217.

Day H W (1972) History of coronary care units. *American Journal of Cardiology,* 30: 405–407.

Department of Health 'Look After Your Heart' (1990) *Beating Heart Disease in the 1990s; A Strategy for 1990–1995.* London: Health Education Authority.

Dickey W and Adgey A A J (1992) Mortality within hospital after resuscitation from ventricular fibrillation outside hospital. *British Heart Journal,* 67: 334–338.

EMIP: the European Myocardial Infarction Project Sub-Committee (1988) Potential time saving with pre-hospital intervention in acute myocardial infarction. *European Heart Journal*, **9**: 118–124.

Fibrinolytic Therapy Trialists' Collaborative Group (1994) Indications for fibrinolytic therapy in suspected acute myocardial infarction: collaborative overview of early and major mortality from all randomised trials of more than 1000 patients. *Lancet*, **343**: 311–322.

Fitzpatrick B, Watt G C M and Tunstall-Pedoe H (1992) Potential impact of emergency intervention on sudden deaths from coronary heart disease in Glasgow. *British Heart Journal*, **67**: 250–254.

Gillum R F, Folsom M R and Blackburn H (1984) Decline in coronary heart disease mortality. *American Journal of Medicine*, **76**: 1055–1065.

Goldman L and Cook E E F (1984) The decline in ischaemic heart disease mortality rates. *Annals of Internal Medicine*, **101**: 825–836.

Graboys T B (1975) In-hospital sudden death after coronary care unit discharge. *Archives of Internal Medicine*, **135**: 512–514.

GREAT study group (1992) Feasibility, safety, and efficacy of domiciliary thrombolysis by general practitioners: the Grampian Regional Early Anistreplase Trial. *British Medical Journal*, **305**: 548–553.

Henderson V (1980) Preserving the essence of nursing in a technological age. *Journal of Advanced Nursing*, **5**: 245–260.

Horgan J, Bethell H, Carson P, Davidson C, Julian D, Mayou R A and Nagle R (1992) Working party report on cardiac rehabilitation. *British Heart Journal*, **67**: 412–418.

ISIS-1 Collaborative Group (1988) Mechanisms for the early mortality reduction produced by beta-blockade started early in acute myocardial infarction. *Lancet*, **1**: 921–923.

ISIS-2 Collaborative Group (1988) Randomised trial of intravenous streptokinase, oral aspirin, both or neither amongst 17,187 cases of suspected acute myocardial infarction. *Lancet*, **2**: 349–360.

ISIS-3 Collaborative Group (1992) A randomised comparison of streptokinase vs TPA vs anistreplase and of aspirin alone among 41,299 cases of suspected acute myocardial infarction. *Lancet*, **339**: 753–770.

ISIS-4 Collaborative Group (1995) A randomised factorial trial assessing early oral Captopril, oral mononitrate and intravenous magnesium sulphate in 58,050 patients with suspected acute myocardial infarction. *Lancet*, **345**: 669–685.

Jowett N I (1984) *Recombinant DNA Gene-specific Probes and the Genetic Analysis of Diabetes, Hyperlipidaemia and Coronary Heart Disease*. MD thesis, University of London.

Jowett N I (1986) The junior doctor on the intensive care unit. *Intensive Care Nursing*, **1**: 177–179.

Julian D G (1961) Treatment of cardiac arrest in acute myocardial ischaemia and infarction. *Lancet*, **ii**: 840–844.

Julian D G (1987) The history of coronary care units. *British Heart Journal*, **57**: 497–502.

Kannel W B and Thom T J (1984) Declining cardiovascular mortality. *Circulation*, **70**: 331–336.

Kuchar D L, Thorburn C W and Sammel N L (1987) Prediction of serious arrhythmic events after myocardial infarction: signal averaged ECG, Holter monitoring and radionuclide ventriculography. *Journal of the American College of Cardiology*, **9**: 531–538.

Lewis S J, Holmberg S, Quinn E, Baker K, Grainger R, Vincent R and Chamberlain D A (1993) Out-of-hospital resuscitation in East Sussex: 1981–1989. *British Heart Journal*, **70**: 568-573.

Mann J I and Marmot M G (1987) Epidemiology of ischaemic heart disease. In *Oxford Textbook of Medicine*, 2nd edn, Weatherall D J, Ledingham J G G and Warrell D A (eds), p. 13.143. Oxford: Oxford Medical Publications.

Mathewson Z M, McCloskey B G, Evans A E, Russell C J and Wilson C (1985) Mobile coronary care and community mortality from myocardial infarction. *Lancet*, **1**: 441–443.

Moher M and Johnson N (1994) Use of aspirin by general practitioners in suspected acute myocardial infarction. *British Medical Journal*, **308**: 760.

Monpere C, Francois G and Broudier M (1988) Effect of comprehensive rehabilitation programme in patients with 3 vessel coronary artery disease. *European Heart Journal*, **9** (supplement M): 28–31.

Mulcahy R, Mulcahy H and Hickey N (1993) Is the coronary epidemic on the wane? *British Journal of Cardiology*, **1**: 35–39.

Office of Health Economics (1990) *Coronary Heart Disease. The Need for Action*. London: Office of Health Economics.

Osmond C and Barker D J P (1991) Ischaemic heart disease in England and Wales around the year 2000. *Journal of Epidemiology and Community Health*, **45**: 71–72.

Pantridge J F and Geddes J S (1967) A mobile intensive care unit in the management of myocardial infarction. *Lancet*, **ii**: 271–273.

Rawles J M (1992) General practitioners and emergency treatment for patients with suspected myocardial infarction: last chance for excellence? *British Journal of General Practice*, **42**: 525–528.

Ridker P M, O'Donnell C, Marder V J and Hennekens C H (1993) Large scale trials of thrombolytic therapy for acute myocardial infarction: GISSI-2, ISIS-3 and GUSTO-1. *Annals of Internal Medicine*, **119**: 530–532.

Secretary of State for Health (1992) *The Health of the Nation* (Cmnd 1523). London: HMSO.

Stamler J (1985) The marked decline in CHD mortality rates in the United States 1968–1981. *Cardiology*, **72**: 11–22.

Thompson D R (1990) *Counselling the Coronary Patient and Partner*. London: Scutari Press

Thompson D R (1994) Cardiac rehabilitation services: the need to develop guidelines. *Quality in Health Care*, **3**: 169–172.

Thompson R G, Hallstrom A P and Cobb L A (1979) By-stander initiated cardiopulmonary resuscitation in the management of ventricular fibrillation. *Annals of Internal Medicine*, **90**: 737–740.

Waine C, Hannaford P and Kay C (1993) Early thrombolysis therapy: some issues facing general practitioners. *British Heart Journal*, **70**: 218.

Webster R A and Thompson D R (1992) *Comprehensive Coronary Care*. Oxford: Butterworth Heinemann.

Weston C F M, Penny W J and Julian D G, on behalf of the British Heart Foundation Working Group (1994) Guidelines for the early management of patients with myocardial infarction. *British Medical Journal*, **308**: 767–771.

Wiseman M N, Whimster F and Skinner D V (1989) Resuscitation skills among the general public in London. *British Medical Journal*, **299**: 434.

World Health Organization Working Group on the Development of Coronary Care in the Community (1979) *Review of Developments in Coronary Care in the Last 5 Years*. ICP/ CVD 003(9). Geneva: WHO.

Wyllie H R and Dunn F G (1994) Pre-hospital opiate and aspirin administration in patients with suspected myocardial infarction. *British Medical Journal*, **308**: 760–761.

2

Anatomy and Physiology

THE ANATOMY OF THE HEART

The heart is a hollow muscular organ located behind the costal cartilages in the middle mediastinum. The size of the heart corresponds quite accurately with the size of the patient's clenched fist and it weighs about 280–340 g. It lies obliquely in the chest and resembles an inverted cone, with the base facing upwards and the apex pointing downwards, forwards and to the left (Figure 2.1). About two-thirds of the heart lies to the left, and one third to the right, of the median plane. The apex lies a little below and medial to the left nipple in the 5th intercostal space and can usually be seen as the apex beat.

At the junction of the upper one third and lower two-thirds of the heart, a deep oblique *atrioventricular groove* passes round the heart, separating the atria from the ventricles. From this, two other grooves extend towards the apex, anteriorly (the *anterior interventricular groove*) and posteriorly (the *posterior interventricular groove*). These mark the position of the *interventricular septum*, which separates the right and left ventricles internally. The junction of the posterior interventricular and posterior atrioventricular grooves is known as the *crux*. Internally, at this junction, the *interatrial septum* joins the interventricular septum.

The tough, fibrous pericardium encloses the heart and serves to limit any sudden cardiac distension. Within the fibrous pericardium and extending onto the surface

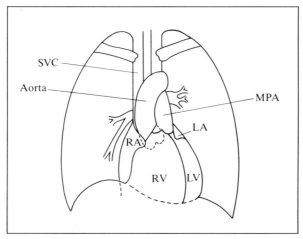

Fig. 2.1   Anterior view of the heart
RA = right atrium; LA = left atrium; RV = right ventricle; LV = left ventricle;
MPA = main pulmonary artery; SVC = superior vena cava.

of the heart is a thin, delicate membrane, the *serous pericardium*. This has been invaginated by the heart during development, to form a two-layered structure. The outer parietal layer lines the inner surface of the fibrous pericardium, and the inner visceral layer (*epicardium*) covers the outer surface of the heart and the adjoining portions of the great vessels. Where the great vessels pass through the fibrous pericardium, the two layers of the serous pericardium are reflected back and become continuous with one another. Between the two layers is a potential space, the *pericardial cavity*. This normally contains a small amount of fluid secreted by the serous pericardium, which acts as a lubricant to facilitate movement of the heart within the pericardial cavity.

The fibrous pericardium blends with the tunica adventitia of the great vessels and is firmly attached to the central tendon of the diaphragm below, and to the back of the sternum by the sternopericardial ligaments.

The chambers and valves of the heart

The heart consists of four chambers: two *atria* above and two *ventricles* below (Figure 2.2). The right and left sides of the heart are separated by an interatrial

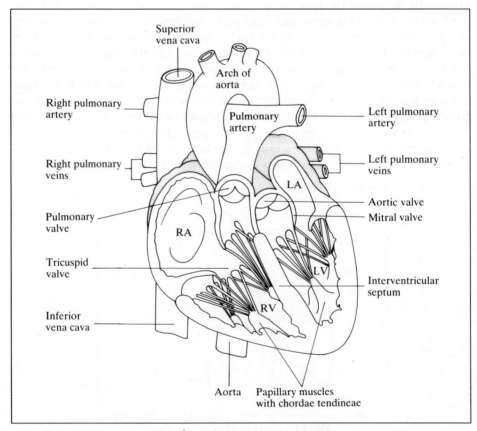

Fig. 2.2   The internal anatomy of the heart
RA = right atrium; LA = left atrium; RV = right ventricle; LV = left ventricle

septum and an interventricular septum. The main valves of the heart are the *mitral* and *aortic* valves on the left side of the heart, and the *tricuspid* and *pulmonary* valves on the right side of the heart. They are complex avascular structures and are very strong. During a normal lifetime, they will open and close some 2700 million times.

The right atrium

The right atrium lies to the right of and slightly behind the right ventricle, and anterior and to the right of the left atrium. It forms the lower right lateral heart border on the chest radiograph.

The right atrium is a thin-walled (2 mm) chamber that receives the venous return to the heart from the two largest veins in the body, the *superior and inferior venae cavae*. The right atrium also drains the coronary sinus and the anterior cardiac veins. The opening of the superior vena cava is valveless, but the inferior vena cava and the opening of the coronary sinus have rudimentary valves. The inner surfaces of the posterior and septal walls are smooth, whilst the surfaces of the lateral wall and the right atrial appendage are composed of parallel muscle fibres known as the *pectinate muscles*. Posteriorly, they end on a longitudinal elevation (the *crista terminalis*), which runs from the right side of the opening of the superior vena cava to the right side of the orifice of the inferior vena cava. This is marked externally on the surface of the right atrium by a shallow groove, the *sulcus terminalis*. On the interatrial septum is a depression known as the *fossa ovalis*, which marks the site of the foetal foramen ovale. The floor of the right atrium is perforated by the right atrioventricular orifice and the tricuspid valve. This has three triangular cusps: septal, anterior and posterior.

The right ventricle

The right ventricle is located directly beneath the sternum. It is the most anteriorly-located chamber, its inferior border located beneath the xiphoid process. The crescent-shaped chamber has a relatively thin outer wall (5 mm), which is approximately one third the thickness of the left ventricular wall. The pulmonary trunk rises from a cone-shaped area at the base of the ventricle, called the *infundibulum*. Blood entering the infundibulum is ejected superiorly and to the right, through the pulmonary valve and into the pulmonary artery. The pulmonary valve has three semilunar cusps: anterior, right and left. On the inner surface of the right ventricular wall are a number of irregular projections of raised muscle bundles (*trabeculae carneae*). The *papillary muscles* project into the ventricular cavity to become continuous with the *chordae tendineae*, which are attached to the free border of the cusps of the tricuspid valve. Contraction of the ventricle not only opposes the tricuspid valve cusps, but also prevents the valve being pushed back into the atrium, by maintaining tension on the chordae tendineae. A large, rounded muscle bundle, the *moderator band*, crosses the cavity of the right ventricle from the interventricular septum to the anterior wall. This conveys the right bundle branch of conducting tissue to the ventricular muscle. The right ventricle receives venous blood from the right atrium during ventricular diastole and expels it against low resistance (25–32 mmHg pressure) into the pulmonary circulation during ventricular systole.

The left atrium

The left atrium is the most posterior chamber and lies to the midline behind the right ventricle. It is the only cardiac chamber not normally visible on the chest X-ray. The left atrium receives blood from the pulmonary veins. It serves as a reservoir during left ventricular systole and as a conduit during left ventricular filling.

The chamber is irregularly cuboidal in shape and somewhat smaller than the right atrium, with slightly thicker walls (about 3 mm). A small conical pouch (the *auricle*) projects from the upper left corner. It receives the four pulmonary veins, arranged in pairs on each side, and all four orifices are devoid of valves.

The interior of the left atrium is smooth, except in the auricle, where the ridges of the pectinate muscles occur. The left atrial aspect of the septum is roughened, being the flap valve of the fossa ovalis. In the floor is the circular left atrioventricular orifice, guarded by the mitral valve. The latter is so called because it possesses two unequal triangular cusps, arranged like a Bishop's mitre.

The left ventricle

The left ventricle receives blood from the left atrium during ventricular diastole and ejects blood against high resistance into the systemic circulation during ventricular systole. It forms the lower left lateral cardiac border and lies posteriorly and to the left of the right ventricle, and below and to the left of the left atrium.

The chamber is conical, and its apex lies approximately in the 5th intercostal space within the midclavicular line. As it normally expels blood against a much higher resistance than the right ventricle, the walls of the left ventricle are much more muscular than those of the right ventricle (8–15 mm). The interventricular septum is also thick and muscular, except for a small membranous area. The septum separates the two ventricles, and its upper portion additionally separates the right atrium from the left ventricle.

Below and posteriorly, the left ventricle communicates with the left atrium through the left atrioventricular orifice and the mitral valve. The two papillary muscles are much larger than those of the right ventricle, and, from these, chordae tendineae are attached to both cusps of the mitral valve. Above and anteriorly, the left ventricle opens into the aorta. The portion of the ventricular chamber immediately adjoining the aorta is known as the *vestibule*. The aortic valve is in continuity with the mitral valve by a fibrous, double-looped band, shaped like a figure 8. The aortic valve has three semilunar cusps (right, left and posterior), which are stronger than those of the pulmonary valve. At the origin of each cusp, the walls of the aorta show a slight dilatation or *sinus*. The right coronary artery arises from the right aortic sinus and the left coronary artery from the left aortic sinus, the orifice of each artery arising above the level of the cusp. These three aortic sinuses are known collectively as the *sinuses of Valsalva*.

The atrioventricular junction

There is no muscular continuity between the atria and the ventricles except through the conducting tissue of the *atrioventricular (AV) node* and *AV bundle*. The aortic and mitral valves have strong fibrous rings that prevent the orifices from stretching and rendering the valves incompetent. These rings are continuous with a dense fibrocartilaginous mass, sometimes called the heart skeleton. This framework affords a firm anchorage for the attachment of the atrial and ventricular musculature, as well as the valvular tissue. The pulmonary valve does not have a ring, and that of the tricuspid valve is only partially formed.

The tissues of the heart

The main mass of the heart consists of muscular tissue (the *myocardium*), which is lined by the *endocardium* and covered by the visceral layer of serous pericardium (the *epicardium*). Blood and lymphatic vessels, nerves and specialised conducting tissues lie within the myocardial mass.

The epicardium

The epicardium consists of a single layer of mesothelial cells covering a thin layer of loose connective tissue, which contains elastic fibres, small blood vessels and nerves. It is in places separated from the myocardium by a layer of adipose tissue, which carries the coronary blood vessels.

The myocardium

The myocardium is composed of specialised involuntary cardiac muscle. Individual myocardial cells are grouped in bundles in a connective tissue framework, which carries small blood and lymphatic vessels and autonomic nerve fibres. The density of capillaries in cardiac muscle cells is much greater than in skeletal muscle, because of its higher blood requirements. The myocardium is thickest towards the apex and thins towards the base.

The myocardium consists of a network of muscle fibres that show transverse and longitudinal striation and which branch and connect with each other. The ends of the cells are in very close contact with adjacent cells, and the 'joints' can be seen as thick dark striations called *intercalated discs*. Because of the close relationship of one muscle fibre with the next, once contraction starts in any part, it cannot remain localised and spreads throughout the entire network of muscle cells.

The endocardium

The endocardium is in continuity with the lining of the blood vessels (*tunica intima*). It is much thinner than the epicardium and consists of a lining of endothelial cells, a middle layer of dense connective tissue containing many elastic fibres and an outer layer of loose connective tissue, in which there are small blood vessels and specialised conducting tissue. The heart valves are formed by folds of endocardium, thickened by a core of fibrous tissue extending in from the tissue of the sulcus. The endocardium and myocardium are firmly bound together by connective tissue.

The conducting system

In addition to the purely contractile muscle fibres comprising the atria and ventricles, the heart possesses certain specialised muscle cells that form the conducting system. These cells initiate and conduct electrical impulses within the heart, to produce myocardial contraction. The conducting system comprises:

- The sinus node
- The atrioventricular (AV) node
- The bundle of His
- The right and left bundle branches
- The peripheral ramifications of the bundle branches (Purkinje fibres)

The sinus node

The sinus node is the normal site of initiation of the heart beat. It is situated at the junction of the superior vena cava with the right atrium (Figure 2.3). This junction is marked internally by the top end of the crista terminalis. The node is spindle-shaped, about 25 mm in length and about 3 mm in width. The framework of the node is collagenous, interlaced by bundles of small conduction fibres. There are numerous autonomic nerve endings in the node, with parasympathetic fibres derived from the right vagus nerve. The blood supply is via the nodal artery, which in 60% of people arises from the right coronary artery. In the remaining 40%, it arises from the left coronary artery.

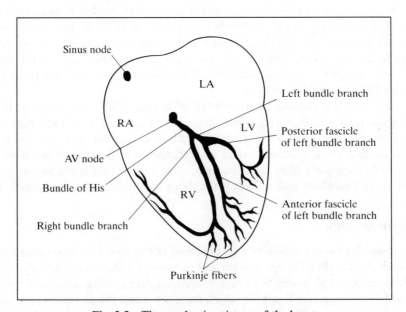

Fig. 2.3 The conducting tissues of the heart

Specialised pathways (*internodal tracts*) may exist in the atria, linking the sinus and the AV nodes, but there is no histological evidence of this. Conduction seems to occur preferentially along the thick muscle bundle of the right atrium.

The atrioventricular (AV) junction

The AV junction comprises the AV node and AV bundle (of His). The AV node lies between the opening of the coronary sinus and the posterior border of the membranous interventricular septum. The node is divided into a transitional zone and a compact portion. Its function is to cause a delay in transmission of the cardiac impulse from the atria to the ventricles, so that the atria have time to expel their contents into the ventricles before systole.

The AV node has a structure similar to that of the sinus node, but there is much less collagen in the framework, and the conduction fibres are thicker and shorter than those of the sinus node. There is a rich autonomic nerve supply, the parasympathetic fibres being derived from the left vagus nerve. The blood supply is from a specific nodal artery (*ramus septi fibrosi*), which arises from the right coronary artery in 90% of cases and from the left circumflex artery in the remaining 10%. The AV bundle extends from the AV node, along the posterior margin of the membranous portion of the interventricular septum, to the crest of the muscular septum. Here it bifurcates into the *right and left bundle branches*. The AV bundle is oval or triangular in cross-section. The fibres of the bundle run parallel to one another, unlike the fibres of the sinus and AV nodes, which interweave. The AV bundle and the proximal few millimetres of both bundle branches are supplied by the terminal branch of the AV nodal artery and from the septal branches of the left anterior descending artery.

The bundle branches

The right and left bundle branches extend subendocardially along both sides of the interventricular septum. The right bundle is a cord-like structure that passes down the right side of the interventricular septum towards the apex, lying more deeply beneath the endocardium than does the left main bundle. It then runs in the free edge of the moderator band, to reach the base of the anterior papillary muscle, where it ramifies amongst the right ventricular musculature.

The left bundle branch is an extensive sheet of fibres that passes down the left side of the interventricular septum. The initial part of the left bundle is fan shaped and breaks up into two interconnecting left and right hemifascicles (see Figure 2.3). The terminal branches of the bundle branches are the *Purkinje fibres*, which ramify within the ventricular myocardium.

The bundle branches are supplied by septal arteries from the left anterior descending artery.

The coronary circulation

The heart and proximal portion of the great vessels receive their blood supply from the two *coronary arteries*, which originate from the sinuses of Valsalva (Figure 2.4).

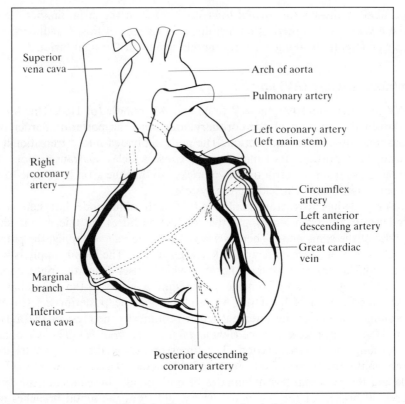

Fig. 2.4 The coronary circulation

The right coronary artery

The right coronary artery arises from the right coronary sinus of the aorta and runs forward to the atrioventricular groove, giving off a small branch to the sinus node. It follows the sulcus downwards and round the inferior margin of the heart, giving off a marginal branch to supply the right ventricular wall. It then winds around the heart to the posterior aspect and passes down in the interventricular groove as the *posterior descending coronary artery*, which supplies the ventricles and interventricular septum. Frequently, a transverse branch continues in the posterior AV groove, supplying branches of the left atrium before anastomosing with the circumflex branch of the left coronary artery. Branches of the right coronary artery supply the conducting tissues, the right ventricle and the inferior (diaphragmatic) surface of the left ventricular wall.

The left coronary artery

The left coronary artery arises from the left posterior sinus of the aorta, runs to the left behind the pulmonary trunk and then runs forwards between it and the left auricle to the AV groove. Here, it divides into two branches: an *anterior descending* branch and a *circumflex* branch.

The left anterior descending (LAD) artery descends in the anterior interventricular groove to the apex of the heart, where it turns round to ascend a short distance up the posterior interventricular groove, anastomosing with the posterior interventricular branch of the right coronary artery. Diagonal branches supply the anterior ventricular wall, and septal branches supply the interventricular septum.

The left circumflex branch passes round the left margin of the heart in the AV groove under the left atrial appendage, supplying branches to the left atrium and the left surface of the heart. In some individuals, the circumflex artery gives rise to the posterior descending artery, and this is called a left-dominant coronary artery system. Other coronary artery variants include:

- Single coronary artery
- Circumflex branch arising from the right aortic sinus

The *left marginal* branch arises from the circumflex artery and runs down the left margin of the left ventricle.

Within the myocardium, there are rich anastomoses between the right and left coronary arteries, but the vessels involved are small. These anastomoses are genetically determined and can enlarge in the event of a gradual coronary artery occlusion, providing collateral circulation to the affected area of muscle. However, if the occlusion is sudden, necrosis of a segment of cardiac muscle will result, since these vessels cannot enlarge acutely.

The coronary veins

Most of the venous drainage of the heart is from veins that run with the coronary arteries and drain directly into the right atrium. The *coronary sinus* occupies the posterior part of the AV groove, between the left atrium and left ventricle. It receives the great, middle and small *cardiac veins* and opens directly into the right atrium. One or two large anterior cardiac veins also open directly into the right atrium, whilst smaller veins (*venae cordis minimae*) open directly into the heart chambers.

Lymphatic drainage

The heart is rich in lymphatic capillaries. Large vessels form the subendocardial and subepicardial lymphatic plexuses. The main collecting trunks accompany the larger blood vessels in the grooves of the heart. One large trunk ascends on each side of the heart to end in anterior mediastinal lymph nodes below the arch of the aorta and at the bifurcation of the trachea. The final drainage is to the thoracic duct, although there may be a connection with the bronchomediastinal trunk on the right side.

The nerve supply to the heart

Because of 'intrinsic rhythmicity', the heart can beat even if removed completely from the body. However, the heart is well supplied with both sympathetic and parasympathetic nerve fibres, which can modify cardiac function by changing the heart rate and strength of myocardial contraction. Control of the autonomic nerves is via the cardiac centre in the medulla oblongata of the brain.

The sympathetic fibres derive from the cervical and upper thoracic sympathetic ganglia, via the superficial and deep cardiac plexuses. The parasympathetic supply is from the vagus. Sympathetic nerve fibres supply the SA node, atrial muscle, AV node, specialised conduction tissue and ventricular muscle. Parasympathetic nerve fibres supply mainly the sinus node and AV node and, to a lesser extent, the atrial and ventricular muscle.

Vagal stimulation to the heart is mediated by acetylcholine, which decreases heart rate and, probably, strength of ventricular contraction. The main action on the AV node is to slow conduction and lengthen the refractory period. In contrast, stimulation of the sympathetic fibres leads to the release of noradrenaline, which acts specifically on beta-1 adrenergic receptors in cardiac muscle. Circulating adrenaline from the adrenal medulla may also elicit cardiac responses. Adrenergic stimulation increases both heart rate and force of contraction. Conduction velocity increases, and there is shortening of the refractory period in the AV node.

The vagal and sympathetic nerves are distributed to the heart by the cardiac plexus, which lies between the concavity of the aortic arch and the tracheal bifurcation. Pressure changes in the aorta and carotid arteries can affect cardiac performance. Sensory receptors (*baroreceptors*) can detect increased pressure in the aorta and carotid arteries. Sensory impulses travel via the vagus and glossopharyngeal nerves and pass to the vasomotor centre in the medulla, causing slowing of the heart rate (Marey's reflex). These baroreceptors can be artificially stimulated by carotid sinus massage.

It is thought that most of the cardiac fibres of the right vagus terminate in the sinus node, while the majority of the fibres of the left vagus terminate in the AV node. Some vagal fibres probably terminate in the walls of the great veins near their entrance to the right atrium and are responsible for the cardiac acceleration that accompanies increased venous return to the heart (Bainbridge reflex).

Chemoreceptors

Chemosensitive cells are located in two *carotid bodies* (at the carotid bifurcation) and several *aortic bodies* adjacent to the aortic arch. They detect changes in blood Po_2, Pco_2 and pH. The afferent impulses arising in these fibres alter respiration, heart rate and vasomotor tone. The efferent impulses from the chemoreceptors pass with the afferent fibres from the pressor receptors via the glossopharyngeal and vagus nerves to the vasomotor centre in the medulla.

CARDIAC PHYSIOLOGY

The heart is a double pump that maintains two circulations: the pulmonary circulation and the systemic circulation. These serve to transport oxygen and other nutrients to the body cells, remove metabolic waste products from them and convey substances (e.g. hormones) from one part of the body to another. At rest, the heart beats at about 70–80 beats per minute and pumps about 5 litres of blood. During exercise, the rate may approach 200 beats per minute and the cardiac output may increase to as much as 20 litres.

Histology

The heart comprises two major types of cell:

- Myocardial cells specialised for contraction
- Automatic cells specialised for impulse formation

Myocardial cells

The myocardial cells provide the mechanical pumping action of the heart by short-ening in response to electrical stimulation. Each cell is about 100 μm long and 15 μm wide, containing a central nucleus and numerous (about 150) myofibrils aligned along the cell's axis. Each fibril runs the length of the cell and is made up of repeat-ing functional subunits, or *sarcomeres*, containing actin and myosin arranged hexa-gonally. The thin *actin* filaments are attached to a limiting membrane (*Z-line*) and interdigitate with the thicker central *myosin* fibres. The sarcomeres of adjacent myofibrils are aligned at the Z-line. During contraction, the actin filaments slide

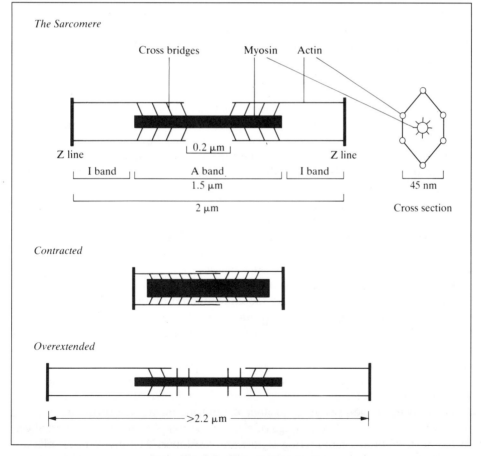

Fig. 2.5 The sarcomere

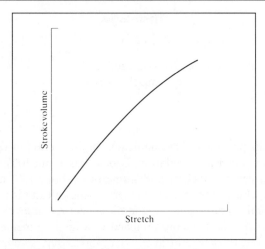

Fig. 2.6   Ventricular function (Starling's) curve

together, bringing the Z-lines closer together. The forces that generate sliding (i.e. contraction) occur at bridges between the actin and myosin (Figure 2.5). It is the heads of the myosin molecules that form these bridges and contain the enzyme ATPase responsible for breaking down ATP (adenosine triphosphate) to provide the energy for contraction. It is likely that the greater the number of bridges, the more forceful the contraction. The thicker myosin filaments (seen as the *A* band on microscopy) are 1.5 μm in length and have a central portion (0.2 μm) that is devoid of bridges. The thin actin filaments (seen as lateral *I bands*) are shorter (1 μm), so it can be seen that maximum bridging takes place when the overall sarcomere length is between 2.0 and 2.2 μm. If the sarcomere is stretched beyond these limits, some bridges become disengaged, which will limit the force of contraction. Starling's Law of the heart (Starling, 1918) states that, within physiological limits, the greater the diastolic volume of the heart, the greater the energy of contraction. This is why the graphs demonstrating Starling's Law fall off at the upper limits of myocardial stretching (Figure 2.6). However, this simplified concept is modified by the action of another contractile protein, *troponin*. This is attached to the actin filaments and has an inhibitory effect that must be counteracted before actin and myosin can produce contraction. This is mediated by free calcium ions.

A large number of mitochondria are present (one third of the cell volume), which are responsible for generating the large amount of energy required to maintain cardiac contraction. Energy is produced by the process known as oxidative phosphorylation, in which substrates such as glucose, lactate and free fatty acids are oxidised to replenish the energy sources adenosine triphosphate (ATP) and creatine phosphate (CP).

The limiting cell membrane is known as the *sarcolemma*, and adjacent cells are held together by intercalated discs. Electrical resistance through these discs is about 1/400th of the resistance through the outside membrane of the myocardial fibre, allowing virtually free passage of electrical currents from one myocardial cell to the next, without encountering significant resistance. The myocardial cells are so tightly bound together that stimulation of any single cell causes the action potential (AP) to spread to all adjacent cells, eventually spreading throughout the entire myocardial network. This is why the cardiac muscle is described as a syncytium (Guyton, 1986).

Automatic cells

Automaticity describes the ability of specialised cardiac tissue to initiate electrical impulses. The cells responsible are known as *pacemaker* or *automatic* cells. In the sinus node, these will discharge spontaneously about 80 times per minute, although automatic cells elsewhere will have a slower discharge rate. In the AV node, for example, this may be 60 times per minute, and in the ventricles, 40 times per minute. This system of 'escape rhythms' exists to prevent rhythm failure should the sinus node fail to discharge. Sometimes the rate of discharge will increase in places other than the sinus node, and these regions then take over the pacemaker function of the heart. This is often seen following acute myocardial infarction (e.g. accelerated idionodal or idioventricular rhythms).

Both myocardial cells and automatic cells can transmit impulses, but the specialised conducting tissues are used preferentially since they allow a more rapid and ordered carriage of impulses through the heart.

Cardiac electrophysiology

The electrolyte concentrations within cardiac cells and in the extracellular fluid are of major importance for electrical stimulation of the heart. The ions primarily involved in the generation of a cardiac action potential are sodium (Na^+), potassium (K^+) and calcium (Ca^{2+}). The predominant intracellular ion is potassium (K^+), and the predominant extracellular ions are sodium (Na^+) and calcium (Ca^{2+}). There are also negatively charged ions present: protein (Pr^-) within the cell and chloride (Cl^-) and bicarbonate (HCO_3^-) outside.

In the normal resting state, the potential across the myocardial cell membrane is about $-90\,mV$. The relative concentration of Na^+ and K^+, and thus the electrical difference across the cell membrane, is maintained by an active, energy-consuming, 'sodium pump'. The pump transfers K^+ ions into the cell up to five times more rapidly than it extrudes Na^+ ions. Within the cell, the concentrations of potassium and sodium are 140 and 10 mmol/l respectively, whereas outside the concentrations are 4 and 140 mmol/l. This ionic imbalance helps to maintain the resting membrane potential at $-90\,mV$, and the cells are then said to be 'polarised'. Should an electrical stimulus reach the cell membrane, permeability is altered, allowing a change in ionic concentrations and depolarisation of the cell.

There are distinct phases of electrical activity in myocardial cells during the generation of an action potential (Figure 2.7).

1. *Polarisation (phase 4).* In the resting (inactive) state, where the cell has a membrane potential of $-90\,mV$, the cell is said to be polarised. The cell interior is negatively charged with respect to the exterior.

2. *Depolarisation (phase 0).* When electrical activation of the cell occurs, changes in the cell membrane permeability result in marked shifts in ionic concentrations. There

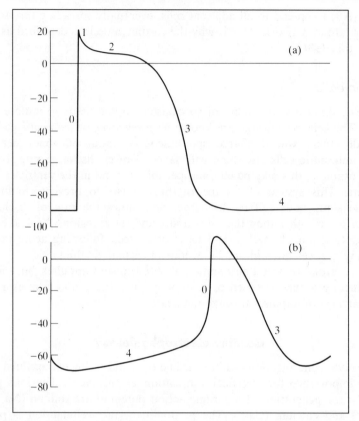

Fig. 2.7 The action potential in (a) myocardial and (b) pacemaker cells

is a rapid influx of positively charged Na⁺ into the cell (the fast sodium current) until a threshold potential of −60 mV is reached. At this critical potential, membrane permeability is further increased, with a secondary rapid intracellular passage of Na⁺ ions, accompanied by a moderate but more sustained influx of Ca²⁺ ions. Depolarisation is represented by the upstroke or spike on the action potential curve.

It can be seen that, after excitation, the polarity of the membrane has been reversed, the membrane potential changing rapidly from −90 mV to a slightly positive value of +20 mV. The cell now has a net positive intracellular charge and negative extracellular charge (Figure 2.8). Since this is the reverse pattern to that of the surrounding cells, a potential difference exists, and an electrical current will flow from one cell to the next, and so on.

3. *Repolarisation (phases 1–3).* Repolarisation is the process whereby the cell is returned to its normal resting state. This has three phases, the first of which is the 'overshoot' when chloride ions re-enter the cell and there is a slow fall in intracellular charge to +10 mV (phase 1 of the action potential). After the initial spike, the membrane remains depolarised (for 0.15 second in atrial muscle and 0.3 second in ventricular muscle), exhibiting a plateau, followed by the abrupt descent that represents repolarisation. The plateau phase (phase 2) of the action potential

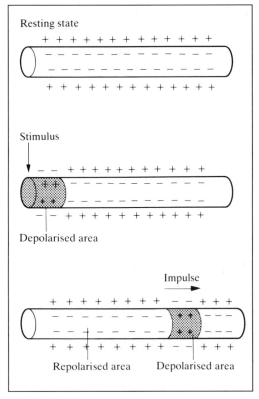

Fig. 2.8 Myocardial cell transmembrane potential (a) at rest, (b) during depolarisation and (c) during repolarisation

reflects a moderate and sustained slow influx of Ca^{2+}, which accompanies the more marked but less sustained influx of Na^+. The calcium entry into the cell is essential for excitation–contraction coupling (see below). The calcium and sodium influx is balanced by an efflux of K^+. Thus, the net effect is a relative balance of positive charges, which gives rise to the plateau.

The downstroke of phase 3 represents the rapid efflux of K^+ from the cell, when membrane permeability to K^+ increases markedly.

Following repolarisation, phase 4 recovery ensues, whereby sodium is actively pumped out again and potassium in so that the cell becomes repolarised. The transmembrane potential returns to its resting level of −90 mV, and the action potential ends.

Once depolarisation has started, it is inevitably transmitted along the length of the cell to the adjacent cells. In this manner, a single electrical stimulus can depolarise the whole heart.

The action potential in automatic cells

The action potential in automatic cells differs from that in myocardial cells. The specialised fibres of the conduction system have the inherent ability to initiate an electrical impulse spontaneously without external influence. Because these cells are responsible for initiating the electrical impulse, phase 4 of the action potential does not properly exist and the cells have an unstable resting phase, with slow spontaneous phase 4 (diastolic) depolarisation (see Figure 2.7). This slow depolarisation is produced by a slow continuous movement of sodium ions into the cells during diastole, which reduces the intracellular negative charge until a threshold potential is reached and full depolarisation takes place.

The refractory period

The myocardium is normally refractory to restimulation during the initial phase of systole. The normal *effective refractory period* of the ventricle is 0.25–0.3 second and occurs when the potential lies at about −55 mV. Stimulation, no matter how strong, does not produce an action potential. Certain antidysrhythmic agents act by lengthening or shortening this refractory period.

Following the effective refractory period there is a *relative refractory period* of about 0.05 second, during which the muscle can be stimulated but with difficulty. Just after this is a vulnerable period, when even a very weak stimulus can evoke a potential.

The normal refractory period of the atrium is about half that of the ventricles, and the relative refractory period is an additional 0.03 second. As a result, the atria can beat much faster than the ventricles.

Myocardial contraction

The mechanism by which the action potential causes the myofibrils to contract is known as *excitation–contraction coupling*. Electrical excitation produces mechanical activation, leading to myocardial contraction.

Electrical excitation

The function of the automatic cells is to regulate the contraction of the myocardial cells by providing the initial electrical stimulation. Their contractile elements are sparse and do not contribute significantly to the cardiac contraction.

Normally, the activating impulse spreads from the sinus node in all directions. It travels at a rate of about 1 m/s, thus reaching the most distant parts of the atrium in only 0.08 second. A delay of approximately 0.04 second in AV transmission occurs during passage through the node, which allows atrial systole to be completed. From the atria, the wave of electrical excitement passes rapidly along the specialised muscle fibres of the AV bundle, bundle branches and peripheral ramifications of these branches. The spread of excitation causes contraction of the ventricular musculature.

Mechanical activation and myocardial contraction

The unit of contraction is the sarcomere, which contains the two contractile proteins, actin and myosin (see above). The contractile process is initiated when the nerve impulse reaches the cardiac cell and travels along the sarcolemma. A series of fine branching T-tubules (the *sarcoplasmic reticulum*) runs from the sarcolemma to the inner contractile elements. These allow any electrical changes occurring at the cell membrane to be rapidly transmitted to the myofibrils and provide the link between the electrical and mechanical activities of the heart.

When an action potential reaches the cardiac muscle membrane, it spreads to the interior of the cell via the sarcoplasmic reticulum. This releases calcium ions from pouches (*cisternae*) in the T-tubules. These diffuse into the myofibrils to catalyse a chemical reaction that activates the sliding of the actin and myosin filaments along each other, to effect contraction. The strength of myocardial contraction is dependent upon the concentration of Ca^{2+} ions, as well as the rate of ATP production. At the end of contraction, the calcium ions in the sarcoplasm are rapidly pumped back into the cisternae.

The cardiac cycle

The function of the heart is to maintain a constant circulation of blood through the body. It acts as a pump whose cyclical contraction (*systole*) and relaxation (*diastole*) is known as the *cardiac cycle*. This cyclical activity is normally initiated by spontaneous generation of an action potential at the sinus node. The impulse travels at about 1 m/s through the atrial muscle to produce atrial systole. Tissues at the atrioventricular groove prevent transmission from atrial to ventricular muscle, and conduction can take place only through specialised tissues in the AV junction. The duration of the cardiac cycle is about 0.8 second, producing an average heart rate of 75 beats per minute. Provided the heart receives excitation along the normal pathways, the heart rate remains constant; each successive cardiac cycle follows the same pattern of systole and diastole.

The duration of atrial systole is about 0.1 second and that of ventricular systole 0.3 second. Thus, the combined duration of atrial and ventricular systole is approximately 0.4 second. The timing remains fairly constant at fast heart rates, so that any increase in heart rate decreases diastolic timing. Complete cardiac diastole normally lasts 0.4 second, but as the pulse rate increases, the diastolic interval decreases. Since coronary perfusion takes place in diastole, fast heart rates may critically impair the myocardial blood supply.

Atrial function

Atrial diastole lasts for 0.3 second, during which venous blood drains into the atria, which act as a reservoir, storing the blood. The AV ring moves upwards at the end of ventricular systole, causing a rise in atrial pressure (the '*v*' wave). The AV valves then open, and the ventricles rapidly begin to fill, allowing the valve cusps to float upwards into opposition. The atria then contract (the right usually very slightly before the left), a process taking 0.1 second. Blood is forced through the AV valves into the ventricles, increasing ventricular filling by about 10–20% and priming the ventricles for contraction.

Since there are no valves between the right atrium and the venae cavae, some blood is also expelled backwards during atrial contraction, causing a transient rise in the central venous pressure: the *'a' wave* (Figure 2.9). The delay of electrical transmission at the AV node allows the atria to empty completely before ventricular contraction starts.

Ventricular function

The pressure of blood in the ventricles begins to rise whilst that in the relaxing atria is falling. The cusps of the AV valves snap shut (causing the first heart sound, *S1*) and are held in opposition by the pull of the papillary muscles on the chordae tendineae. After closure of the AV valves, the blood pressure rises because of isometric contraction of the ventricular muscle. During this phase, the ventricles alter their shape (becoming shorter and fatter), although not their volume (this is called isovolumetric contraction). This momentarily causes a backward bulging of the AV valve cusps into the atria and produces a transient increase in atrial pressure (the *'c' wave*).

When the rising ventricular pressure exceeds the pressure in the aorta and pulmonary artery, the semilunar aortic and pulmonary valves open. The isotonic phase of contraction then begins, and the ventricular contents are ejected. Descent of the AV ring during ventricular systole causes a fall in right atrial pressure (the *'x' descent*).

As the ventricular muscle relaxes and the pressure falls below that in the aorta and pulmonary artery, the semilunar valves close (the second heart sound, *S2*), producing the dicrotic notch on arterial pressure traces. The aortic valve closes slightly before the pulmonary valve. Simultaneously, blood enters the atria and the intra-atrial pressure gradually rises, so that when the AV valves open, blood flows rapidly from the atria to the ventricles, producing the third heart sound (*S3*), heard in some children and young adults.

Haemodynamics

The circulation is a continuous circuit, although it is often conveniently subdivided into the systemic and pulmonary circuits.

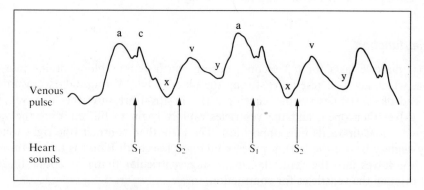

Fig. 2.9 The venous pulse waveform

The pulmonary circulation

The pulmonary circuit is a low-pressure system with short, wide, thin-walled vessels and a small capacity (500–900 ml). The mean pressure in the circuit in the adult is approximately 15 mmHg – less than one sixth of that in the systemic circulation. It circulates all the blood from the right ventricle to the left atrium. As blood is carried through the pulmonary vascular bed, carbon dioxide diffuses outwards into the lungs and oxygen is absorbed.

The pulmonary trunk carrying deoxygenated blood passes upwards from the right ventricle and divides into two main *pulmonary arteries*, one passing to each lung. Within the lungs, the arteries divide and subdivide to form the pulmonary capillary bed where gaseous exchange takes place. Eventually, these capillaries join up to form two main *pulmonary veins*, carrying oxygenated blood to the left atrium.

The systemic circulation

The systemic circulation is a high-pressure system that supplies all the tissues of the body (except the lungs) with blood. The aorta is elastic in nature, which helps it function both as a reservoir for blood during the rapid ejection phase from the left ventricle and as a compression chamber to help propel the blood forward. As the branches arising from the aorta divide, the total cross-sectional area of the arteries, arterioles and capillaries increases and the average velocity of blood flow decreases. The arterioles offer the largest resistance to flow. In the capillary bed, there is often stasis of flow in some capillaries and an active flow in others. The normal systemic capillary pressure is about 24–25 mmHg, and the normal systemic capillary blood volume at rest is about 5% of the total volume (250 ml).

Coronary blood flow

The primary function of the coronary circulation is to provide an adequate supply of oxygen to support the metabolic demands of the heart. The rate of oxygen consumption is the major factor that determines coronary blood flow. Myocardial oxygen consumption (MVO_2) is related to myocardial work in response to exercise or other stimuli, including drugs such as adrenaline, noradrenaline, calcium, thyroxine and digitalis.

About 4% of cardiac output passes into the coronary vessels (about 225 ml/min), which fill in diastole. During systole, the coronary vessels are compressed so that the resistance to flow at that time is sharply increased. Coronary blood flow is largely determined by the calibre of the coronary arteries themselves and is regulated almost entirely by the local metabolic needs of the working cardiac muscle.

Regulation of myocardial function

The normal adult blood volume is about 5 litres; about 3.5 litres are in the systemic (predominantly venous) circulation. The volume in the heart is about 0.6 litre, bringing the total central circulation in the heart and lungs to about 1.5 litres. Not all blood is expelled from the left ventricle at the end of systole. The residual volume, the *left ventricular end diastolic volume* (LVEDV), is about 140 ml. The quantity of blood ejected during ventricular systole (the *stroke volume*) is only about 80 ml, and hence the *ejection fraction* (EF) is approximately $80/140 = 60\%$. If the heart rate is 70 beats per minute, then:

$$\text{Cardiac output} = \text{Heart rate} \times \text{Stroke volume}$$
$$(\text{beats/min}) \quad (\text{ml/beat})$$
$$= \text{about } 5.6 \text{ litres}$$

The cardiac output may increase up to 20 litres during heavy exertion. To alter cardiac output to meet changing bodily demands for tissue perfusion, the heart rate or stroke volume (or both) must be altered. These mechanisms normally operate together to increase the cardiac output as required.

The main determinants of cardiac output are stroke volume and heart rate. If the stroke volume is constant, cardiac output will linearly follow heart rate. However, stroke volume varies constantly, and thus the heart rate must alter to maintain the cardiac output.

Stroke volume is determined by:

- Preload (filling of the heart during diastole)
- Afterload (resistance against which the heart must pump)
- Contractility of the heart muscle

Preload

Preload is the tension exerted on cardiac muscle at the end of diastole, usually expressed as the *left ventricular end diastolic pressure* (LVEDP). This is determined by the volume of blood in the left ventricle at the end of diastole (LVEDV). The Frank–Starling law of 1918 states that, within physiological limits, increases in LVEDV are accompanied by an increase in stroke work. Hence, although the volume of blood passing through the heart may vary considerably, cardiac muscle fibres can contract more forcefully to cope with increased loads. This intrinsic ability of the heart to adapt to changing loads of inflowing blood may be shown graphically (see Figure 2.6) and is approximately linear. Unfortunately, once the load increases beyond physiological limits, the heart begins to fail. Preload can be estimated by measurement of left and right atrial pressures. Clinically, this is done either by a central venous pressure (CVP) line in the right atrium or by a Swan–Ganz catheter measuring the pulmonary capillary wedge pressure to approximate the pressure in the left atrium.

Afterload

Afterload is the force opposing ventricular ejection and is a function of both arterial pressure and left ventricular size. Two major determinants of left ventricular afterload are the resistance of the aortic valve and systemic vascular resistance. Conditions that increase afterload include those causing obstruction to ventricular outflow (e.g. aortic stenosis) and those causing high systemic vascular resistance (e.g. hypertension).

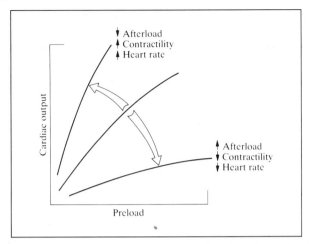

Fig. 2.10 Ventricular function (Starling's) curves showing the effects of preload, afterload, contractility and heart rate

Contractility

Contractility is an intrinsic property of the heart and exists independently of loading. The speed and force of contraction can be increased by sympathetic nervous stimulation or drugs such as adrenaline, noradrenaline or dopamine. These improve the speed and strength of contraction (i.e. they have positive inotropic and chronotropic effects) by increasing ATP production and calcium (Ca^{2+}) fluxes. Myocardial hypoxia, ischaemia and beta-blocking agents have the reverse effect and decrease cardiac contractility (negative inotropic and chronotropic effects). The contractile state can be gauged by the size of the EF or ejection fraction. The normal EF is 0.60–0.75, i.e. the left ventricle ejects about 60–75% of its contents during systole. This may be estimated by echocardiography or nuclear scanning or at cardiac catheterisation. Using the Frank–Starling graphs, contractility can be represented by different curves; higher degrees of contractility displace the curve upwards and to the left (Figure 2.10).

Blood pressure

Blood pressure may be defined as the force or pressure that the blood exerts upon the vessel walls. When the ventricle contracts, blood is forced into an already full aorta, and the pressure wave produces a systolic blood pressure of about 120 mmHg (16 kilopascals [kPa]). During complete cardiac diastole, the arterial pressure falls to about 80 mmHg (11 kPa).

Blood pressure is maintained through many variables, including:

● Cardiac output
● Blood volume
● Peripheral resistance
● Elasticity of the vessel walls
● Venous return

Cardiac output is controlled by pulse rate and stroke volume. An increase in cardiac output raises both systolic and diastolic blood pressure, but an increase in stroke volume increases the systolic pressure to a greater degree. Blood volume is obviously important, as can be seen by the fact that blood pressure falls in shock. This may be due to an absolute loss of blood volume (e.g. haemorrhage) or a relative loss of circulating volume when there is widespread vasodilatation (e.g. septicaemic shock).

Peripheral resistance is controlled via sympathetic vasoconstrictor nerves originating in the vasomotor centre of the medulla oblongata. Normally, the artery walls are in a state of mild constriction, giving rise to 'resting tone'. Selective vasoconstriction and vasodilatation can take place around the body, to ensure a constant blood supply to the vital organs, especially the heart and brain.

The elasticity of the arterial walls is important to propel the blood forwards. Distension and recoil occur throughout the arterial system. During diastole, arterial recoil maintains the diastolic blood pressure. As the arterial tree ages, atheromatous deposits cause 'hardening of the arteries'. Elasticity is lost and the systolic blood pressure rises, since the arterial walls are unable to buffer the effect of the ventricular systolic shock wave.

Venous return via the superior and inferior venae cavae also plays an important role in maintenance of the blood pressure. The force of the left ventricle is not sufficient on its own to force blood round the body. It is, therefore, assisted by muscular contraction and respiration. Contraction of skeletal muscle puts pressure on the veins and squeezes blood forwards. Backward flow is prevented by valves. The negative intrathoracic pressure caused by inspiration also helps, by sucking blood into the heart. In addition, diaphragmatic movement raises the intra-abdominal pressure, squeezing blood out of the abdominal vessels.

References

Guyton A C (1986) *Textbook of Medical Physiology*. Philadelphia: W B Saunders.
Starling E H (1918) *The Linacre Lecture on the Law of the Heart*. London: Longmans Green.

3

Coronary Heart Disease: Risk Factors and Pathology

Coronary heart disease (CHD) is the single major cause of death in most Western industrialised countries and closely relates to what may be defined as 'life-style'. In England and Wales, it accounts for over 163 000 deaths each year (Figure 3.1). Thirty per cent of all male deaths and 22% of female deaths are attributable to coronary heart disease, well over one third of these occurring in people aged less than 70 years.

RISK FACTORS IN CORONARY HEART DISEASE

Epidemiological studies have sought associations between the occurrence of coronary heart disease and physical, biochemical and environmental characteristics of

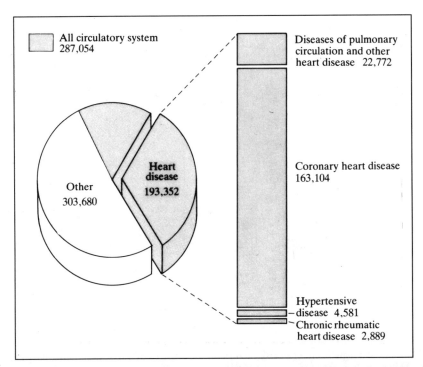

All circulatory system 287,054

Diseases of pulmonary circulation and other heart disease 22,772

Other 303,680

Heart disease 193,352

Coronary heart disease 163,104

Hypertensive disease 4,581

Chronic rheumatic heart disease 2,889

Fig. 3.1 Mortality in England and Wales in 1985 (From Wells, 1987. Reproduced by kind permission of the Office of Health Economics)

populations and individuals. As a result, predictive variables, termed *risk factors*, have been defined, which have been shown to associate with the development of coronary heart disease; these include, for example, male gender, increasing age and a positive family history of coronary heart disease. These are, of course, unavoidable. However, many other treatable risk factors have been defined, the most important of which are hypercholesterolaemia, cigarette smoking and hypertension. In addition, diabetes mellitus is an important risk factor for both small and large vessel disease. Such risk factors are extremely common in the UK; nearly three-quarters of the population have a total serum cholesterol greater than 5.2 mmol/l, a quarter of the adult population smoke and two-thirds get little or no exercise. As might be expected from the frequency of these risk factors, they tend to 'cluster' in individuals, and an important feature of the different risk factors is that where they occur together, the cumulative risk is not just additive but synergistic (Criqui, 1986), one factor multiplying the risk of another (Figure 3.2). The Multiple Risk Factor Intervention Trial (MRFIT) showed that a high risk of coronary heart disease is associated with multiple risk factors (often not severe), rather than a single severe risk factor (Neaton and Wentworth, 1992).

Although, by definition, each risk factor associates positively with the risk of coronary heart disease, it by no means follows that risk factors are causal (Burch, 1980). Indeed, many patients presenting with coronary heart disease do not have identifiable risk factors. In addition, there is no relationship between particular

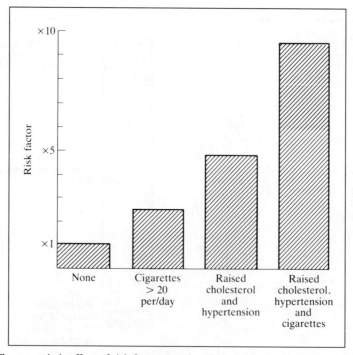

Fig. 3.2   The synergistic effect of risk factors on the chances of a first major coronary episode, where blood cholesterol level is greater than 6.5 mmol/l and blood pressure is greater than 160/95 mmHg

risk factors and the severity or extent of atheroma. Risk factors are weak predictors of coronary heart disease for individuals, and there are probably many other mechanisms that can precipitate the clinical syndromes of coronary heart disease (Oliver, 1987).

Age, sex and race

Mortality from coronary heart disease rises steeply with increasing age, which is primarily due to a cumulative effect of exposure to known risk factors (especially smoking, dyslipidaemia and hypertension) over the years. Women seem to be relatively protected against coronary heart disease; on average, similar death rates do not occur in women until about 10 years after those in men.

Atherosclerosis and coronary heart disease affect all races, but there are marked international differences in the occurrence of coronary heart disease, even allowing for the differences made in disease classification by different countries. In the Seven Countries study (Keys, 1980), the incidence of coronary heart disease varied between 0.15% in Japan and 1.98% in Finland. Migrants who move from low-risk to high-risk areas increase their risk of cardiovascular disease to that of the host country.

Genetic predisposition

Mortality from cardiovascular disease has changed dramatically in many countries over the last 30 years. For example, in the USA, there have been falls in mortality from coronary heart disease (down 39%), stroke (down 54%) and other cardiovascular diseases (down 19%) in the 20-year period from 1964 to 1984, compared to a reduction of only 12% in non-cardiovascular disorders (National Center for Health Statistics, 1984). This decline can only be explained by changes in environmental or nutritional factors. Alterations in the genetic structure of such populations cannot have taken place sufficiently fast to account for such dramatic changes. Nevertheless, it is clear that genetic influences are of importance in the aetiology of coronary heart disease. Coronary heart disease often aggregates in families, especially in those with maternal histories (Rissanen and Nikkila, 1979). The presence of coronary heart disease in a first-degree relative with an onset before the age of 50 years (55 years in women) is a strong risk factor and seems to be independent of the other risk factors. Studies of identical and non-identical twins indicate that coronary heart disease is more often found in both identical twins than in both non-identical twins, which supports the evidence for the genetic influence (Berg, 1983). Genetic factors affecting this susceptibility to coronary heart disease may operate through known risk factors that run in families, such as dyslipidaemia, diabetes and hypertension, or through as yet undefined genetic mechanisms.

Obesity

There are many causes of obesity, and, unfortunately, virtually all are environmental. Affluence, familial obesity (due to role modelling and eating habits) and the

Western sedentary life-style all contribute. The instant food market has led to instant obesity. The increasing consumption of alcohol is also a major factor. Hormonal imbalance, although a popular excuse, is not an underlying cause, and endocrine disorders such as hypothyroidism and Cushing's syndrome invariably present with other symptoms.

Acceptable ranges for body weight have been defined by the Royal College of Physicians of London (1983), although distinction should be made between 'average' weights and 'ideal' weights. *Average weights* are always higher in the West, where we overeat. *Ideal weights* are based on the pooled experience of life assurance companies, who have calculated desirable weight based on excess mortality figures.

Obesity may be defined by the body mass index (BMI) given by:

$$BMI = \frac{\text{Weight (kg)}}{[\text{Height (m)}]^2}$$

BMI values for non-obese individuals lie between 20 and 25. Obesity is viewed as starting at a value of 30 and gross obesity at 40. About 3 million people (6% of men and 8% of women) in the UK have a body mass index of over 30. Obesity is a more important risk factor in men than women, since abdominal fat seems to relate more strongly to coronary heart disease than does fat on the limbs or hips. The waist:hip ratio may be a better predictor of cardiovascular mortality than the body mass index (Jarret, 1986).

Obesity increases the risk of coronary heart disease by about 35%, although the pathogenesis is complex. Obesity is associated with increased blood pressure, blood volume, resting cardiac output, left ventricular filling pressure and vascular resistance. All these factors lead to an increased cardiac workload. Hypertension and hypercholesterolaemia are very common associates of obesity and compound the cardiovascular risk.

Other risks of obesity are diabetes (135% increased risk), cerebrovascular disease (53% increase), accidents (18% increase) and cancer (16% increase). On average, life expectancy is decreased by 15% for every 10% excess of ideal body weight. Other coexisting problems that frequently occur are respiratory disease, arthritis, varicose veins, hernias and gallstones.

Blood lipids and lipoproteins

Lipids play an essential physiological role in the cardiovascular system. The major lipids are triglycerides and cholesterol. The former are found predominantly in adipose tissue as stored energy reserves. In addition, they are the main vehicle for the transport of fatty acids from the liver and intestine to the tissues (including the myocardium), for energy, and to the endothelium, for prostaglandin synthesis. Cholesterol (with phospholipids) forms an integral cell membrane component. Lipids are insoluble in water, and in order for them to be transported in blood, they are converted to water-soluble complexes called lipoproteins. The main lipoproteins are chylomicrons, low-density lipoprotein (LDL), very low-density lipoprotein (VLDL) and high-density lipoprotein (HDL).

Chylomicrons are the largest lipoproteins and consist mainly of exogenous (dietary) triglyceride that has been absorbed from the small intestine. *VLDL* is a small, triglyceride-rich lipoprotein, bearing lipids synthesised mainly in the liver. *LDL* is the main transport vehicle for cholesterol. *HDL* is the smallest lipoprotein and contains cholesterol, which is transported away from cells to the liver.

There is persuasive evidence that high blood cholesterol concentrations are causally related to atherosclerosis and its complications, and there is a clear correlation between raised serum cholesterol levels and the risk of coronary heart disease (Rose and Shipley, 1980), the relationship being virtually linear (Figure 3.3). There is no such thing as 'normal' serum lipid levels; few constituents in the blood vary between populations as much as cholesterol. Mean levels of total cholesterol in New Guinea are only 2.5 mmol/l, as opposed to, for example, east Finland, where the level is 7.5 mmol/l. The mean serum cholesterol in middle-aged men in Britain is 6.3 mmol/l (Mann et al, 1988).

The average level of serum cholesterol in different populations roughly predicts the risk of coronary heart disease in that population: the higher the average cholesterol, the higher the risk. Furthermore, populations with high numbers of other risk factors but a low serum cholesterol have a low incidence of coronary heart disease. For example, the prevalence of smoking and hypertension is very high in Japan, but serum cholesterol is low, as is the mortality from coronary heart disease.

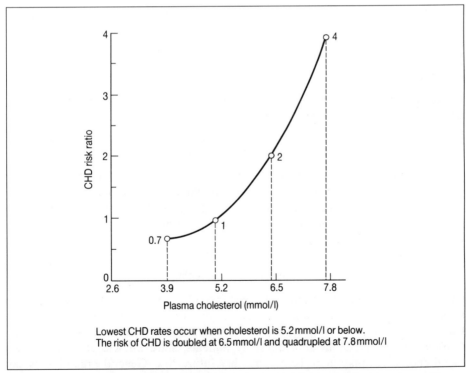

Fig. 3.3 Relationship of plasma cholesterol concentrations to mortality, based on a $7\frac{1}{2}$ year follow-up of 17 718 men in the Whitehall study (data from Rose and Shipley, 1980)

Whilst high total plasma cholesterol concentrations are a very strong risk factor for coronary heart disease, the atherogenic effect actually reflects the concentration of LDL cholesterol. Low levels of HDL cholesterol also independently predict coronary mortality; high levels of HDL cholesterol (particularly the HDL2 subfraction) are negatively correlated with atheromatous disease. Low levels of HDL are often associated with other risk factors, such as lack of exercise, diabetes, obesity and cigarette smoking, whilst raised HDL levels are often found in premenopausal women, joggers and moderate, regular drinkers of alcohol.

The hyperlipidaemias are a common group of metabolic disorders, many of which have been shown to predispose to coronary heart disease (the dyslipidaemias). Hyperlipidaemias may be classified as either primary (idiopathic) or, more commonly, secondary. The former are often familial and should only be diagnosed by exclusion of known underlying causes, the most common of which are diabetes, thyroid disease, renal disease, cholestasis, alcohol and other drugs (Jowett and Galton, 1987). Atheromatous plaques progress more quickly in the presence of a high serum cholesterol, and successful lowering of the cholesterol level can lead to regression of atheroma (Thompson, 1992). Reducing very high cholesterol levels may additionally reduce the incidence of coronary heart disease, coronary death, myocardial infarction, angina and the need for coronary artery bypass surgery (Oliver, 1984). The role of hypertriglyceridaemia in the aetiology of coronary heart disease is a little harder to interpret. Whilst high levels associate with the risk of ischaemic heart disease, they are not an independent risk factor. This is because they are normally associated with raised LDL cholesterol and reduced HDL cholesterol. However, hypertriglyceridaemia can cause acute pancreatitis or may draw attention to other cardiovascular risk factors, such as diabetes.

Screening

Hyperlipidaemia is usually asymptomatic and is commonly detected by screening, either opportunistically or selectively.

Selective screening

This should include all patients who have cardiovascular disease, particularly those with positive family histories. This is especially important in those who have had a heart attack, bypass surgery or coronary angioplasty. Selective screening is also desirable in those with other cardiovascular risk factors, including diabetes, hypertension or renal disease.

Opportunistic screening

Opportunistic screening includes all other individuals who may have their cholesterol levels estimated when attending the surgery for other reasons. In the UK, the Coronary Prevention Group (1987) recommends that estimation of serum cholesterol should be available on request by patients, since knowledge of their own blood cholesterol may help them to modify future risk. General practitioners can play a major role here in risk factor identification and preventative care. Risk factor counselling can take place at the same time as blood is taken for cholesterol estimation, along with blood pressure measurement. However, knowledge of one's cholesterol concentration may have unpredictable results. A study of male factory workers found that only half those who were found to have raised concentrations on routine screening were willing to accept that their result was abnormal (Irvine and Logan, 1994). The remainder responded by denial and refused to make changes to their diet or life-style.

Family screening

Many of the primary hyperlipidaemias are familial, and lipoprotein abnormalities may be found in the patient's relations. Measurement of serum lipids should always be offered to first-degree relatives, particularly younger males, for whom early therapy will be of most value. This is especially important in monogenic familial hypercholesterolaemia (FH), a dominantly-inherited disorder that carries a high risk of early cardiovascular morbidity and death. Early diagnosis and therapy offers the best hope of improving the prognosis.

Screening tests

The most commonly employed screening test is a random serum cholesterol estimation. If this is less than 5.2 mmol/l, there is no need for further analysis, unless there is a high suspicion of another abnormality, such as low HDL cholesterol or hypertriglyceridaemia. If the random cholesterol is greater than 5.2 mmol/l, or if there is likely to be another lipid abnormality, total cholesterol, HDL cholesterol and triglyceride levels should be measured in a sample of venous blood, taken, preferably without venous stasis, after an overnight (12-hour) fast.

The LDL cholesterol (LDL-C) concentration can be measured directly but is usually estimated by the Friedewald formula:

$$\text{LDL-C (mmol/l)} = \text{Total cholesterol} - \text{HDL-C} - \left(\frac{\text{triglyceride}}{2.2} \right)$$

Low HDL-C levels (less than 1.0 mmol/l) and high LDL-C levels (more than 5.0 mmol/l) are the major associates of atherosclerotic disease, and a ratio of these two lipoproteins of less than 0.2 appears to be an important predictor of coronary heart disease.

Further investigation must serve to exclude secondary causes of hyperlipid- aemia, by assessing alcohol intake and drug ingestion and by performing thyroid, liver and renal function tests, plus a fasting blood sugar.

It should be noted that acute illness such as infection, trauma (including surgery) and myocardial infarction may alter serum lipoprotein concentrations. For example, for about 3 months after acute myocardial infarction, plasma tri- glycerides may be higher and total cholesterol lower than pre-infarction levels (Ryder et al, 1984).

The recommended threshold for medical intervention is now suggested to be 5.2 mmol/l (*Lancet*, 1987), since at this plasma cholesterol level the risk of coronary heart disease is comparatively small (Martin et al, 1986). Above this level, there is a directly proportional rise in atherosclerotic cardiovascular events, notably coronary heart disease (see Figure 3.3). More than two-thirds of the adult population of the UK have serum cholesterol levels above the recommended level of 5.2 mmol/l. The average serum total cholesterol in middle-aged British men carries a two-fold risk of major coronary events, compared with those with lower concentrations.

The British Hyperlipidaemia Association (Betteridge et al, 1993) classifies total cholesterol levels as:

- Desirable (less than 5.2 mmol/l)
- Borderline (5.2–6.4 mmol/l)
- Abnormal (6.5–7.8 mmol/l)
- High (above 7.8 mmol/l)

If abnormal values are discovered, the Association recommends that fasting levels are remeasured on three occasions at weekly intervals before a diagnosis of hyperlipidaemia is established. Lipoprotein and triglyceride concentrations should then be assessed.

Generally, abnormal values are:

- LDL cholesterol >4.9 mmol/l
- HDL cholesterol <0.9 mmol/l
- Triglyceride >2.3 mmol/l
- Total:HDL cholesterol ratio >6.5
- LDL:HDL cholesterol ratio >5

If the HDL cholesterol level is high, the threshold for treatment should be based upon the LDL cholesterol level, which is the most important cholesterol determinant upon which to base therapy. The total:HDL cholesterol or LDL:HDL ratios may, additionally, be used to overcome this problem.

Some centres would further explore the index of risk by measuring lipoprotein (a). This lipoprotein is structurally similar to fibrinogen, and high levels are an independent risk factor for cardiovascular disease, probably by promoting thrombosis.

Smoking

Tobacco smoke is a complex aerosol containing (in addition to tar) two implicated cardiovascular toxins: nicotine and carbon monoxide.

1. *Nicotine.* Nicotine absorption during smoking varies from about 5 to 100%, depending upon smoking patterns, and a heavy smoker may absorb about 100 mg of nicotine per day. Its pharmacological action is to stimulate catecholamine release, which raises the heart rate, blood pressure and force of myocardial contraction, leading to increased myocardial work. Additionally, there is a thrombogenic action caused by inhibition of fibrinolysis, release of free fatty acids and an increase in platelet aggregation and stickiness.

2. *Carbon monoxide.* Carbon monoxide is a cellular poison and makes up about 3–6% of inhaled cigarette smoke (eight times the maximum air pollution allowed in industry!). It binds 200 times more readily with haemoglobin than does oxygen, which it displaces to form carboxyhaemoglobin. Typically, a heavy smoker will have 20% of his haemoglobin carboxylated, which shifts the oxygen dissociation curve to the left, thereby impairing oxygen release in tissues. Oxygenation is, therefore, reduced, despite increased myocardial requirements, due to nicotinic stimulation. Carbon monoxide may, additionally, increase endothelial permeability, predisposing to atheroma.

Pipe and cigar smoke have effects identical to those of cigarette smoke if inhaled, but no increased risk has been seen in those who smoke cigars or pipes and have never smoked cigarettes. This is probably because smoking patterns in this group of patients usually differ, with reduced intake of smoke into the lungs. Former cigarette smokers who switch to these forms of smoking maintain an increased risk of cardiovascular events; this probably relates to the smoking pattern, with the tendency to inhale. It is worth noting too, that self-reports on the depth of inhalation of smoke are extremely inaccurate.

Smoking is almost certainly causally related to coronary heart disease (Dawber, 1980). In absolute numbers, coronary heart disease is a far greater problem than lung cancer, a fact not appreciated by most smokers. Smoking is probably the single most important risk factor for both first and subsequent heart attacks. In the UK, about 111 000 men and women die prematurely from smoking-related diseases every year, including about 10 000 men and women under the age of 65 who die from coronary heart disease attributable to smoking. It is directly implicated in 25% of coronary deaths in patients under the age of 65 years and 80% of men under the age of 45 years. Those with additional risk factors, such as hypertension and diabetes, are especially at risk. Myocardial infarction and sudden death occur two to four times more frequently in smokers than in non-smokers (Friedman et al, 1979), and, overall, the risk of death from coronary heart disease is twice that of non-smokers. Those who start smoking before the age of 20 years and those smoking more than 20 cigarettes per day increase their risk by three to five times (Ball and Turner, 1974). Additionally, smoking contributes to the 24 000 deaths due to bronchitis and to the 40 000 lung cancers that occur annually in the UK, as well as to an estimated 21 million lost working days due to sickness every year. In Pembrokeshire, we have estimated that 1 in 6 of all deaths are smoking related. Nearly 500 patients are admitted annually to our hospital because of an illness caused by smoking, at a cost of £770 000.

Passive smoking, or second-hand smoking, is a term applied to breathing other people's smoke, and this is now a significant public health issue. This is why non-smoking should be considered the norm, and special provision should be made for smokers, rather than vice versa. It has been estimated that 300 of the 40 000 lung cancer deaths in the UK each year are due to passive smoking. One overview study suggests that passive smoking may increase the risk of coronary heart disease by as much as 25% (Beaglehole, 1990). Children living in smoking households may 'smoke' up to 150 cigarettes each year, contributing to asthma, chronic chest infections and middle ear infections and probably predisposing them to atheroma.

In 1991, 97 billion cigarettes were sold in the UK, earning the government in excess of £7000 million. This is probably why successive British governments have been unwilling to act more effectively in the fight against smoking.

Hypertension

The justification for regarding hypertension as a disease requiring therapy is that blood pressures at the upper limits of the population distribution of blood pressure are associated with atherosclerotic, thrombotic and haemorrhagic vascular

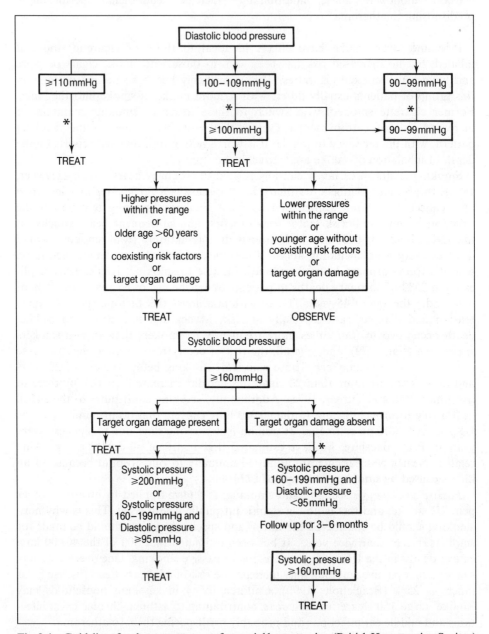

Fig. 3.4 Guidelines for the management of essential hypertension (British Hypertension Society)

All patients given non-pharmacological measures
* Repeated measurements

disease, with increased morbidity and mortality due to strokes, myocardial infarction and peripheral vascular disease. The major cause of death attributable to raised blood pressure is coronary heart disease. Whilst increasing levels of both systolic and diastolic blood pressure increase the risk of death, the systolic blood pressure is the better predictor of subsequent cardiovascular disease. The risk is not uniform but is higher in those with other risk factors, such as smoking and hypercholesterolaemia. Once hypertension has induced target organ damage, the risks associated with hypertension are greater, and left ventricular hypertrophy carries a particularly poor prognosis.

The distribution of blood pressure values in the population is a continuum, and the cut-off point above which patients are considered hypertensive is arbitrary. Blood pressure rises with age, and the increase usually accelerates after the age of 45 years. Guidelines from the British Hypertension Society (Severs et al, 1993) state that average systolic blood pressures greater than 160 mmHg and diastolic pressures greater than 100 mmHg (90 mmHg in the elderly) are abnormal. The guidelines are summarised in Figure 3.4. As with other factors, attributed risk should be individualised.

In general, most people are unaware of the risks of hypertension, and one third of those admitted to our coronary care unit report never having had their blood pressure taken. Fortunately, the attitude to hypertension has changed dramatically over the last 30 years, which is reflected in terms of awareness, screening, investigation and management. Over 75% of American patients with hypertension are aware of their diagnosis, and, what is more, the number taking effective antihypertensive treatment has risen from 4 million to 12 million. This kind of increased awareness and intervention has contributed to the fall in American cardiovascular mortality. The situation in Europe may not be so good. A major audit of hypertension in seven European countries (Britain not included) found a wide divergence between opinions and actual practices of physicians (World Health Organization, 1994). As a result of this, nearly half the patients with hypertension are either untreated or poorly controlled.

Stress

The definition and measurement of stress are not easy, and although many sufferers from coronary heart disease believe that stress must have played a part in their illness, we really do not know its role. Certainly, acute mental stress, anger or excitement can precipitate angina or dysrhythmias. It may be that this and similar events could lead to transient elevation of blood pressure, which could be the stimulus for producing a dysrhythmia or plaque rupture and hence myocardial infarction, heart failure or sudden death. Stressful life-events often precede admission to coronary care (Solomon et al, 1969).

The influence of personality factors on coronary heart disease has become a subject of increasing interest. Among the personality traits related to ischaemic heart disease are aggression, hostility and anxiety, or so-called 'Type A' behaviour (Friedman and Rosenman, 1959; Rissanen and Nikkila, 1979). Type A characteristics include abrupt gestures, hurried speech, impatience, tenseness and rapid, illegible handwriting. There is an intense striving for achievement, competitiveness, time-urgency, being easily provoked and impatience, with overcommitment to vocation or profession and excessive drive. 'Type B' behaviour, in contrast, is characterised by a relaxed, unhurried, satisfied life-style. Neither are fixed personality traits. Whilst Type A behaviour pattern may constitute an independent risk factor for coronary heart disease, there is no relation between Type A behaviour and the course of coronary heart disease following acute myocardial infarction (Case et al, 1985). In addition, Type A behaviour has not been found to relate to new cardiac events in British men, although it is more common in those with ECG or questionnaire evidence of coronary heart disease (Johnston et al, 1987). It might be that Type A behaviour confers a risk only in collaboration with other behavioural or psychological factors that result in increased sympathetic (catecholamine) activity.

Diabetes and glucose intolerance

Glucose tolerance may be formally assessed by measurement of the blood sugar and a subsequent oral glucose tolerance test, if indicated (Figure 3.5). In the developing world, where diabetes is a relatively common disorder, it is usually not associated with an increased risk of coronary heart disease. However, in those

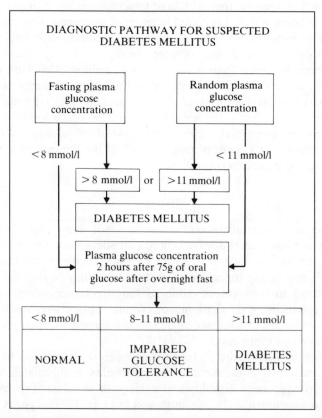

Fig. 3.5 Diagnostic pathways for suspected diabetes mellitus (Reproduced by kind permission of Current Medical Literature Ltd)

countries where coronary heart disease is common, there is a linear trend between the degree of carbohydrate intolerance and the subsequent development of ischaemic heart disease. Whilst part of this risk is mediated by the association of diabetes with obesity, hypertension and dyslipidaemia, it is clear that diabetes independently increases the cardiovascular risk. The incidence of coronary heart disease in these diabetics is approximately twice that of the age-matched population, and it is even higher in diabetic women, who seem to lose the protection that their gender normally affords. Even those patients with impaired glucose tolerance (IGT) run twice the risk of developing large vessel atheroma when compared to those with normal glucose tolerance (WHO Expert Committee on Diabetes Mellitus, 1980). The British Regional Heart Study (Shaper et al, 1985) suggests that asymptomatic hyperglycaemia is an independent risk factor for major coronary events.

Exercise

It is perhaps inevitable that the availability of modern technology has been implicated in the rise in coronary deaths. Whereas the manual worker in the past was protected from the effects of a sedentary occupation, the advent of mechanical aids, including the car, conveyor belts, lifts and other labour-saving devices, has minimised the amount of exercise taken at work. It is hard to demonstrate the benefits of exercise, since observations may simply reflect a generally healthier life-style in those who take regular exercise. However, those who engage in vigorous sports and keep-fit exercises have half the incidence of fatal and non-fatal coronary events, compared with those who do not (Morris et al, 1980). This remains the case, regardless of age or the presence of other risk factors. The protective effect seems to be particularly related to current exercise habits, suggesting perhaps a modification of the acute thrombogenic phase of myocardial infarction.

Acute myocardial infarction is more likely to occur at rest than during exercise; only one third of cases occur during physical exertion.

Other risk factors

Uric acid

A high blood uric acid level (with or without gout) is possibly an independent risk factor for coronary heart disease. However, those prone to hyperuricaemia are usually overweight, with hyperlipidaemia and glucose intolerance.

Alcohol

Alcoholics and heavy drinkers have an increased cardiac mortality, although moderate drinkers (particularly of wine) appear to be less prone than even those who do not drink. This may be because alcohol ingestion raises HDL levels and can ameliorate stress.

Hormonal factors

A study from the Royal College of General Practitioners (1974) found that the incidence of myocardial infarction was three times higher in women taking the oral contraceptive pill, the problem being greater in those with other risk factors, particularly smoking. This may in part be due to alteration of plasma lipid concentrations or perhaps changes in blood clotting factors; raised levels of factors VII and VIII and fibrinogen have been found to be predictors of ischaemic heart disease mortality. The effect of hormone replacement therapy (HRT) on cardiovascular risk is unclear (Findlay et al, 1994). Work since the 1950s has supported the role of oestrogen in the prevention of atherosclerosis, but most recent trials (e.g. Stampfer and Colditz, 1992) have been based upon unopposed oestrogen, that is, oestrogen given without progesterone as in usual HRT. Although no large randomised controlled trial has yet been carried out, current opinion is that hormone replacement therapy probably helps to prevent coronary heart disease. Decisions regarding HRT must be individualised, depending on the competing risks of coronary heart disease, osteoporosis, menopausal symptoms and endometrial and breast cancer.

Fibrinogen

Fibrinogen is the source of fibrin, the main protein involved in thrombus formation. As expected, elevated plasma fibrinogen levels are an independent risk factor for coronary heart disease. Higher concentrations of fibrinogen are found in patients with unstable angina, particularly smokers; smoking increases fibrinogen levels.

Hyperinsulinaemia

High levels of plasma insulin are a risk factor for coronary heart disease. These are found in patients with non-insulin-dependent diabetes and obesity. The insulin resistance syndrome (Reaven's Syndrome) describes patients with hyperinsulinaemia, central obesity, glucose intolerance, hypertension, hypertriglyceridaemia and depressed HDL levels. Small wonder that such patients are at risk of coronary heart disease (Reaven, 1993).

THE RELATIONSHIP BETWEEN ATHEROSCLEROSIS AND CORONARY HEART DISEASE

The term coronary heart disease is used to describe the effects of impaired or absent blood supply on the myocardium. In the majority of cases, this is caused by atheromatous obstruction of the coronary arteries (Davies, 1987). Epidemiological and clinical studies have consistently linked the presence of atherosclerosis to coronary heart disease (Bulkley, 1986; Factor and Kirk, 1986), and coronary angiography reveals atherosclerotic changes in over 97% of patients with acute myocardial infarction (Pichard et al, 1983).

Although coronary atheroma is responsible for virtually all cases of coronary heart disease, many more people have coronary atheroma than have clinical evidence of myocardial ischaemia, which suggests that the association between coronary atherosclerosis and the clinical manifestations of coronary heart disease is not direct. In addition, the severity of symptoms has a poor correlation with both the severity and distribution of coronary atherosclerosis. About 10% of patients with angina pectoris or myocardial infarction have either normal coronary arteries or exhibit no critical stenoses in their coronary arteries (Betriu et al, 1981). This is often the case in young patients (Brecker et al, 1993). Hence, it appears that the clinical manifestations of coronary heart disease are precipitated by additional, transient factors that interfere with coronary blood supply, occurring against a background of varying degrees of coronary atherosclerosis (Maseri, 1982).

ATHEROSCLEROSIS

Atherosclerosis is a complex disease, characterised by proliferation of smooth muscle cells and accumulation of lipid within the intima of large and medium arteries. An important feature is the focal distribution of the lesion as plaques. There is a predilection for these plaques to occur around branching vessels or areas of arterial curvature, suggesting that haemodynamic stresses may play an important initiating role (Ross, 1986).

Although several theories have been postulated to explain the pathogenesis of atheroma, the aetiology remains unclear. The role of repeated endothelial injury, such as from toxins (e.g. from smoking), vasospasm and other haemodynamic stresses, is generally assumed to be central to the initiation and progression of these lesions. Endothelial injury exposes subendothelial collagen and causes adenosine triphosphate (ATP) and adenosine diphosphate (ADP) to be released from damaged cells. This activates platelets, causing them to adhere to the vessel wall. In turn, these platelets release thromboxane A2 and ADP, which cause a secondary aggregation of platelets and contraction of vascular smooth muscle. Platelet-derived growth factor (PDGF) is also released, which stimulates smooth muscle cells to migrate from the arterial media into the intima and then proliferate. If the injury is minor and brief, the endothelium will heal and regress, leaving an irregular and slightly thickened intima. Repeated injury, however, may lead to lipid accumulation and further proliferation of smooth muscle cells.

Atherosclerotic plaques may be classified into three general types:

1. *Fatty streaks.* The process of atherosclerosis begins in childhood, with the development of flat, lipid-rich lesions, termed fatty streaks. These consist of lipid-laden macrophages (foam cells) and smooth muscle cells within the intima. The lesions are yellowish in appearance and cause little or no obstruction of the affected artery. They are thought to be benign in themselves but may be precursors of advanced atheromatous lesions.

2. *Fibrous plaques.* These are white lesions that become elevated, so that they

protrude into the lumen of the artery. They are uncommon in the first 20 or 30 years of life. During the development of the plaque there is a proliferation of smooth muscle cells to form a fibrous cap. The deposition of a new connective tissue matrix and the accumulation of lipids released when foam cells die lead to layers of varying amounts of extracellular lipid and cell debris (the 'lipid pool'). The fibrous plaque often progresses, with potential for luminal narrowing, or it may degenerate.

3. *Advanced (complicated) lesions.* These are degenerative lesions composed of fibrous tissue, fibrin, intracellular and extracellular lipid and, often, extravasated blood. The necrotic, lipid-rich core increases in size and often becomes calcified. The atheromatous plaques cause narrowing of the lumen and may become fissured. The cause of this fissuring is unknown but could be arterial spasm.

Plaque rupture with thrombosis seems to be a common pathogenic mechanism in many acute coronary events, including sudden death, unstable angina and non-transmural and transmural myocardial infarction (Davies and Thomas, 1985). Plaque fissuring is a random and unpredictable event, occurring in response to mechanical stresses, coronary artery spasm and other factors acting on the coronary vasculature. Plaque rupture exposes collagen, which triggers platelet activity and initiates thrombosis. Some plaques are more prone to rupture than others and high-risk plaques seem to have larger lipid pools (>40% of plaque volume).

Angiographic studies during acute cardiac events have led to the classification of coronary artery lesions into type I and type II (Davies, 1992).

Type I lesions appear to have smooth, regular edges at angiography, but visual inspection shows intimal damage, with endothelial loss. Although the integrity of the fibrous cap and lipid pool is unaltered, the loss of endothelium may lead to thrombus formation. This mechanism is responsible for one quarter of sudden deaths.

Type II lesions are more common and have ragged, irregular edges, often showing a filling defect on angiography. There is deep intimal injury, with plaque fissures in the fibrous cap that allow blood to dissect inwards, forming a platelet-rich thrombus within the intima. If the fissure heals, a large plaque-containing thrombus remains, which partially or completely occludes the coronary lumen. Alternatively, fresh thrombus may extend into the lumen and may cause complete obstruction (Figure 3.6). This dynamic process occurs over a period of hours to days preceding an acute coronary event.

Slow endogenous fibrinolysis can take place, leading to recanalisation (which may be enhanced by aspirin and fibrinolytic therapy), and up to 60% of patients with stable angina, and 85% of those with previous myocardial infarction and angina, have segments of artery in which the original channel is replaced by several small channels, suggesting recanalisation through a previously occlusive thrombus.

The symptoms of myocardial ischaemia result from an imbalance between myocardial oxygen demand and supply. Critical restriction to ordinary flow occurs when the diameter of the lumen is reduced by more than 50% (equivalent to a 75% stenosis if the vessel is circular), usually resulting in angina. An abrupt diminution or total loss of coronary blood supply will result in acute myocardial infarction.

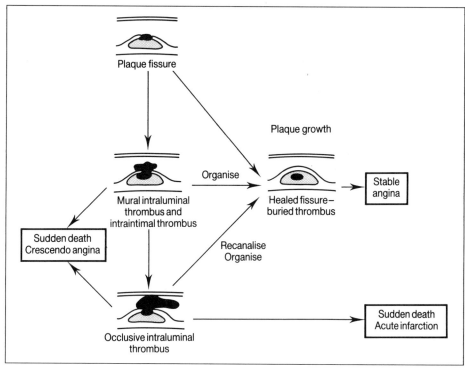

Plaque fissure

Plaque growth

Organise

Mural intraluminal
thrombus and
intraintimal thrombus

Healed fissure—
buried thrombus

Stable
angina

Sudden death
Crescendo angina

Recanalise
Organise

Occlusive intraluminal
thrombus

Sudden death
Acute infarction

Fig. 3.6   Relationship between the clinical expressions of coronary heart disease and the stages of plaque fissuring

Oxygen demand depends mainly upon heart rate, strength of myocardial contraction and left ventricular wall tension. When the heart rate increases, systolic timing does not alter by very much, and the increased heart rate occurs at the expense of diastolic timing. As a result, there is a reduction in coronary perfusion time (which takes place in diastole), despite the higher demands placed upon it by the increased heart rate. Additionally, sympathetic stimulation leads to an increase in the force of contraction, which increases myocardial oxygen demand. Increased wall tension will also increase myocardial work and is determined by intracardiac pressures and volumes secondary to changes in preload and afterload.

In general, the delivery of oxygen to the myocardium varies with coronary blood flow, which is in turn determined by perfusion pressure. Perfusion pressure may be compromised by abnormalities of the vessel wall, abnormalities in blood flow or abnormalities in the blood itself.

1.   *Abnormalities of the coronary vessel wall.* Coronary blood supply may be impaired by fixed or reversible lesions. Atheroma is the most common cause of coronary stenosis, although congenital lesions, such as coronary ectasia, may be responsible. In most cases of stable angina, there is a 50% stenosis in one or more of the coronary arteries, and in between one half and two-thirds of cases, the original lumen is replaced by several smaller channels, where recanalisation has occurred in a previous thrombosis. Coronary artery spasm gives rise to intermittent, reversible stenoses and is the underlying abnormality in 'variant angina', described by Prinzmetal et al (1959).

Both spasm and atheroma are usually present in patients with symptomatic coronary heart disease, although their precise contribution to impairing myocardial perfusion at any given time will differ (Maseri, 1982). Coronary artery spasm occurs in about one third of patients with unstable angina and may also follow the sudden withdrawal of nitrate therapy. The usual situation is for spasm and fixed stenosis to act in combination, that is, vascular contraction takes place around a fixed obstruction, causing a critical reduction in flow, which leads to regional ischaemia. However, temporary occlusion of coronary flow by spasm, even in the absence of atheroma, can lead to angina or even myocardial infarction.

Rarely, the coronary vessel wall may be involved in inflammatory diseases, such as systemic lupus erythematosus (SLE) and polyarteritis nodosa (PAN), which may cause symptomatic occlusion.

2. *Abnormalities in blood flow.* Valvular heart disease, especially aortic stenosis, will impede blood flow from the left ventricle and reduce perfusion of the coronary arteries. This may provoke angina, even in the absence of coronary atheroma.

3. *Abnormalities in the blood.* Anaemia will prevent adequate oxygen carriage and may provoke angina. Hyperviscosity syndromes, such as polycythaemia and myeloma, may result in myocardial ischaemia by slowing blood flow.

It can be seen that the heart can be rendered ischaemic by mechanisms other than fixed atherosclerotic lesions in the coronary arteries. Myocardial infarction and unstable angina often occur at times when there is little or no demand placed upon the heart (at rest or during minimal exertion). The precipitating cause would, therefore, seem to be decreased oxygen supply to the heart, rather than increased oxygen demand. The rapid onset of symptoms suggests that there is a precipitating event occurring in the presence of advanced coronary atherosclerosis, and it is now known that several mechanisms – atherosclerosis, platelet adhesion, coronary thrombosis and coronary artery spasm – interact in the pathogenesis of coronary heart disease and its clinical manifestations.

THE MANIFESTATION OF CORONARY HEART DISEASE

The main clinical manifestations of coronary heart disease are angina (stable or unstable), myocardial infarction (non-transmural and transmural) and sudden death. Cardiac failure and acute dysrhythmias are also usually attributable to myocardial ischaemia.

Angina

Angina is a symptom and not a disease. It may be broadly defined as a discomfort located in the chest or adjacent areas that is caused by myocardial hypoxia secondary to inadequate coronary blood flow and which is not associated with myocardial necrosis.

Post mortem studies on patients with stable angina usually reveal more than 75% stenosis (cross-sectional) of two or more coronary vessels. In life, however, patients with angina show much less evidence of atheroma, and the myocardium is, remarkably, usually spared.

In patients with unstable angina, the vessels show type II plaques undergoing fissuring, often with non-occlusive luminal thrombus. Distal micro-embolisation into small myocardial vessels is very common, although the effect on left ventricular function has not been determined. Arterial spasm is another mechanism for unstable angina, often in association with eccentric type I atheromatous stenoses.

Myocardial infarction

Myocardial infarction refers to necrosis of myocardial cells caused by cessation of or reduction in their blood supply. It is usually associated with an occlusive thrombus in one or more of the coronary arteries, superimposed on a discrete and fissured atherosclerotic plaque (*Lancet*, 1985), leading to what is termed regional acute myocardial infarction. If more than two-thirds of the ventricular wall is involved, the infarction is termed 'transmural'. If it involves less than this, it is termed 'subendocardial' infarction. A more diffuse pattern of myocardial infarction is sometimes seen in patients with left ventricular hypertrophy or cardiogenic shock and is the result of prolonged hypoperfusion. The whole of the left ventricle is then involved, and, occasionally, there is little evidence of coronary atheroma.

Coronary occlusion quickly leads to transmural myocardial ischaemia. Pain is experienced within 1 minute, and the ECG changes within 30 seconds. Left ventricular contractility degenerates rapidly. After about 20–30 minutes, necrosis begins and progresses in a wavefront from endocardium to epicardium. If reperfusion is re-established early, there is the potential for full recovery. The infarcted area is at first red because of 'stuffing in' of the red cells (infarct = stuffed in). The area later becomes pale as the necrotic muscle swells and squeezes out the extravasated blood. Finally, the infarcted area is gradually replaced by fibrous scar tissue over the course of 1 week to 3 months.

Although occlusive thrombi are found in up to 90% of patients immediately following myocardial infarction, this frequency diminishes as time passes because of spontaneous thrombolysis (Mandelkorn et al, 1983; Rentrop, 1985). The speed with which some arteries reopen suggests that spasm may play an important role. About 1% of patients with acute myocardial infarction have normal coronary arteriograms, and the cause of the infarction remains speculative (Arnett and Roberts, 1976).

Subendocardial (non-Q wave) infarction probably results from intermittent or partial coronary artery occlusion, reperfusion of the vessel being re-established within 1 or 2 hours, or by collateral circulation in the subpericardial zone. Subendocardial infarction often leads to reinfarction in the same area and has a higher late mortality. This is probably due to the presence of viable, but ischaemic, myocardium, which acts as a focus of electrical instability and hence dysrhythmias.

Sudden death

A sudden death is one occurring from natural causes, in which the patient dies within 6 hours of developing symptoms (often immediately). Coronary heart disease is responsible for about 70% of sudden deaths, but about half will have had no previously recognised heart disease. If a coronary artery is ligated experimentally, histological changes do not occur for 4–6 hours, so that patients who die suddenly often do not have firm morphological, enzyme or electrocardiographic evidence of myocardial infarction.

Sudden death has two major underlying causes: vascular (haemorrhagic or thromboembolic) and dysrhythmic. These may occur alone or, more commonly, together. Ambulatory electrocardiography in patients dying suddenly suggests that an acute ventricular dysrhythmia (ventricular tachycardia or ventricular fibrillation) is the most common cause of death (Milner et al, 1985). Most cases are presumed to be initiated by an acute event, such as coronary artery spasm, acute plaque fissuring or perhaps coronary emboli arising from ulcerated plaques, producing distal 'micro-infarcts'. Post mortem evidence usually shows type II plaque fissuring, often in association with fresh coronary thrombus. In 40% of cases, this would have led to myocardial infarction had the victim lived longer. About one third of cases have smaller intraluminal thrombosis, which seems to embolise distally, creating micro-infarcts, rather like transient cerebral ischaemic attacks (Stehbens, 1985). In 20% of cases, there is a fissure associated with intra-intimal thrombus, which may be responsible for initiating spasm, or intraluminal coronary thrombosis. In those with no evidence of fissures or acute coronary artery thrombosis, the cause of the dysrhythmias is probably left ventricular dysfunction secondary to myocardial ischaemia (Glover and Littler, 1987).

LEFT VENTRICULAR REMODELLING AFTER MYOCARDIAL INFARCTION

The complex structural changes in the left ventricular myocardium that follow acute myocardial infarction have an important effect on subsequent left ventricular function and, hence, prognosis. Left ventricular remodelling takes place during the first 6 weeks following acute myocardial infarction, as a result of expansion of the infarcted area and global left ventricular dilatation. Late remodelling, with progressive ventricular dilatation, can occur over the subsequent year. Those patients with extensive myocardial infarction and persistent occlusion of the infarct-related artery are most at risk of ventricular remodelling. The area of infarct expansion develops within hours of injury and provides a site for left ventricular thrombus formation. As infarct expansion proceeds over the first 3 weeks, there is the possibility of aneurysm formation and subsequent left ventricular rupture. Global ventricular dilatation, with distortion of the cavity, results in an increase in left ventricular volume and defines overall prognosis: the bigger the volume, the greater the mortality (Vannan and Taylor, 1992). Early and complete reperfusion of the infarct-related artery will limit infarct expansion, which may be aided by unloading the heart with nitrates and calcium-channel blocking agents. Recently, the role of ACE-inhibitors has been studied, and evidence suggests that their early and long-term use following myocardial infarction will prevent ventricular remodelling and its sequelae (St John Sutton, 1994).

References

Arnett E N and Roberts W C (1976) Acute myocardial infarction and angiographically normal coronary arteries: an unproven combination. *Circulation*, **53:** 395–400.

Ball K and Turner R (1974) Smoking and the heart. The basis for action. *Lancet*, **ii:** 822–826.

Beaglehole R (1990) Does passive smoking cause heart disease? *British Medical Journal*, **301:** 1343–1344.

Berg K (1983) The genetics of coronary heart disease. In *Progress in Medical Genetics*, Vol. V, Steinberg A G, Bearner A G, Motulsky A G and Childs B (eds), pp. 52–68. Philadelphia: W B Saunders.

Betriu A, Pare J C, Sanz G A, Casals F, Magrina J, Castaner A and Navarro-Lopes F (1981) Myocardial infarction with normal coronary arteries: a clinical–angiographic study. *American Journal of Cardiology*, **48:** 28–32.

Betteridge D J, Dodson P M, Durrington P N, Hughes E A, Laker M F, Nicholls D P, Rees J A E, Seymour C A, Thompson G R, Winder A F, Wincour P H and Wray R (1993) Management of hyperlipidaemia: guidelines of the British Hyperlipidaemia Association. *Postgraduate Medical Journal*, **69:** 359–369.

Brecker S J D, Stevenson R N, Roberts R, Uthayakumar S, Timmis A D and Balcon R (1993) Acute myocardial infarction in patients with normal coronary arteries. *British Medical Journal*, **307:** 1255–1256.

Bulkley B H (1986) Pathology of coronary atherosclerotic heart disease. In *The Heart*, 6th edn., Hurst J W (ed.), pp. 839–856. New York: McGraw-Hill.

Burch P R J (1980) Ischaemic heart disease; epidemiology, risk factors and cause. *Cardiovascular Research*, **14:** 307–338.

Case R B, Heller S S and Case N B (1985) Type A behaviour and survival after acute myocardial infarction. *New England Journal of Medicine*, **312:** 737–741.

Coronary Prevention Group (1987) Risk assessment: its role in the prevention of coronary heart disease. *British Medical Journal*, **295:** 1246.

Criqui M H (1986) Epidemiology of atherosclerosis: an updated overview. *American Journal of Cardiology*, **57:** 18C–23C.

Davies M J (1987) Pathology of ischaemic heart disease. In *Ischaemic Heart Disease*, Fox K M (ed.), pp. 33–68. Lancaster: MTP Press.

Davies M J (1992) Anatomic features in victims of sudden coronary death. *Circulation*, **85**(supplement 1): 19–24.

Davies M J and Thomas A C (1985) The cause of acute myocardial infarction, sudden ischaemic death and crescendo angina. *British Heart Journal*, **53:** 363–373.

Dawber T R (1980) *The Framingham Study. The Epidemiology of Atherosclerotic Disease.* Cambridge, Massachusetts: Harvard International Press.

Factor S M and Kirk E S (1986) Pathophysiology of myocardial ischaemia. In *The Heart*, 6th edn., Hurst J W (ed.), p. 856. New York: McGraw-Hill.

Findlay I, Cunningham D and Dargie H J (1994) Coronary heart disease, the menopause and hormone replacement therapy. *British Heart Journal*, **71:** 213–214.

Friedman D G, Dales L G and Ury H K (1979) Mortality in middle aged smokers and non-smokers. *New England Journal of Medicine*, **300:** 213–217.

Friedman M and Rosenman R H (1959) Association of specific overt behaviour pattern with blood and cardiovascular findings. *Journal of the American Medical Association*, **169:** 1286–1296.

Glover D R and Littler W A (1987) Factors influencing the survival and mode of death in severe ischaemic heart disease. *British Heart Journal*, **57:** 125–132.

Irvine M J and Logan A G (1994) Is knowing your cholesterol number harmful? *Journal of Clinical Epidemiology*, **47:** 131–145.

Jarrett R J (1986) Is there an ideal body weight? *British Medical Journal*, **293:** 493–495.

Johnston D W, Cook D G and Shaper A G (1987) Type A behaviour and ischaemic heart disease in middle aged British men. *British Medical Journal*, **295:** 86–89.

Jowett N I and Galton D J (1987) The management of the hyperlipidaemias. In *Drugs for Heart Disease*, 2nd edn., Hamer J (ed). London: Chapman & Hall.

Keys A (1980) *Seven Countries*. London: Harvard University Press.

Lancet (1985) Treatment of coronary thrombosis. *Lancet*, **i:** 375–376.

Lancet (1987) Prevention of coronary heart disease. *Lancet*, **i:** 601–602.

Mandelkorn J B, Wolf N M, Singh S, Shechter J A, Kersh R I, Rodgers D M, Workman M B, Bentivoglio L G, LaPorte S M and Meister S G (1983) Intra-coronary thrombus in nontransmural myocardial infarction and in unstable angina pectoris. *American Journal of Cardiology*, **52:** 1–6.

Mann J I, Lewis B, Shepherd J, Winder A F, Fenster S, Rose L and Morgan B (1988) Blood lipid concentrations and other cardiovascular risk factors: distribution, prevalence and detection in Britain. *British Medical Journal*, **296:** 1702–1706.

Martin M J, Hulley S B, Browner W S, Kuller L H and Wentworth D (1986) Serum cholesterol, blood pressure and mortality: implications from a cohort of 361 662 men. *Lancet*, **ii:** 933–936.

Maseri A (1982) Expanding views on ischaemic heart disease: a perspective for the 1980s. *Clinical Science*, **62:** 119–123.

Milner P G, Platia E V, Reid P R and Griffith L P C (1985) Ambulatory electrocardiographic recordings at the time of fatal cardiac arrest. *American Journal of Cardiology*, **56:** 588–592.

Morris J N, Everitt M G, Pollard R, Chave S P W and Semmence A M (1980) Vigorous exercise in leisure time: protection against coronary heart disease. *Lancet*, **ii:** 1207–1210.

National Center for Health Statistics (1984) Advance report of final mortality statistics. *Monthly Vital Statistics Report* **33,** Supplement, 1–43.

Neaton J D and Wentworth D (1992) Serum cholesterol, blood pressure, cigarette smoking and death from coronary heart disease. Overall findings and differences by age for 316,099 white men. Multiple Risk Factor Intervention Trial Research Group. *Archives of Internal Medicine*, **152:** 56–64.

Oliver M F (1984) Hypercholesterolaemia and coronary heart disease: an answer. *British Medical Journal*, **288:** 423–424.

Oliver M F (1987) Problems and limitations. In *Screening for Risk of Coronary Heart Disease*, Oliver M F, Ashley-Miller M and Wood D (eds), pp. 3–9. Chichester: John Wiley & Sons.

Pichard A D, Ziff C, Rentrop P, Holt J, Blanke H and Smith H (1983) Angiographic study of the infarct-related coronary artery in the chronic stage of acute myocardial infarction. *American Heart Journal*, **106:** 687–692.

Prinzmetal M, Kennamer R, Merliss R, Wada T and Bor N (1959) Angina pectoris. I. A variant form of angina pectoris: preliminary report. *American Journal of Medicine*, **27:** 375–388.

Reaven G M (1993) Role of insulin resistance in human disease (syndrome X): an expanded definition. *Annual Review of Medicine*, **44:** 121–131.

Rentrop K P (1985) Thrombolytic therapy in patients with acute myocardial infarction. *Circulation*, **71:** 627–631.

Rissanen A M and Nikkila E A (1979) Aggregation of coronary risk factors in families of young men with fatal and non-fatal coronary heart disease. *British Heart Journal*, **42:** 373–380.

Rose G and Shipley M J (1980) Plasma lipids and mortality: a source of error. *Lancet*, **i:** 523–526.

Ross R (1986) The pathogenesis of atherosclerosis – an update. *New England Journal of Medicine*, **314:** 488–500.

Royal College of General Practitioners (1974) *Oral Contraceptives and Health*. London: Pitman.

Royal College of Physicians of London (1983) Report on obesity. *Journal of the Royal College of Physicians of London*, **17:** 3–58.

Ryder R E, Hayes T M, Mulligan I P, Kingswood J C, Williams S and Ownes D R (1984) How soon after myocardial infarction should plasma lipid values be assessed? *British Medical Journal*, **286:** 1651–1653.

Severs P, Beevers G, Bulpitt C, Lever A, Ramsay L, Reid J and Swales J (1993) Management guidelines in essential hypertension: report of the second working party of the British Hypertension Society. *British Medical Journal*, **306:** 983–987.

Shaper A G, Pocock S J, Walker M, Phillips A N, Whitehead T P and Macfarlane P W (1985) Risk factors for ischaemic heart disease: the prospective phase of the British Regional Heart Study. *Journal of Epidemiology and Community Health*, **39:** 197–209.

Solomon H A, Edwards A L and Killip T (1969) Prodromata in acute myocardial infarction. *Circulation*, **40:** 463–471.

Stampfer M J and Colditz G A (1992) Estrogen replacement therapy and coronary disease: a quantitative assessment of epidemiological evidence. *Preventive Medicine*, **20:** 47–63.

Stehbens W E (1985) Relationship of coronary artery thrombosis to myocardial infarction. *Lancet*, **ii:** 639–642.

St John Sutton M (1994) Should ACE inhibitors be used routinely after infarction? Perspectives from the SAVE trial. *British Heart Journal*, **71:** 115–118.

Thompson G R (1992) Progression and regression of coronary artery disease. *Current Opinions in Lipidology*, **3:** 263–267.

Vannan M A and Taylor D J E (1992) Ventricular modelling after myocardial infarction. *British Heart Journal*, **68:** 257–259.

Wells N (1987) *Coronary Heart Disease: The Need for Action.* London: Office of Health Economics.

World Health Organization (1994) *Assessing Hypertension Control and Management.* WHO European Series No. 47. Geneva: WHO.

WHO Expert Committee on Diabetes Mellitus (1980) *Second Report.* WHO Technical Report Series No. 646. Geneva: WHO.

4

Assessment of the Patient

The initial contact with a patient suspected of having coronary heart disease may be either in an outpatient department or following an acute admission to hospital. Clinical appraisal will include taking a history, making an examination and carrying out special investigations. These initial steps often take place on the coronary care unit and may necessarily have to be brief. The immediate decisions to be made are: does the patient have a cardiovascular illness and, if so, what needs to be done (either therapeutically or diagnostically)? As many as two-thirds of patients admitted to coronary care may later be shown not to have suffered a myocardial infarction (Table 4.1), so that the coronary care unit has a diagnostic as well as a therapeutic role.

In the medical clinic, patients may present with many symptoms other than chest pain. Equally, not all patients presenting with chest pain will be found to have coronary heart disease. Although the diagnosis of myocardial ischaemia may

Table 4.1 Primary discharge diagnosis in patients admitted to our coronary care unit in one year

	Percentage
Cardiovascular (78.9%)	
Myocardial infarction	37.3
Angina	18.4
Dysrhythmias	12.8
Left ventricular failure	5.7
Pericarditis	2.4
Post cardiac arrest	2.3
Non-cardiac (21.1%)	
Chest pain of uncertain origin	6.7
Gastrointestinal causes	2.1
Respiratory tract infection	2.0
Musculoskeletal	2.0
Viral infection	1.7
Pulmonary embolus	1.3
Anxiety/hyperventilation	0.9
Cerebrovascular accident	0.7
Aortic dissection	0.4
Asthma	0.3
Others – pancreatitis, pneumothorax, carcinoma of lung, anaemia, gastrointestinal haemorrhage, constipation, cervical spondylitis, Munchausen's syndrome, etc.	<0.5

be easy, this is frequently not the case. The clinician must be aware of the methods available for confirming or refuting the diagnosis. If coronary heart disease is suspected, full assessment is required to plan therapy and predict prognosis.

Patient assessment may be divided into:

● Defining the symptoms
● Demonstration of clinical signs
● Organising appropriate investigations (see Chapter 5)

Assessment entails the collection and interpretation of information, which is usually factual but may, to some extent, be based upon the impression of the patient.

The clinical history provides subjective information that defines the severity of the illness and how it affects the patient. A quick initial assessment usually gives significant clues to the diagnosis; rapid triage is often essential to ensure that the patient receives thrombolysis for acute myocardial infarction. As it is nurses who are often the first point of contact with the patient, they are in a unique position to utilise their clinical skills to help to identify patients suitable for immediate therapy (Albarran and Kapeluch, 1994). An audit of thrombolysis in elderly patients has recently shown that nursing staff can usefully influence treatment (Hendra and Marshall, 1992), and indeed there are many advantages in using nursing skills for triage (Caunt, 1992).

History-taking improves with experience. Initial details may need to be brief and may be supplemented from the family, past and existing medical notes and nursing reports in a continuous accumulation of data.

SYMPTOMS OF CORONARY HEART DISEASE

Chest pain and breathlessness are two of the most common complaints that lead to a patient seeking medical advice. Causes of chest pain are many and diverse (Table 4.2). Patients suspected of having acute myocardial infarction are admitted to a coronary care unit, so that prognosis may be improved by early intensive care. Unfortunately, the coronary care unit can be a dangerous place for patients who have non-cardiac chest pain; all too often it is assumed that ill patients attached to cardiac monitors have had a heart attack, and it is important for the unit staff to consider alternative or concomitant diagnoses. The frequency with which non-cardiac pain appears on coronary care units demonstrates how difficult it is to determine the origin of chest pain (see Table 4.2).

Chest pain can originate from most tissues in the chest, including the heart and pericardium, the lungs and pleura, the oesophagus, the vertebrae and ribs and the skin. A full diagnosis is often difficult, because the pain can originate from more than one of these tissues. For example, many patients presenting with angina often have concurrent oesophageal reflux. Obtaining the full clinical history acutely may also be difficult; the patient may be in pain or simply frightened. Clinical examination may also be difficult when signs (hypotension, sweating) may reflect pain and not be the underlying problem.

Table 4.2 Some causes of chest pain

Cardiovascular causes	Non-cardiac causes
Myocardial ischaemia	Herpes zoster
Coronary artery spasm	Oesophageal reflux
Myocardial infarction	Oesophageal spasm
Pericarditis	Hiatus hernia
Dissecting aortic aneurysm	Pneumonia
Pulmonary embolism	Pneumothorax
Mitral valve prolapse	Pleurisy
	Peptic ulceration
	Gall-bladder disease
	Musculoskeletal pain
	Da Costa's syndrome (cardioneurosis)

Chest pain

The most important diagnosis not to be missed is coronary heart disease, but the differential diagnosis of chest pain must always be considered. Differentiation from oesophageal pain is usually the most difficult, and both sources of pain may coexist. The radiation of chest pain was assessed in 200 of our patients recently. The results are shown in Table 4.3.

Myocardial ischaemia

About half the patients presenting with myocardial infarction suffer from angina or will have had a previous heart attack. This is useful diagnostically, since the patient is often able correctly to identify the cause of his pain. The differentiation of angina from myocardial infarction is often difficult, unless the pain is particularly severe or is accompanied by sweating, faintness and vomiting. It is, therefore,

Table 4.3 Site of chest pain and radiation in 200 consecutive medical patients with cardiac and oesophageal pain (Withybush General Hospital, 1991)

Radiation	Primary source of pain	
	Cardiac (%)	Oesophageal (%)
Chest	100	100
Left arm		
All	55	20
To elbow	60	25
Right arm		
All	33	4
To elbow	40	12
Throat/jaw	33	8
Epigastrium	7	35

wise to assume that myocardial infarction has occurred if the pain lasts longer than half an hour or does not respond to two active glyceryl trinitrate (GTN) tablets. The action of GTN takes only a few seconds or at most 2–3 minutes. The tablets have a limited active life, and any carried in pockets for years will not relieve any sort of pain.

Anginal pain is usually described as a constricting ache in the chest, frequently radiating to the jaw, the neck, the back and one or both arms. It is precipitated by exercise (including sexual intercourse), particularly in the cold. It is relieved quickly by rest and GTN. Nocturnal angina (angina decubitus) is often relieved by sitting up. Angina is often atypical, and 10% of patients do not have central chest pain as a leading symptom. The origin of anginal pain is probably the myocardium itself, a phenomenon analogous to cramp taking place. The impulses travel from the myocardium via sympathetic fibres to the thoracic sympathetic ganglia to nerve roots T1–5. These spinal nerves supply the anterior chest wall and the inner aspect of the arm and hand. For that reason, the pain is felt in the region bounded by these thoracic nerves. Even in its atypical presentation, ischaemic pain rarely extends beyond the region between the lower jaw and the epigastrium (roots C3–T6). The location is never so sharply localised that it may be identified with a pointing finger.

Chest pain in women is very common, and nearly half subsequently turn out not to have coronary heart disease. The clinical, investigative and prognostic features in men with chest pain are not necessarily applicable to women (Sullivan et al, 1994).

Sudden onset of severe chest pain should be managed as myocardial infarction until proved otherwise. Fifty per cent of deaths from heart attack occur in the first 2 hours: 25% immediately or within 15 minutes, 15% in the next 45 minutes, and 10% in the second hour. Rapid hospital admission is usually indicated, and most coronary care units offer an open direct admissions policy, whilst accepting that many admissions may be inappropriate.

There is a high prevalence of asymptomatic myocardial ischaemia in diabetics (Koistinen, 1990).

Pericardial pain

Pain is the usual presenting feature of pericarditis and arises from the parietal pericardium (the visceral pericardium being insensitive). Pericardial pain is sharp, aching and usually made worse by lying back or swallowing. The diagnosis is confirmed by the presence of a pericardial friction rub. The most common underlying cause is acute myocardial infarction. The next most frequent cause is a viral infection, especially in the young patient who has often had a recent flu-like illness. Other causes include connective tissue disorders (e.g. systemic lupus erythematosus or sarcoidosis), tuberculosis and renal failure. The ECG classically (but not always) shows widespread concave ST segment elevation.

Aortic dissection

The chest pain of aortic dissection classically radiates through to the back, and the condition presents with shock and loss of peripheral pulses. Myocardial infarction may result if blood tracks round to occlude the coronary arteries, and pericarditis as well if blood leaks through to the pericardium. The mixture of pains coming from these different tissues can make diagnosis difficult.

Chest pain from the lungs

Pleuritic pain is localised and associated with respiration (especially deep inspiration). It usually complicates lobar pneumonia or viral chest infections.

Pulmonary emboli cause dyspnoea, pleuritic pain and haemoptysis, but large emboli may mimic myocardial infarction, presenting with shock and central chest pain. It is worth remembering that patients with pulmonary emboli may also have critical myocardial ischaemia. The embolus may cause so much additional strain upon the heart that angina may be the presenting complaint.

A left-sided pneumothorax can be confused with myocardial pain, particularly in tension pneumothorax when shock is present.

Oesophageal pain

Oesophageal pain ('indigestion and heartburn') is the most common cause of chest discomfort in the general population. The pain may be very difficult to distinguish from the pain of myocardial ischaemia, and the denial response makes sufferers more likely to self-diagnose indigestion, rather than heart attack. Post mortem examination of patients dying from acute myocardial infarction often reveals one or two antacid tablets in the stomach, taken shortly before death. The main problem is that about 40% of the population have a degree of oesophageal reflux, and symptoms are bound to coexist with other causes of chest pain. A confident diagnosis of oesophageal reflux does not rule out the presence of other pathologies.

Mucosal (Mallory–Weiss) tears may occur after bouts of vomiting, as may oesophageal rupture. Both present with chest pain and the latter with shock. Other gastrointestinal disorders, such as peptic ulceration and gall-bladder disease, often cause difficulty with differential diagnosis. An upper gastrointestinal bleed may present with lower chest pain and shock.

Musculoskeletal pain

Fractures of the ribs, vertebral collapse and other muscular strains can cause chest pain. Bornholm's disease (intercostal myalgia) and Tietz's syndrome (sternal costochondritis) may be severe and are usually associated with a flu-like illness in the younger patient.

Skin

Herpes zoster often presents with pain a day or two before the rash appears. If this affects a thoracic nerve root, chest pain that is often indistinguishable from the pain of myocardial infarction may be the leading symptom.

Chest pain of unknown origin

This is a proper diagnosis, which may be applied to a patient presenting with chest pain in whom myocardial ischaemia seems unlikely and no other cause can be found. The typical patient is a middle-aged male presenting with chronic, intermittent stabbing pain in the left breast, lasting for a few seconds, often radiating down the left arm. GTN has usually been tried and, although claimed to be useful, only works after 30 minutes. The problem is how far to investigate these patients, and many end up having coronary angiography.

Dyspnoea

Dyspnoea means difficulty with breathing, and it is entirely subjective. Many patients who are obviously short of breath at rest will not complain of respiratory difficulties, yet others claim to be short of breath on exertion but are able to complete exercise stress tests with apparent ease. Breathlessness is usually due to cardiorespiratory disorders, obesity or anaemia. Left ventricular failure is the classical cardiac cause of acute breathlessness, with pulmonary oedema causing increased lung rigidity and decreased oxygen transfer. Respiration will, therefore, require greater effort, which is not helped by oedematous narrowing of the larger airways. Dyspnoea may also be caused by a raised left atrial pressure alone, which causes pulmonary venous congestion with few physical signs. The venous congestion reduces vital capacity and stimulates pulmonary stretch receptors, which cause the shortness of breath.

Orthopnoea is difficulty with breathing when lying flat. It is often a early symptom of left ventricular failure but may not be volunteered by the patient who learns to sleep propped up with three or four pillows. The increase in venous return in the recumbent patient reduces vital capacity and lung compliance. Patients with chronic obstructive airways disease often complain of waking with dyspnoea and wheezing. Orthopnoea in this instance is actually due to the loss of the diaphragmatic component of their respiratory pattern, corrected by sitting up. Hence, it can be seen that orthopnoea does not automatically indicate heart failure.

Paroxysmal nocturnal dyspnoea (PND) may be viewed as a delayed form of orthopnoea. Dyspnoea is probably precipitated by the patient sliding down the bed into a horizontal position. The increase in pulmonary congestion leads to dyspnoea, which is reversed by the patient sitting up or standing. Typically, the patient jumps out of bed to an open window, gasping for breath.

In patients with right ventricular failure, an enlarged liver and ascites may contribute to orthopnoea, by diaphragmatic splinting.

Cheyne-Stokes breathing

John Cheyne (1818) and William Stokes (1846) independently described this well-known abnormality of respiration. It consists of a respiratory pattern beginning with hardly perceptible respiratory efforts, gradually increasing in depth (rather like the sound of a wood saw) until very much exaggerated. The effort then dies away, until breathing ceases for a period of about 20–30 seconds. The whole cycle is then repeated, lasting for between 1 and 3 minutes. The mechanism is quite complex, but essentially the pauses in respiration allow the levels of arterial carbon dioxide to rise, which stimulates the respiratory centre to set off a fresh cycle of breathing. Cheyne–Stokes breathing is common in the elderly, especially during sleep. However, it is also found in those with chronic chest disease or following a stroke. In cardiac patients, it is common in heart failure, and it may be associated with heart rhythm disturbances, such as junctional rhythms and heart block.

Syncope

Syncope is a transient loss of consciousness resulting from inadequate cerebral blood flow, leading to cerebral ischaemia. There are many causes of syncope, and only a few are due to cardiac causes, as cerebral blood flow is kept remarkably constant and is not influenced by autonomic control. Vasovagal attacks are the most common cause of syncope and occur following prolonged standing or in response to emotion or pain. The face is pale, the pupils are dilated and the pulse and respiration are slow. Peripheral pulses are often impalpable, leading to the frequent diagnosis of cardiac arrest.

Carotid sinus syncope may result from stimulation of the carotid sinus, either during carotid massage or if the patient's neckwear is too tight.

Micturition syncope occurs in older men with nocturia who lose consciousness whilst voiding. This is either because straining reduces venous return and subsequently cardiac output (Valsalva manoeuvre) or because sudden decompression of an overdilated bladder causes reflex vasodilatation.

Exertion syncope is a characteristic feature of aortic stenosis, when the cardiac output through the narrow valve cannot meet the demands of increased activity.

Dysrhythmia-induced syncope may result from heart rates that are too slow or too fast to maintain cerebral blood flow. Stokes–Adams attacks may be missed if the ECG is normal between attacks. The attack may terminate in a convulsion, leading to an erroneous diagnosis of epilepsy. However, there is no aura, and recovery is prompt and accompanied by flushing, as the blood flows again through vessels dilated by hypoxia. The desire to sleep does not occur, and headache is not as common.

Paroxysmal tachycardias often lead to a marked fall in cardiac output, with resulting syncope.

Oedema

Oedema is an abnormal accumulation of fluid in the interstitial tissues and is usually preceded by weight gain from 3 to 5 kg of extracellular fluid. It is a relatively late manifestation of heart failure. Oedema will preferentially collect in loose tissues, and the distribution of fluid is determined by both gravity and the degree of ambulation. In most patients, the legs and feet are affected, but in those who are confined to bed the fluid accumulates over the sacrum. Greater degrees of oedema will gradually affect the whole of the lower extremities, extending to the torso and eventually the face (*anasarca*). The oedema characteristically pits when pressure is applied (*pitting oedema*).

Normally, fluid is exuded into the tissues because arterial capillary pressure (30 mmHg) exceeds plasma oncotic pressure (25 mmHg). However, the fluid is forced back into circulation at the venous end of the capillaries because pressure here (12 mmHg) is exceeded by the oncotic pressure (25 mmHg). If the venous pressure rises (as in heart failure), the resorption of fluid is impaired and oedema results (Figure 4.1). Effusions into the chest and abdomen (*ascites*) occur later in the course of heart failure, for the same reasons.

Haemoptysis

Coughing up blood is not a common symptom in cardiac disease. When related to circulatory pathology, the volume of blood is small, and the sputum is usually only streaked. When haemoptysis is related to exercise or is heavy, it usually indicates mitral stenosis, with pulmonary veins rupturing under high pressure. However, frank haemoptysis usually indicates pulmonary disease (such as bronchial carcinoma or tuberculosis) or pulmonary infarction.

Palpitations

Palpitation is an awareness of the heart beat, familiar to those awaiting examinations! Most people are aware of their heart beat at some time, especially at night when lying on the left side. As such, palpitation is a common symptom, regardless of any underlying heart disease. It may be felt and described in many different ways. Some complain of a racing heart, others of thumping or feeling a missed beat, and the description frequently does not help with diagnosis.

A thumping or pounding heart is the most common complaint and is usually the awareness of normal beats, sometimes exaggerated in strength and speed by sympathetic overactivity (e.g. stress and anxiety). This frequently occurs for prolonged periods and on a daily basis.

Dropped beats are probably the next most common complaint, and these are more frequent if basic sinus rhythm is slow. Ectopic activity and sinus thumping are more frequent when the heart is overstimulated by anxiety or by drugs, including tobacco, caffeine, alcohol, bronchodilators and nasal decongestant sprays.

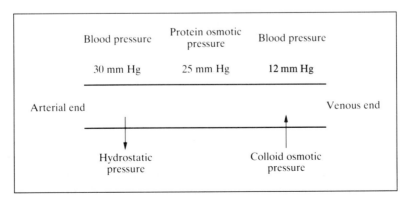

Fig. 4.1 Changing pressures within a capillary

Racing of the heart is usually abnormal if the pulse rate exceeds 130 beats per minute and may be due to supraventricular, junctional or even ventricular tachycardia. The history may go back for many years, although attacks are usually infrequent. If the heart is giving irregular flutters, it is usually due to paroxysmal atrial fibrillation. Frequent ectopic beats may produce the same feeling, and both are common in the elderly.

IMPORTANT CARDIAC SIGNS

In the UK, unlike North America, it is uncommon for nurses to undertake a physical examination of the patient other than by simple observation. However, an appreciation of the techniques involved and what additional information may be gained is often helpful.

Cyanosis

Cyanosis describes the blue (cyan) discoloration imparted to the skin and mucous membranes due to low oxygen content of the blood (less than 85% arterial saturation). It becomes visible when there is more than 5% oxygen-depleted haemoglobin in the vessels being considered. Cyanosis is described as either peripheral or central.

Peripheral cyanosis occurs at the peripheries of the body – the fingers and toes – and is caused by a higher degree of oxygen extraction at those sites. It usually indicates a slowing of peripheral circulation, allowing more oxygen to be extracted as the blood passes through the constricted capillaries. It occurs most commonly in cold weather. In hospital practice, it may be seen in patients with low cardiac output or shock.

Central cyanosis is observed centrally in the body, i.e. the lips and tongue. It is produced by inadequate oxygenation of the blood as it passes through the lungs (as in pulmonary disease) or sometimes when the lungs are bypassed all together (as in right-to-left intracardiac shunts).

The arterial pulse

Arterial pulses should be examined for rate, rhythm, volume and character of the waveform. Although the rate and rhythm are usually assessed by palpation of the radial artery, an artery closer to the heart (e.g. the carotid) is usually better for appreciating pulse width and waveform. In clinical practice, all features may be best assessed by palpation of the right brachial artery.

Rate

The pulse should be counted over 30 seconds, unless irregular, when it should not be assessed for less than 1 minute. The normal adult pulse rate varies between 60 and 100 beats per minute. Slower rates are found in patients taking beta-adrenergic blocking agents but otherwise usually indicate a bradydysrhythmia. Pulse rates in excess of 100 are often associated with anxiety or pain, and those above 130 beats per minute usually indicate an abnormal tachycardia.

Rhythm

The normal pulse is regular, or very slightly irregular if there is a sinus arrhythmia, when the heart quickens on inspiration.

An occasional irregularity indicates an ectopic beat, and an irregularly irregular pulse indicates either multifocal ectopic beats or atrial fibrillation. Gently exercising the patient will produce a regular pulse in the former cases (the resulting rise in the pulse rate will abolish the ectopic), whilst it will have no effect on the irregularity produced by atrial fibrillation.

Volume

Pulse volume (width or amplitude) is an appreciation of the pulse pressure (i.e. the difference between systolic and diastolic blood pressures). This is described as normal, small or large. Small volume pulses are typically felt in shocked patients, whereas large volume pulses are found in patients with anaemia, thyrotoxicosis or aortic incompetence.

Waveform

The character of the pulse waveform is not often easily appreciated but can help with diagnosis. Examples of such descriptions include:

- *Pulsus alternans*: alternate high and low volume beats as found in left ventricular failure. It indicates poor left ventricular function
- *Pulsus paradoxus*: an excessive reduction in pulse pressure (> 10 mmHg) on inspiration. It may be found in asthma, pericardial tamponade or pericardial constriction
- *Collapsing pulse*: large volume with rapid rise and fall, as may occur in thyrotoxicosis or aortic incompetence
- *Plateau pulse*: low volume, slow rise and slow fall, as found in aortic stenosis
- *Absent pulse*: due to atherosclerosis, aortic dissection or peripheral embolisation

Jugular venous pressure (JVP)

The pulsation and level of the internal jugular vein are used to assess the central venous pressure (CVP) and may be seen in front of the sternomastoid muscle. With a normal CVP, pulsation of the internal jugular vein is usually only visible when the patient lies flat. When observing for elevation, the height above the sternal angle should be measured with the patient lying at 45°. Confirmation of the level may be made by pressing on the liver, which transiently increases the CVP (by increasing venous return to the heart). This is known as *hepatojugular reflux*. Liver enlargement (as in heart failure) and pulsation (as in tricuspid incompetence) may also be appreciated. An elevated JVP indicates high right-sided cardiac pressures, as in heart failure, pulmonary embolism, tricuspid or pulmonary stenosis or cor pulmonale.

Much has been written about the pulsation in the jugular vein, but clinical interpretation is often difficult. Sometimes 'a' and 'v' waves may be seen, which correspond to right atrial and right ventricular contractions. Very large 'a' waves (cannon waves) may be seen when the right atrium contracts against a closed tricuspid valve, as may occur in complete heart block, when atrial and ventricular contraction are not synchronised. There will be no 'a' waves if the heart is in atrial fibrillation, since the atria do not contract.

Blood pressure

The first recorded measurement of blood pressure was in 1730, by the Reverend Stephen Hales, who measured the height to which a column of blood reached when he inserted a glass tube into the neck veins of a horse. The tube had to be more than 8 feet long! Fortunately, Scipione Riva-Rocci devised the sphygmomanometer in 1896, which greatly cleaned up and simplified blood pressure estimation. Blood pressure is still most commonly measured indirectly with an aneroid or mercury sphygmomanometer, although precise measurement of arterial blood pressure requires a return to 'old-fashioned' invasive monitoring.

The 'Riva-Rocci' or 'auscultatory' method of blood pressure estimation employs a sphygmomanometer to occlude the brachial artery and a stethoscope to detect sounds of turbulent blood flow within the artery following the release of arterial compression. These sounds are known as the Korotkoff sounds, named after Nicholi Korotkoff, a Russian army surgeon who described them in 1905. Mercury sphygmomanometers are widely available in hospital practice and are more useful than the aneroid type, which require frequent recalibration. This auscultatory method of determining blood pressure has now been superseded in some modern machines by an oscillometric technique, which employs a sensing pressure transducer to detect minute oscillations of the blood and vessel wall, which start as the systolic pressure is reached and continue until there is no arterial constriction.

The original units introduced by Poiseuille for the mercury manometer still persist, so that blood pressure continues to be measured in millimetres of mercury (mmHg). However, the International System of Units, adopted by many countries (including the UK), should have led to replacement of millimetres of mercury by kilopascals (kPa), where $1\,\text{mmHg} = 0.13\,\text{kPa}$, or $1\,\text{kPa} = 7.52\,\text{mmHg}$. Hence, a blood pressure of 120/80 mmHg is roughly equivalent to 16/11 kPa.

As yet, the adoption of the kilopascal has not really caught on for routine blood pressure measurement, although it has done so for blood gas analysis.

Measuring the blood pressure

It is important that the equipment is checked thoroughly before blood pressure measurement. The mercury column must be at zero and the column vertical. The valve must not leak, and the cuff must be at the same level as the heart during blood pressure estimation.

The correct selection and application of the pressure cuff is important, especially in small women and obese patients (Geddes and Whistler, 1978). The choice of cuff size should be based upon the measurement of arm circumference, and clear marking of cuff bladder size by the manufacturers would be useful in this respect.

The cuff size selected should be recorded, and the same size should always be used for serial measurements in the same patient. The width of the cuff bladder should be not less than 40% of the midarm circumference (range 40–50%) and should cover more than two-thirds of the circumference of the arm. Do not be misled by terms such as 'paediatric cuffs'; the correct size is solely dependent upon arm circumference. A simple guide can be employed to show the best available cuff width based upon arm size (Figure 4.2).

The cuff should be applied firmly 2 cm above the antecubital fossa, with the bladder overlying the brachial artery. It must not be twisted or in contact with the patient's clothing. The patient should be comfortable and the forearm supported, slightly extended and externally rotated. The midpoint of the cuff is often marked and should rest over the artery. If the arm is small, it may be easier to put the cuff on upside down so that the tubing is well away from the artery and pointing towards the patient's shoulder.

Correct positioning of the arm is required for accurate blood pressure measurement. The blood pressure rises as the arm is lowered below the level of the heart, and vice versa. Additionally, if the arm is unsupported, isometric muscle contraction needed to hold the arm up against gravity will raise the blood pressure. Hence, the arm should be supported horizontal on a level with the nipples.

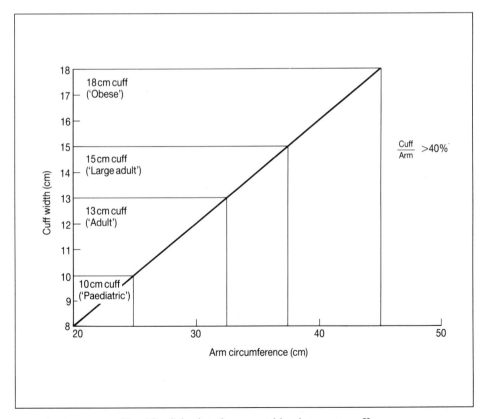

Fig. 4.2   Selecting the correct blood pressure cuff

The cuff should firstly be inflated, whilst the brachial pulse is palpated to determine the systolic pressure. The cuff should then be fully deflated and reinflated to 30–40 mmHg above the previously-determined systolic blood pressure. The mercury column should be observed at eye level and allowed to fall until a faint tapping sound is heard through the stethoscope, which is applied firmly over the brachial artery. This is phase 1 of the Korotkoff sounds and is equivalent to the systolic blood pressure. It should be recorded to the nearest 2 mmHg. As the mercury column continues to fall, there is often a silent gap (phase 2) until the sounds are heard again (phase 3). The sounds then become faint again (phase 4) until they disappear completely (phase 5). Both phase 4 and phase 5 have been used in the past as an indication of diastolic blood pressure. These days, phase 5 should be universally used, unless sounds are heard down to zero. In this instance, both the phase 4 and phase 5 blood pressure should be recorded (e.g. 140/80/0).

Normally, the diastolic blood pressure rises a little on standing, with a slight fall in the systolic blood pressure. In patients with autonomic failure, taking vasodilator medication or in shock, this fall may be very marked (postural or orthostatic hypotension). There is little difference between sitting and lying blood pressure. It is usual to record the blood pressure twice, using the second recording only. The arm used for recording should be noted, and initially, the pressure in both arms should be recorded, so that a subclavian arterial stenosis is not missed.

There are certain occasions on which blood pressure estimation is difficult. This is particularly so in severe hypotension, when indirect readings with the mercury sphygmomanometer are inaccurate. Detection by Doppler or invasive monitoring is then required. If the pulse is irregular, particularly in atrial fibrillation, blood pressure may vary from beat to beat. An average of several estimations is then required.

Automatic blood pressure recorders

Over the last few years, many automatic blood pressure measuring devices have appeared. Most employ a microphone that is positioned over the brachial artery to detect the Korotkoff sounds. Unfortunately, these still have the same limitations as auscultatory methods employing the ear. Additionally, great care is required when using these devices to keep the patient still, or spurious results may be obtained. In general, these machines have not been found to be terribly accurate.

The Doppler principle may be used to detect the return of blood flow when the cuff is deflated, and automated devices are available (e.g. Arteriosond from Hoffman–LaRoche) that sense wall motion of the artery. Again, movement artefact limits its use.

Because of the limitations of auscultatory methodology, and movement artefact, there has been much research in the development of oscillometric systems that can measure systolic, diastolic and mean blood pressures (e.g. Dinamap from Critikon Ltd, Berkshire). Arterial pulsations are transmitted via the whole cuff, rather than a microphone, and hence precise location of the cuff over the artery is not required. It can even measure blood pressure through shirt sleeves. With oscillometric devices, it is important that a correct cuff size is employed and that the cuff fits snugly around the arm. In obese patients, where the arm may be cone shaped, the forearm may be a better choice. The machines need regular calibration and a rigid adherence to the service contract schedule.

The recorded oscillations are transmitted to the recording device, which has a motion-artefact rejection system, such that only when two identical pulses are found will the cuff deflate further. If there has been any external movement vibration, this will be eliminated. Typically, readings take less than half a minute. An automatic cycle mode allows repeated measurements to be made at between 1 and 90 minute intervals. The machine will display pulse rate and systolic, diastolic and mean arterial blood pressures.

There may be several occasions on which blood pressure estimation is difficult (Table 4.4). This is particularly so in hypotensive patients or those with unstable blood pressure; the recordings may not be completely accurate, and invasive blood pressure monitoring is then recommended (see Chapter 5).

The apex beat and cardiac impulse

The apex beat (the maximal thrust of the left ventricle) is normally seen and felt just inside the midclavicular line in the 5th left intercostal space. It may be displaced by abnormalities of the heart, lungs or rib cage. Collapse of the right lung, for example, will move the mediastinum (and heart) to the right, and a thoracic scoliosis may move the mediastinum either way. Seeing, or even feeling, the apex beat is probably only possible in 50% of cases (O'Neill et al, 1989). It is particularly difficult in the obese or in those with hyperinflated chests (e.g. in chronic

Table 4.4 Problems in measuring blood pressure

Problem	Cause	Reasons
False high reading	Cuff too small	Small cuff does not adequately disperse the pressure over the arterial surface
	Bladder not centred over the brachial artery	More external pressure is needed to compress the artery
	Cuff not applied snugly	Uneven and slow inflation results in varying tissue compression
	Arm positioned below heart level	Hydrostatic pressure imposed by weight of blood column above site of auscultation additive to arterial pressure: reposition arm to appropriate level
	Very obese arm	Cuff too small for a large arm will cause too little compression of the artery at the suitable pressure level: apply a large thigh cuff to the upper arm if necessary
False low reading	Cuff too large	Pressure is spread over too large an area and produces a damping effect on the Korotkoff sounds
	Arm positioned above heart level	Hydrostatic pressure in the elevated arm causes resistance to pressure generated by the heart

obstructive airways disease or emphysema). Turning the patient to the left or leaning him forward may then help.

Whilst of limited value in determining mild cardiac dilatation, forceful left and right ventricular contraction or thrills (palpable murmurs) may be felt.

Some diagnostic features of the apex beat

The left ventricle produces a sustained heaving or thrusting apex beat if hypertrophied, but when enlargement is due to dilatation, it is weak and diffuse. It has a 'tapping' quality in mitral stenosis. If there is a left ventricular aneurysm, there may be a double apical beat (rocking or dyskinetic impulse). The right ventricular impulse is usually not palpable in health. When enlarged (owing to pulmonary hypertension or right-sided valve disease), the ventricle gives rise to a parasternal heave. More usually this is due to mitral incompetence.

The heart sounds

The first sound

The first sound (S1) is related to closure of the mitral and tricuspid valves. The mitral component is louder (so it is best heard at the apex) and occurs fractionally before that from closure of the tricuspid valve. At the onset of ventricular systole, the valve cusps have been forced downwards into the ventricle by atrial contraction, and the sound seems to be related to their snapping back up again, the movement being checked by the chordae tendineae.

Loud first heart sounds will occur if the left atrial pressure is abnormally high (mitral stenosis), during fast heart rates or if the atrium contracts very close to ventricular systole (i.e. with a short PR interval). A soft first heart sound occurs if the mitral valve is rigid (e.g. calcified) or does not move well or if left ventricular contraction is poor.

When there is dissociated contraction of the atria and ventricles (as in complete heart block or ventricular tachycardia), the first sound varies in intensity, depending on the position of the valve at the onset of ventricular systole.

The second sound

The second sound (S2) is related to closure of the pulmonary and aortic valves and is best heard in the 2nd left intercostal space. It is louder in pulmonary or systemic hypertension. The sound is normally split because the aortic valve closes before the pulmonary valve on inspiration (the right ventricle takes longer to expel the increased venous return).

Wide splitting is caused when the right ventricle is overloaded and the valve is unable to close quickly (pulmonary stenosis or cor pulmonale), or in right bundle branch block, when there is delayed left ventricular depolarisation.

Reversed splitting (where the splitting is best heard on expiration) occurs if the ventricle is overloaded (aortic stenosis, left ventricular failure or systemic hypertension). It may also occur in left bundle branch block, because the right ventricle is prematurely activated.

Fixed splitting (which does not vary with respiration) occurs when increased venous return affects both ventricles (e.g. atrioseptal defect).

The third sound

The third sound (S3) is associated with the ventricles tensing during rapid filling and implies heart failure or a widely open mitral valve. (It cannot, therefore, occur in severe mitral stenosis.) It is low pitched and best heard at the apex. The third sound may occur normally in the young and in pregnancy but is usually abnormal in patients over the age of 40 years.

The fourth sound

The fourth sound (S4) is heard late in the cardiac cycle (just before the first sound) and is probably produced by rapid atrial emptying into a non-distending ventricle, as may be caused by hypertrophy or cardiomyopathy. It is never heard in health and is usually found in left ventricular hypertrophy or hypertrophic obstructive cardiomyopathy (HOCM).

Gallop rhythm is often heard in heart failure. The addition of a third heart sound with a tachycardia makes the sounds resemble those of a galloping horse. If both third and fourth heart sounds are present, it is called a summation gallop.

Other heart sounds

Ejection clicks occur immediately after the first heart sound at the time of aortic and pulmonary valve opening and are usually associated with stenosis of the valves.

The opening snap of the mitral valve occurs at the time of mitral opening and cannot be heard if the valve is heavily calcified. It may be confused with a third heart sound but is much more widely conducted.

Heart murmurs

Murmurs are sounds caused by turbulent blood flow. This may be either because the blood flow is more rapid or because it is passing through an obstructed pathway. Murmurs are not necessarily pathological.

Innocent murmurs (functional murmurs) are due to minor turbulence unassociated with disease or structural abnormality and may be physiological, as occurs in the hyperdynamic flow of pregnancy, thyrotoxicosis, fever or anaemia. Functional murmurs are very common in children, and most disappear at or about puberty.

Pathological murmurs are indicative of a structural or functional cardiac abnormality.

Murmurs are either systolic or diastolic, and their intensity is classed as grades 1–6 for systolic murmurs and 1–4 for diastolic murmurs; the higher the number, the louder the murmur. Clues to the origin of the murmur may be found by determining when the murmur occurs in the cardiac cycle, where and how it is best heard, how loud it is and, finally, where it radiates to.

Systolic murmurs

These are either pansystolic (i.e. heard throughout systole) or midsystolic (loudest in midsystole). The latter are sometimes called ejection systolic murmurs, as they are usually associated with outflow through a stenosed pulmonary or aortic valve. Innocent and physiological murmurs are virtually always systolic.

Diastolic murmurs

These are either early diastolic, mid-diastolic or late diastolic (presystolic). They are always low pitched.

Continuous murmurs

These start in systole and continue into diastole but not necessarily throughout the whole cardiac cycle.

Features of the different murmurs are shown in Figure 4.3. The more frequent cases are given below.

Pulmonary systolic murmur

This short, 'blowing' murmur is often found in young adults. It may be heard down the left sternal edge and apex. A number of patients will be noted to have a sternal depression or an abnormally straight back ('straight back syndrome'). The mediastinum presumably squashes the heart from front to back, altering blood flow patterns. Although previously considered to be a form of pseudo-heart disease, it may be a familial condition and associated with mitral valve prolapse (Davies et al, 1980).

Aortic ejection murmur

In middle-aged and elderly patients (especially those with hypertension), aortic thickening and dilatation of the ascending aorta are very common. Differentiation from significant aortic stenosis is difficult, and clinical assessment is often unreliable. Hence, all patients should have an echocardiogram, with Doppler assessment of the valve.

Mitral systolic murmur

Fibrosis and calcification of the mitral ring are common in the elderly and produce a murmur identical to that of mitral incompetence. In young women, a short, late systolic murmur is fairly common, and may be due to prolapse of a mitral cusp into the left atrium at the end of ventricular systole. The prognostic significance of this is debatable (Oakley, 1984).

Pericardial friction rub

This is a scratchy sound (rather like sandpaper) produced by the inflamed visceral

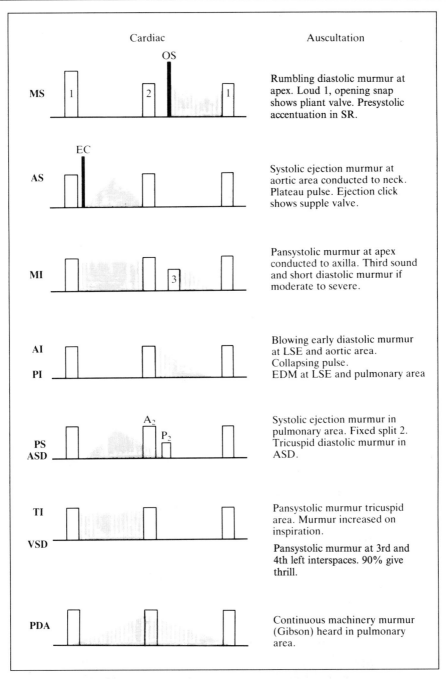

Fig. 4.3 Representation of cardiac murmurs heard on auscultation
MS = mitral stenosis; AS = aortic stenosis; MI = mitral incompetence; AI = aortic incompetence; PI = pulmonary incompetence; EDM = early diastolic murmur; LSE = left sternal edge; PS = pulmonary stenosis; ASD = atrial septal defect; TI = tricuspid incompetence; VSD = ventricular septal defect; PDA = patent ductus arteriosus; 1, 2 = first and second heart sounds

and parietal pericardia rubbing against each other. It may be localised, generalised, long lasting or transient. It is best heard with the patient sitting forward.

Thrills

Thrills are palpable murmurs. The most common are the apical systolic thrills of mitral regurgitation and ventricular septal defects (VSD) and the basal systolic thrill of aortic stenosis.

Signs of hyperlipidaemia

There are three common cutaneous signs of high blood fats, two of which are shown in Figure 4.4.

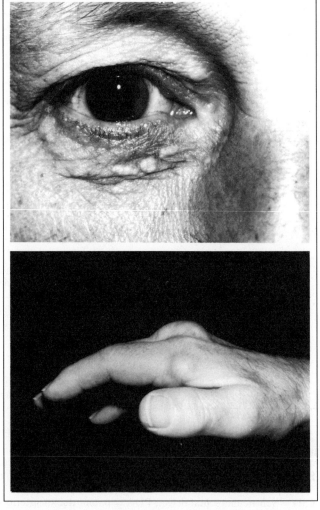

Fig. 4.4 Cutaneous signs of high blood lipids: (a) xanthelasma, (b) tendon xanthoma

Arcus lipidis (senilis)

A white ring surrounding the cornea is very common in the elderly, owing to degenerative changes. However, in patients under the age of 45 years, it is frequently associated with high blood cholesterol levels.

Xanthelasma

These are small, raised, yellow plaques on the eyelids, which contain cholesterol.

Tendon xanthomata

Tendon xanthomata are hard modules found over the knuckles and the patella and in the Achilles tendon. They are an important sign of familial hypercholesterol-aemia (FH), a condition associated with a very high incidence of early and severe coronary heart disease.

The diagonal earlobe crease

An association between coronary heart disease and earlobe creases was described in 1973 (Frank, 1973). This has been substantiated in many studies since, although the cause is not known. The most recent paper (Patel et al, 1992) found a very high correlation between severe coronary atherosclerosis and the presence of the earlobe crease, and it is a clinical sign that should form part of routine clinical examination (Figure 4.5).

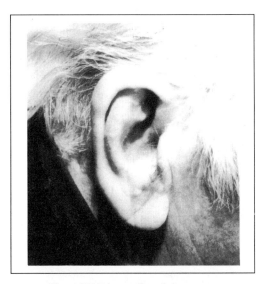

Fig. 4.5 Diagonal earlobe crease

References

Albarran J and Kapeluch H (1994) Role of the nurse in thrombolytic therapy. *British Journal of Nursing*, **3:** 104–109.

Caunt J E (1992) The changing role of coronary care nurses. *Intensive Care Nursing*, **8:** 82–93.

Davies M K, Mackintosh P, Clayton R M, Page A J F, Shiu M F and Littler W A (1980) The straight back syndrome. *Quarterly Journal of Medicine*, **49:** 443–460.

Frank S T (1973) Aural sign of coronary artery disease. *New England Journal of Medicine*, **289:** 327–328.

Geddes L A and Whistler S J (1978) The error in indirect blood pressure measurement with the incorrect size of cuff. *American Heart Journal*, **96:** 4–8.

Hendra T J and Marshall A J (1992) Increased prescription of thrombolytic treatment in elderly patients with suspected myocardial infarction associated with audit. *British Medical Journal*, **304:** 423–425.

Koistinen M J (1990) Prevalence of asymptomatic myocardial ischaemia in diabetic subjects. *British Medical Journal*, **301:** 92–95.

Oakley C M (1984) Mitral valve prolapse: harbinger of death or variant of normal. *British Medical Journal*, **288:** 1853–1854.

O'Neill T W, Barry M, Smith M and Graham I M (1989) Diagnostic value of the apex beat. *Lancet*, **1:** 410–411.

Patel V, Champ C, Andrews P S, Gostelow B E, Gunasekara N P R and Davidson A R (1992) Diagonal earlobe creases and atheromatous disease: a postmortem study. *Journal of the Royal College of Physicians of London*, **26:** 274–277.

Sullivan A K, Holdright D R, Wright C A, Sparrow J L, Cunningham D and Fox K M (1994) Chest pain in women: clinical, investigative and prognostic features. *British Medical Journal*, **308:** 883–886.

5

Investigation of Coronary

Heart Disease

Investigation of patients with coronary heart disease may be required for diagnostic, therapeutic or prognostic reasons. The screening of asymptomatic patients is generally unrewarding, and attention should be directed at those with cardiac symptoms (predominantly chest pain and dyspnoea). The investigation sequence may be:

1. *Preliminary (general practice).* Initial investigations by the primary care team should include a resting (electrocardiogram ECG), chest X-ray and bloods for haemoglobin, ESR, blood sugar, blood lipids and serum urate.

2. *Intermediate (district general hospital).* Most large district general hospitals should be able to perform exercise electrocardiography, 24-hour cardiac taping and echocardiography. Nuclear scanning is available at many of these hospitals.

3. *Specialist (regional cardiac centre).* Specialist investigation facilities and personnel are needed for coronary angiography and cardiac catheterisation.

Apart from the very elderly and infirm, all patients with chest pain compatible with myocardial ischaemia should be referred to hospital for assessment. The prognosis can be influenced by intervention in most cases, and those without coronary heart disease can be reassured. The annual workload of an average district general hospital should include 5000–6000 resting ECGs, 300 exercise stress tests, 250 echocardiograms and 200 ambulatory ECGs per 100 000 population (British Cardiac Society, 1987). Hospitals currently providing lesser numbers may not be offering sufficient support to general practitioners and their patients. There is a need for adequate non-invasive diagnostic facilities for patients of all ages, no matter where they live. Purchasing authorities need to plan for appropriate resources in view of the ageing population. In patients over the age of 65, coronary heart disease is the single most important cause of death (80% of all coronary deaths occur in this age group). In addition, cardiac disease is a major contributory factor to loss of independence of elderly people living at home.

THE ELECTROCARDIOGRAM

The normal electrical impulse originates in the sinus node and is conducted as a wave over the atrium. This wave activates the atrioventricular (AV) node and is then transmitted to the ventricles by the bundles of His. The left bundle perforates the intraventricular septum, and both bundles carry the impulse onwards, the septum being activated from left to right. The impulse then spreads over the endocardial surface of the ventricles via the Purkinje fibres and through the ventricular myocardium, from endocardium to epicardium.

The electrical forces generated by the heart travel in multiple directions simultaneously. The ECG is designed to record these electrical impulses, and the generated waveform has been divided into P, Q, R, S, T and U waves. The *P wave* represents atrial activation, and the *QRS complex* ventricular activation. The *T wave* represents ventricular repolarisation, but the atrial repolarisation wave (T_a) is usually not seen, being buried in the QRS complex.

The signals are amplified, and (by convention) the display is arranged so that impulses moving towards a surface electrode give rise to an upward (positive) deflection, whilst impulses moving away from the electrode give a downward (negative) one. To help to interpret the electrical movement patterns, electrocardiography is carried out in different planes. The three major planes are recorded via electrodes on the right arm (RA), left arm (LA) and left leg (LL). A fourth electrode is traditionally placed on the right leg, but this is not used for recording and serves as a ground (earth) electrode. An electrical triangle is formed by the three planes, with the heart in the centre (Figure 5.1). These three different views of the heart are designated standard leads I, II and III.

The normal ECG consists of recordings from 12 leads. In addition to the three main standard limb leads, there are three 'augmented' unipolar leads (aVR, aVL and aVF). Six unipolar chest (V) leads complete the standard 12-lead ECG and view the heart electrically from the front, as shown in Figure 5.2.

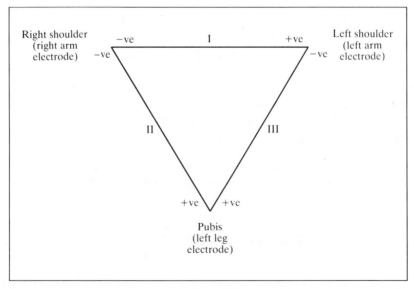

Fig. 5.1   The Einthoven triangle (named after Willem Einthoven, 1860–1927, Professor of Physiology, University of Leiden)

Positioning of the leads

The standard (limb) leads are not often confused as they are usually clearly marked on the electrodes. However, positioning of the chest leads can easily vary

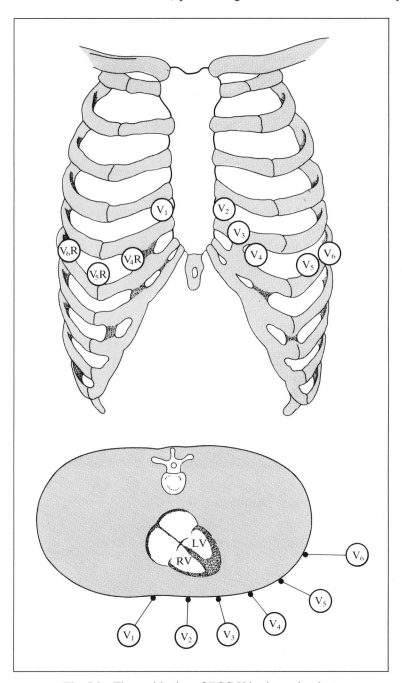

Fig. 5.2 The positioning of ECG V leads on the chest

between serial recordings, and it is important that the correct surface marking is used to prevent artefactual ECG changes between recordings.

- ● V1: 4th intercostal space, immediately to the right of the sternum
- ● V2: 4th intercostal space, immediately to the left of the sternum
- ● V3: Midway between V2 and V4
- ● V4: 5th intercostal space, midclavicular line
- ● V5: Anterior axillary line, on the same horizontal line as V4
- ● V6: Midaxillary line, also horizontal with V4

Many other additional placements can be used to demonstrate particular aspects of the heart (Marriott, 1983), such as V7 and V8 (further laterally) or V3R and V4R (V3 and V4 positions on the right side of the chest).

Assessing the quality of the recording

Before analysing an electrocardiogram, it is essential to ensure that the recording was obtained correctly. Errors in lead placement or connection, paper speed selection, standardisation and lead labelling are very common. Hence, the technical quality of the recording should first be assessed.

1. *Standardisation.* A potential of 1 mV should be represented by a 10 mm vertical deflection. A standard deflection should be recorded at the start and finish of a 12-lead recording.

2. *Speed.* Recordings are usually made at 25 mm/s. Ensure that the machine has not been running at 50 mm/s.

3. *Correct lead placement and labelling.* The net electrical movement in the heart is from lead aVR towards lead II. Hence, in the normal ECG, the complex should be totally positive in lead II (upright P, QRS and T waves) and totally negative in aVR.

4. *Clear tracings.* Too little or too much stylus heat will produce too faint or too thick a tracing. Mains interference may produce a fuzzy trace, as may patient movement caused by cold, shock or fear.

Analysing the ECG

If a standard approach is made towards an ECG, important changes will not be missed. The sequence should be: rate, rhythm, axis, waveform.

Rate

The ECG is recorded at 25 mm/s on standard ECG paper, which has fine lines at 1 mm intervals and heavier divisions every 5 mm. Each millimetre, therefore, represents 0.04 second and each large division is 0.2 second.

To calculate the rate, the number of large squares between two successive complexes should be measured and divided into 300. If the heart rhythm is irregular, a greater number of complexes should be assessed. Special rulers (often provided by manufacturers of cardiac drugs) can simplify the calculation of rate and also give anticipated values for the QT interval.

Rhythm

Normal sinus rhythm should show a normal P wave preceding each QRS complex, with a constant PR interval. If this is not the case, a dysrhythmia is present (dysrhythmias will be discussed later).

Axis

The cardiac axis represents the net electrical direction the impulse takes as it spreads through the myocardium. It does not represent the anatomical position of the heart; right axis deviation does not mean that the heart has swivelled around such that is pointing over the right shoulder!

Axis is usually assessed in the frontal plane, with lead I designated 0°, and the 360° circle surrounding the heart divided into +180° (clockwise) and −180° (anticlockwise). Normally the cardiac axis lies between −30° and +110° and can be quickly determined in the following manner:

1. *Which lead has equal positive and negative QRS components?* This will be at right angles (90°) to the cardiac axis. However, the impulse could be in either direction, which leads to a further question.

2. *Which lead has the predominant QRS vector?* The net electrical movement must be in this direction as movement towards a surface electrode gives a positive deflection.

Waveform

The size of the different waves and the intervals between them are all precisely defined and are subject to biological variability, such as heart rate, age and sex. Values are shown in Figure 5.3.

P wave

The normal P wave results from the spread of activity from the sinus node across atria. This electrical movement is from right to left, so the P wave will be upright in leads I, II and aVF and inverted in aVR. It should not be greater than 0.1 second in duration and should not be taller than 3 mm in the standard leads or 2.5 mm in the V leads.

Abnormalities may be:

1. *Inversion.* This means that the atria are being depolarised from an unusual site, rather than the sinus node (unless there is dextrocardia). The origin may be elsewhere in the atrium, in the AV node or even below this.

2. *Excessive height.* A tall, peaked P wave results from right atrial enlargement. Because this is often secondary to pulmonary hypertension, the wave is sometimes referred to as *P pulmonale.*

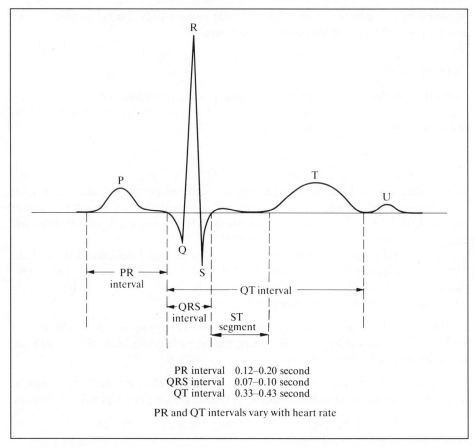

Fig. 5.3 The electrocardiographic cycle showing nomenclature and time intervals

3. *Excessive width.* With left atrial enlargement, the P wave becomes broad and notched, like the letter M. Because this often results from mitral valve disease, the wave is known as *P mitrale*. The P wave is often biphasic in lead V1.

4. *Absent.* The P wave is missing during AV nodal rhythm or may be replaced by flutter or fibrillation waves.

PR interval

This represents the time taken for atrial activation and AV nodal delay and increases with age. It is measured from the start of the P wave to the beginning of the QRS complex and is normally 0.12–0.20 second long (three to five little ECG strip squares). A shortened PR interval is seen when the impulse originates in junctional tissue or when there are accessory conduction pathways (e.g. Wolff–Parkinson–White syndrome). The PR interval lengthens if there is atrioventricular block.

QRS interval

This represents ventricular activation and is measured from the onset of the Q to the end of the S wave. A value greater than 0.12 second (three little squares) is abnormal and usually indicates an intraventricular conduction disorder.

QT interval

This represents the complete electrical activity time of ventricular stimulation and recovery (depolarisation and repolarisation). It is measured from the beginning of the QRS complex to the end of the T wave and varies with heart rate (the QT interval shortens as the heart rate increases). The corrected QT interval (QT_c) may be calculated by the formula:

$$QT_c = \frac{QT}{\sqrt{RR}}$$

where QT is the QT interval and RR is the RR interval. Practically, the QT interval should be less than 50% of the preceding cycle length and seldom exceeds 0.44 second.

The QT interval lengthens in heart failure, following myocardial infarction, with hypocalcaemia and with some drugs. It is shortened in hypercalcaemia and hyperkalaemia.

T wave

The *T wave* results from repolarisation of the ventricles and might, therefore, be assumed to produce a negative deflection. However, because repolarisation takes place in the opposite direction to depolarisation, i.e. from epicardium to endocardium, the T wave is usually positive and has the same axis as the QRS complex. The T wave may be inverted in leads V1 and V2 in healthy individuals and in V3 in negroes.

T waves are normally no greater than 5 mm tall in the standard leads (10 mm in the V leads) but may be taller in hyperkalaemia, myocardial infarction or ischaemia. Flattening or slight inversion is a non-specific abnormality but may reflect hypothyroidism or a low serum potassium. T wave inversion may be found in myocardial infarction, ventricular hypertrophy or bundle branch block.

ST interval

The *ST segment* is measured from the *J point* (at the junction of the S wave and the ST segment) to the start of the T wave. It is very slightly curved upwards but isoelectric. ST displacement or changes in shape are of major importance in electrocardiographic interpretation. Horizontal displacement beyond 1–2 mm upwards or 0.5 mm downwards is abnormal. ST elevation typically occurs in myocardial infarction (when the segment is convex upwards) and pericarditis (when the segment is concave upwards). ST depression is found in myocardial ischaemia and with digoxin therapy.

Frequent mistakes in interpretation of ST morphology are:

1. *High ST take-off.* This frequently occurs in young patients, particularly negroes, and can be up to 2 mm in leads V1 and V2. It is often accompanied by a slight notch on the downstroke of the preceding R wave.

2. *ST depression.*
   a. ST sag during digoxin therapy.
   b. Downward sloping from the J point during sinus tachycardia. Erroneous diagnoses of myocardial ischaemia may be made during exercise stress tests if the ST shift is not measured 40 ms from the J point.
   c. Ventricular hypertrophy leads to ST depression over the relevant ventricle.

U wave

These are low-voltage, broad waves following the T wave. Their origin is not known, but they are especially prominent in hypokalaemia and during digoxin therapy.

Intraventricular conduction blocks

Intraventricular conduction blocks are often found in patients with or without cardiac disease. The term refers to an impairment or block of conduction in one or more of the fascicles of the conducting tissue distal to the bundle of His. Conduction disturbance may also occur within the ventricles.

Bundle branch block

The main bundle of His divides into two main bundle branches (left and right), which depolarise the ventricles, the left ventricle slightly before the right. Either of these bundles may become blocked, resulting in asynchronous ventricular depolarisation and contraction. As a consequence, the morphology of the QRS complex will alter, and the duration of the QRS complex will lengthen to more than 0.12 second. Bundle branch block may complicate 10–20% of cases of acute myocardial infarction and is more common with anterior myocardial infarction.

Left bundle branch block (LBBB)

When the left bundle branch is blocked, septal depolarisation commences from right to left, instead of left to right as normally occurs. Hence, the initial Q wave in the left ventricular leads is lost and is replaced by a small, upright R wave. The right ventricle is depolarised before the left (in contrast to normal), which produces an initial R wave in chest lead V1 and an S wave in lead V6. The left ventricle then depolarises, producing an S wave in V1 and a second R wave (R′) in V6. The delay in biventricular activation prolongs the QRS duration to >0.12 second and alters the QRS morphology, such that a W-shaped complex appears in V1 and an M-shaped complex in V6 (Figure 5.4).

Right bundle branch block (RBBB)

Because of right bundle branch block, right ventricular depolarisation is delayed and follows that of the left ventricle. This late depolarisation produces a secondary R wave (R') in the right chest leads and a deep S wave in the left chest leads. The QRS complex is again prolonged to greater than 0.12 second, and the morphology is reversed, such that in V1 there is an M-shaped complex and in V6 W-shaped

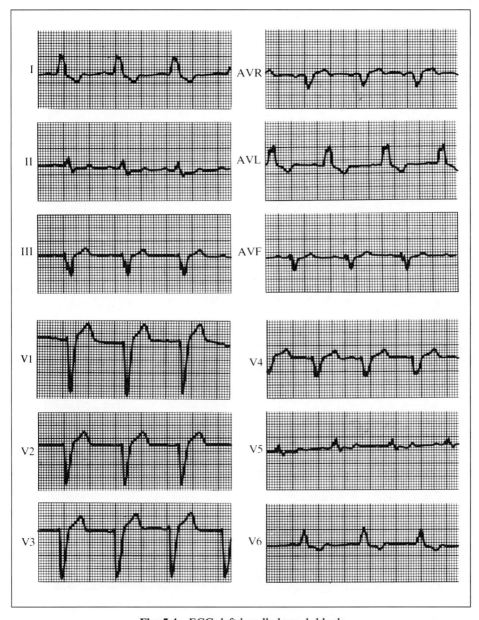

Fig. 5.4 ECG: left bundle branch block

complex (Figure 5.5). **RBBB** complicates about 2% of myocardial infarcts and is associated with the later development of complete heart block.

Hemiblocks

The left bundle divides into two hemifascicles, an anterior one running superio-laterally and a posterior one running inferomedially. Each of these may become blocked, either on its own or in addition to the right and left bundles.

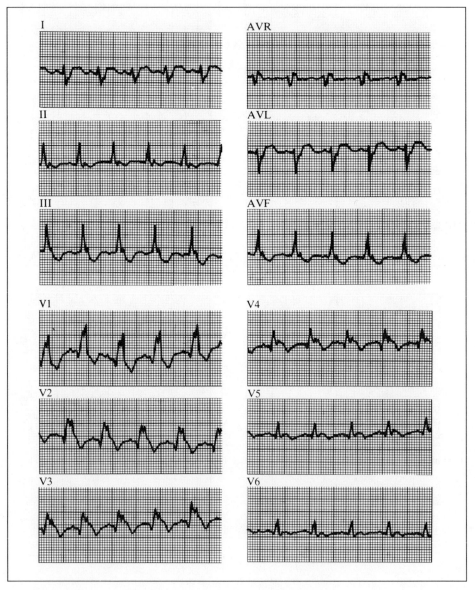

Fig. 5.5   ECG: right bundle branch block

Although hemiblock leads to a slight prolongation of the QRS duration, this is usually not appreciated because the duration is still less than 0.12 second. Recognition is by a change in the frontal QRS axis that cannot be explained by any other cause.

The more common left anterior hemiblock is manifest by left axis deviation to less than $-30°$, whilst left posterior hemiblock produces right axis deviation in excess of $+110°$. Additionally, QRS morphology may alter to show an RS pattern in lead I and a QR in lead III if there is left posterior hemiblock, whilst the reverse is seen in left anterior hemiblock.

Left anterior hemiblock (LAHB) complicating myocardial infarction is considered benign, but left posterior hemiblock (LPHB) is usually only seen with extensive myocardial infarction, and is, therefore, associated with a high mortality.

Bifascicular block means block affecting any two hemifascicles, such as RBBB + LAHB/LPHB or LAHB + LPHB. Bifascicular block after myocardial infarction commonly leads to complete heart block, and prophylactic temporary pacing is sometimes carried out.

Incomplete bundle branch block

This term is commonly used when the morphology of the QRS complex is similar to that observed in established bundle branch block but the QRS duration is within normal limits (<0.12 second). The changes are not thought to be due to actual conduction block but are more indicative of delays caused by depolarisation of enlarged ventricles.

Bundle of His electrocardiography

Invasive electrophysiological techniques are sometimes needed to locate the site of heart block, since the normal ECG does not yield much information about electrical activity within the AV node. Wires are passed and placed in and around the AV node, and electrical spikes of sequential depolarising activity are recorded (A spikes, H spikes and V spikes). Such information is used to plan treatment.

Ventricular hypertrophy

Ventricular hypertrophy increases the amplitude of the QRS complex. Hypertrophy of the left ventricle increases the height of the R waves in the left chest leads, whilst that of the right ventricle increases the height of the R waves in the right ventricular leads. Septal hypertrophy produces a large, narrow Q wave in the left chest leads.

Unfortunately, many factors can influence the magnitude of the QRS complex, including age, thickness of the chest wall, expanded chests (in chronic obstructive airways disease), hypothyroidism and pericardial effusions. However, the following measurements are useful for the diagnosis of ventricular hypertrophy on voltage criteria:

1. *Left ventricular hypertrophy*
   a. The R wave in V5 or V6 is greater than 25 mm.
   b. The R wave in V5 or V6 plus the S wave in V1 is greater than 35 mm (40 mm in the young).
   c. The R wave in aVF is greater than 20 mm.
   Confirmatory evidence is provided by left axis deviation ($< 0°$), ST depression and T wave inversion in V4–V6 and possible P mitrale.

2. *Right ventricular hypertrophy*
   a. An R wave > S wave in V1, and measures more than 5 mm.
   b. The R wave in V1 plus the S wave in V5 or V6 is greater than 10 mm.
   Confirmatory evidence is right axis deviation ($> +110°$), ST depression and T wave inversion in V1–V3 and possible P pulmonale.

THE CHEST RADIOGRAPH

The plain chest radiograph or X-ray is one of the most important aids to the diagnosis of cardiovascular disease. The alveolar air provides an excellent radiographic contrast medium upon which to outline the heart, the great vessels and the pulmonary vasculature. The standard posteroanterior (PA) chest X-ray is taken at full inspiration, with the patient standing facing the film, which is 1.5 m from the X-ray tube focus. High-kilovoltage exposures (120–150 kV) are often preferable for visualising the mediastinum and lung vasculature, although conventional kilovoltage (70–80 kV) allows the bony skeleton and calcified lesions to be seen. In the standard PA view, the right border of the heart consists (from top to bottom) of the superior vena cava, the ascending aorta and the right atrium. The left border is formed by the aortic arch, the descending aorta, the pulmonary artery and its left main branch, and the left ventricle (Figure 5.6). Standard PA chest films are desirable whenever possible because:

- The diaphragm is flattened and allows the bases of the lungs to be seen
- The erect position lowers hydrostatic pressure in the low-pressure pulmonary vascular tree
- The scapulae are slid away from the lung fields
- The PA projection reduces magnification of the heart shadow

However, the patient on coronary care is often too ill to stand, and a recumbent portable AP film is usually taken, with consequent interpretation problems, as might be anticipated from the preceding remarks.

Interpretation

The radiograph should be assessed in a routine method so that nothing is missed.

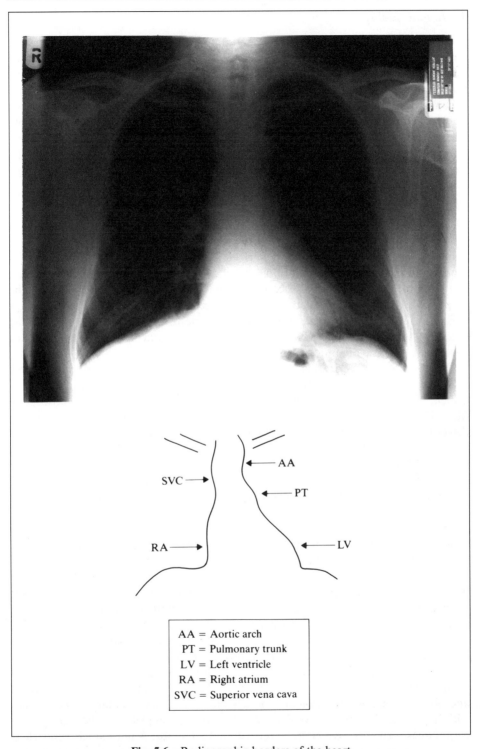

Fig. 5.6 Radiographic borders of the heart

Technical quality

All films should be correctly identified and dated. Right and left markers will avoid a missed diagnosis of dextrocardia. If the film is taken straight, the medial ends of the clavicles should be equidistant from the midline (marked by the spinous processes of the vertebrae). Too low a kilovoltage will underpenetrate the film and enhance lung markings. This is particularly common in the obese patient, often leading to an erroneous diagnosis of pulmonary congestion. It is important to note what kilovoltage has been employed, particularly in coronary care, where interpretation of pulmonary congestion is important. A change to a higher kilovoltage on a subsequent chest film will show the apparent clearing of pulmonary oedema.

The heart

The cardiac size is assessed by determining the cardiothoracic ratio (CTR). This is the ratio of the widest part of the heart shadow to the widest transverse thoracic diameter (measured from the inner surface of the ribs). The CTR should be less than 0.5 in adults. This method of assessing cardiac size is not infallible, however. For example, in aortic valve disease, left ventricular enlargement is towards the diaphragm, and the cardiac diameter is not affected.

Enlargement of the cardiac shadow may be due to pericardial effusion, cardiac dilatation or hypertrophy. Cardiomegaly is common in athletes and does not necessarily indicate dilatation or hypertrophy.

The diagnosis of pericardial effusion is not always easy on the standard chest film, because it cannot readily be distinguished from other causes of cardiac enlargement. If it has formed rapidly, cardiac dilatation may be seen on consecutive films. Large effusions make the heart outline globular; small effusions are hard to detect radiologically and are best detected by echocardiography.

The most frequent cause of cardiac enlargement is dilatation due to volume overload. Hypertrophy normally leads to a volume reduction within the heart chambers, so that the overall cardiac diameters are only very slightly increased. Dilatation and hypertrophy frequently coexist and are probably best differentiated by echocardiography.

Although a good knowledge of radiographic anatomy is useful to distinguish which part of the heart is responsible for the cardiac enlargement, the same final picture can be produced by different underlying processes. Enlargement of the left atrium is the most easy to recognise, gives a projection of 2 cm below the left pulmonary artery shadow and causes a convex bulge immediately below the left main bronchus. In extreme enlargement, the left atrium will protrude above the right atrium, causing a double density at the right border of the heart. Right atrial enlargement simply makes the right border look more prominent, and it produces a long continuous convexity of the right heart border.

Enlargement of the ventricles may be difficult to distinguish on the conventional chest X-ray. Left ventricular enlargement pushes the cardiac shadow downwards and outwards below the cupola of the left diaphragm and is found in association with hypertension, aortic valve disease and mitral incompetence. The right ventricle enlarges forwards, reducing the retrosternal air space. A normal left ventricle is sometimes pushed posteriorly by right ventricular enlargement (due to pulmonary hypertension or pulmonary stenosis), and the cardiac apex is rounded and lifted up above the left diaphragm.

The lung fields

The normal pulmonary artery divisions can be traced to within about a centimetre of the lung edge. The pulmonary veins are large and horizontal in the lower lung fields, but are seen as smaller linear opacities draining towards the left atrium in the upper lung fields.

Increased pulmonary capillary pressures and diminished cardiac output are the final common pathways for the production of pulmonary oedema. As pressure in the pulmonary veins rises, radiological manifestations follow a specific pattern until a critical pressure of about 30 mmHg is reached:

- 18–20 mmHg: onset of pulmonary congestion
- 20–30 mmHg: increasing congestion
- > 30 mmHg: onset of pulmonary oedema

Radiological evidence of pulmonary oedema occurs first in the lower pulmonary veins, where perivascular interstitial oedema develops. This results in local hypoxia and reflex vasoconstriction in the affected vessels. The blood is then diverted to the upper lung vessels (upper lobe diversion), producing the characteristic radiological picture (Figure 5.7). The interstitial oedema collects around hilar vessels to produce the 'bat wing' sign, and collection in and around the pulmonary lympha-

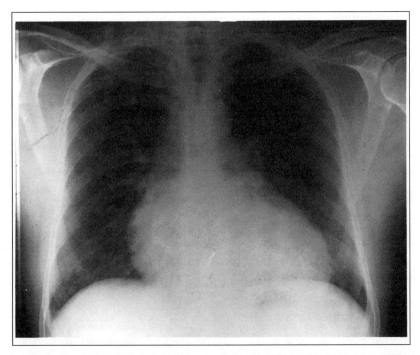

Fig. 5.7   The chest radiograph in left ventricular failure. Note the enlarged heart and upper lobe diversion of blood

tics gives rise to thin linear opacities called Kerley lines. The *Kerley A lines* (engorged intralobular lymphatics) run from the periphery to the hilum, and the more common *Kerley B lines* of interstitial oedema are short parallel lines that run horizontally at the lung peripheries, particularly in the costophrenic angles. As the pulmonary oedema worsens, fluid collects in the alveoli of the lower zones, producing opacities, and later outside the lung to produce pleural effusions.

Rapid response to therapy in patients with early pulmonary congestion may produce a difference in clinical and radiological interpretation of the current haemodynamic position. Features are labile and may clear within a few hours of therapy. However, there may sometimes be a lag of up to 48 hours between haemodynamic stabilisation and resolution of radiological signs. In patients with long-standing pulmonary hypertension and heart failure, there may be thickening of the pulmonary vessel walls, allowing substantial elevation of pulmonary capillary pressures without clinical congestion.

Pulmonary oligaemia may be seen with large pulmonary emboli and emphysema.

The diaphragm

The diaphragm should expand to the level of the 5th rib anteriorly on full inspiration. A fat pad is sometimes seen adjacent to the cardiac border in the obese, and a slight hump of the right diaphragm is frequent in the elderly.

The mediastinum

The position and size of the aorta should be noted. Unfolding is common in the elderly and in the hypertensive patient. Other radiological abnormalities of the aorta commonly found in the elderly are due to degenerative changes and include calcification (especially of the aortic knuckle) and dilatation. An increase in the size of the aortic outline (particularly on serial films) may indicate aortic dissection, particularly in the presence of a small left pleural effusion. The shadow is often calcified.

Bones

The heart will be displaced if there is a thoracic scoliosis. Large aortic aneurysms may erode the anterior surface of adjacent vertebrae. Rib lesions (fractures or metastases) may be a cause of chest pain and should be looked for.

Sternal depression may displace the heart and is the cause of a systolic murmur with apparent cardiac enlargement (the 'straight back' syndrome). This may only be visible with a lateral chest film.

The neck and upper abdomen

Retrosternal extension of a goitre may be misdiagnosed as an aortic aneurysm. The presence of intraperitoneal air (air under the diaphragm) should be excluded, since peritonitis may present with chest and shoulder tip pain.

ECHOCARDIOGRAPHY

Ultrasound imaging (echocardiography) allows the heart to be studied non-invasively and is a powerful tool for assessing cardiac anatomy, pathology and function. The echocardiogram uses a transducer that generates high-frequency pulses of short duration, which travel through the body at different velocities (depending upon the tissues encountered) and are echoed back, to be recorded by the same transducer. Cardiac ultrasound uses frequencies of 2.5–5.0 MHz, and the higher the frequency, the better the resolution (although the worse the penetration).

The two main techniques used are M-mode and cross-sectional (two-dimensional or real-time) echocardiography. The Doppler shift effect during ultrasound can be combined with these techniques to provide information on the velocity and direction of blood flow. Colour flow-mapping uses a multigated, pulsed Doppler technique to estimate the mean velocity of blood cells within the heart and can identify patterns of blood flow and abnormal jets.

Transthoracic echocardiography is the usual method of obtaining cardiac images. The transducer is placed on the chest wall to obtain different views of heart through anatomical 'windows'. The technique is limited by the size of these windows found between the ribs and lungs, since ultrasound does not travel through bone or air. Technical difficulties may be encountered in up to one quarter of recordings.

Transoesophageal echocardiography (TOE) uses a miniature transducer mounted on a modified endoscope, which may be swallowed and positioned directly behind the heart. The image quality is much better because of the proximity of the structures as well as the absence of bone. Biplane probes incorporate two transducers at right angles to each other, and multiplane probes can permit a 180° view of the heart. The probe frequency is extended up to 7.5 MHz (since depth is not so important), which allows very high resolution.

Cross-sectional echocardiography (CSE)

Two-dimensional images are built up by the ultrasound beam being swept through a 90° sector of the heart, producing up to 50 cross-sections per second and generating a recognisable two-dimensional moving image of the heart. Multiple views from different sites on the chest can be used to build up a complete picture of the heart. The images are usually recorded on super-VHS videotape or on laser discs. Photographs can be obtained as a hard copy to file with the notes. On-line computers can be used to measure cardiac dimensions and calculate various parameters, such as ejection fraction and cardiac output. Fall-off in signal can sometimes produce poor images and often makes exact measurement of cardiac function inaccurate.

M-mode echocardiography

M-mode echocardiography is a technique that essentially produces a graph of depth of tissues against time. A single 1 cm ultrasound beam is directed through the heart using a scan line selected from the two-dimensional image. The graph is recorded on rapidly-moving paper, which allows measurement of intracardiac structures (such as wall thickness and cavity dimensions) with timing of events. The M-mode trace does not demonstrate cardiac anatomy and probably should not be interpreted without reference to the cross-sectional image.

Doppler echocardiography

Blood velocity can be calculated by using the Doppler effect on red cells, either by pulsed or continuous wave ultrasound. Pulsed wave (PW) Doppler assesses the velocity of blood at one site, selected by a cursor superimposed on the two-dimensional image. Continuous wave (CW) Doppler emits a constant stream of ultrasound along a single line and superimposes all velocities along that line. CW Doppler can resolve very high velocities (e.g. through stenosed valves), whilst PW Doppler can measure flow at precise depths in conjunction with the two-dimensional image. The machine software is able to display calculated flow velocities and is very useful in assessing obstructive lesions and septal defects.

Colour flow echocardiography

Colour Doppler flow-mapping has been one of the most important developments in cardiac ultrasound since cross-sectional echocardiography. It has allowed a better understanding of flow physiology in health and disease. Colour flow-mapping uses a multigated Doppler system to display blood flow information over the two-dimensional image. By convention, flow towards the transducer is displayed red, flow away from the transducer is coloured blue and turbulence produces a mosaic of different colours. The technique is very sensitive and can detect the trivial regurgitation that occurs through normal valves when they close. Overinterpretation of the images is a common mistake; for example, we now know that 90% of the normal population has physiological tricuspid and pulmonary regurgitation and one third have mitral regurgitation (Houston, 1993).

Colour flow may be combined with M-mode echocardiography and is useful for timing flow events and distinguishing between systolic and diastolic abnormalities.

Echocardiography and coronary care

A modern, two-dimensional ultrasound machine is an essential piece of equipment for the coronary care unit. Its value in emergency coronary care is enormous. In patients with cardiovascular collapse of unknown cause, echocardiography can differentiate at the bedside between hypovolaemia, severe left ventricular dysfunction, pulmonary embolism and pericardial effusion with tamponade. The intimal flap of an aortic dissection can be seen in many cases of aortic dissection, particularly with trans-oesophageal echocardiography, and critical aortic stenosis can also be demonstrated and quantified.

Other frequent applications of echocardiography in patients on coronary care include:

1. *Defining the aetiology of cardiomegaly.* Clinical and radiological cardiomegaly may be due to ventricular dilatation, ventricular hypertrophy or pericardial effusion. Echocardiography allows the correct interpretation.

2. *Supporting the diagnosis of ischaemic chest pain.* Regional left ventricular wall dyskinesia is a feature of myocardial ischaemia and may occur before there are any ECG changes. Stress echocardiography, using dynamic exercise or pharmacological stress (dobutamine), may be used to detect wall motion abnormalities.

3. *Assessing complications of myocardial infarction.* Echocardiography is essential for the prompt diagnosis of the complications of acute myocardial infarction. It can quickly distinguish between acute mitral incompetence and an acquired ventriculoseptal defect. It is an essential investigation in patients with cardiogenic shock, to distinguish severe left ventricular damage from right ventricular infarction or cardiac rupture with tamponade.

4. *Assessment of cardiac failure.* Echocardiography should be carried out in all patients presenting with heart failure to establish the aetiology. The estimation of ejection fraction is of importance in determining which patients will benefit from acute administration of ACE-inhibitors following myocardial infarction (St John Sutton, 1994).

5. *Miscellaneous problems*

   a. *Vegetations* over 3 mm in size may be demonstrable in over half the patients with infective endocarditis. They are seen as rapidly moving masses attached to, or replacing, normal cardiac tissue. TOE is the best approach for confirmation and to show complications, such as mycotic abscesses.

   b. *Mitral valve prolapse* is common (depending upon precise definitions) and is easily identifiable with echocardiography. It may present with dysrhythmias, atypical chest pain or peripheral emboli (Oakley, 1984).

   c. *Hypertrophic cardiomyopathy (HOCM)* may present with chest pain and dysrhythmias. The diagnosis may be established with echocardiography.

   d. *Prosthetic valve function* may need to be assessed in coronary care admissions in case dysfunction is the source of symptoms.

EXERCISE STRESS TESTING

Many patients with cardiac disease have no signs, symptoms or abnormal investigations at rest, and exercise stress testing may reveal hitherto undocumented abnormalities. The main aims of stress testing are:

- To provoke symptoms, such as chest pain and dyspnoea
- To demonstrate ECG changes with progressive workload
- To determine maximum workload
- To assess prognosis

The procedure has a low complication rate, although any investigation of patients with myocardial disease carries a risk of cardiac arrest or myocardial infarction. It is, therefore, usual for such tests to be carried out by trained staff, with a doctor in attendance and with resuscitation facilities available. Sudden death may occur, although in a series of 20 000 tests in Seattle, there were only six cases of ventricular fibrillation, which occurred in the first 5 minutes following cessation of the test (Irving et al, 1977). All these patients had myocardial disease, were hypotensive during exercise and were resuscitated. High-risk patients include those with aortic stenosis, hypertrophic cardiomyopathy, unstable angina, recent myocardial infarction or ventricular dysrhythmias. Close monitoring of these patients, and those with highly abnormal tests, is required, with overnight admission to hospital if there is any concern about delayed response to exercise. The British Cardiac Society (1993) has drawn up guidelines for performing exercise tests in the absence of direct medical supervision.

Despite a wealth of experience, and a great deal of published work on the investigation, controversy still surrounds the interpretation of the test. For example, if ST depression of 1 mm is used to diagnose ischaemia, the false positive rate may be as high as 64% (Epstein, 1978). It is more important perhaps to look at symptoms, pulse and blood pressure response and recovery time following exercise. In general, early onset of angina, marked and widespread ST depression, slow recovery and a poor blood pressure response are indicative of severe ischaemic heart disease.

Methods of stress testing

The original step tests have now been replaced by treadmill and bicycle tests, the choice being largely determined by cost and available space. There are several contraindications to stress testing, which are shown in Table 5.1.

The different recommended lead systems for detecting regional myocardial ischaemia employ from two to 20 electrodes. The simplest and most useful lead for recording is MCL5 (the positive lead in the V5 interspace and the negative on the manubrium), which will demonstrate up to 90% of detectable abnormalities. However, the most common lead system uses the normal 12-lead recording positions. The torso rather than the limbs is used for the limb leads, to prevent entanglement and to reduce movement artefact.

Table 5.1   Contraindications to ECG stress testing

Cardiac
Unstable angina
Severe hypertension
Myocarditis or pericarditis
Aortic stenosis
Serious dysrhythmias

Non-cardiac
Anaemia
Elderly or infirm patient
Gross obesity
Severe respiratory disease

Drugs/electrolytes
Digoxin toxicity
Electrolyte imbalance
Unstable antidysrhythmic therapy

There are many different protocols designed for different circumstances and available equipment (Fletcher et al, 1990). The ideal protocol should offer:

- An appropriate workload for the patient, which will not cause excessive stress
- A gradually increasing workload, with enough time at each level to attain steady state
- Continuous ECG, heart rate and blood pressure recording
- Medical supervision and resuscitation facilities

The most common tests employ the Bruce protocol (Bruce et al, 1963) and the Naughton protocol (Naughton et al, 1964). The Bruce protocol is suitable for routine use and produces a fast increase in progressive workload (Table 5.2). The Naughton protocol is much slower, taking 24 minutes to reach the 12-minute equivalent of the Bruce protocol (Table 5.3) and is more suited to patients known to have cardiac disease, particularly those with recent myocardial infarction.

Table 5.2 Bruce protocol for exercise (treadmill) ECG test

Stage	Speed (mph)	Grade (%)	Duration (min)	METs (units)	Total time elapsed (min)
1	1.7	10	3	4	3
2	2.5	12	3	6–7	6
3	3.4	14	3	8–9	9
4	4.2	16	3	15–16	12
5	5.0	18	3	21	15
6	5.5	20	3	–	18
7	6.0	22	3	–	21

Table 5.3 Naughton protocol for exercise (treadmill) ECG test

Stage	2.0 mph Grade (%)	3.0 mph Grade (%)	3.4 mph Grade (%)	Duration (min)	METs (units)	Total time elapsed (min)
1	–	–	–	2	1.0	2
2	0.0	–	–	2	2.0	4
3	3.5	0.0	–	2	3.0	6
4	7.0	2.5	2.0	2	4.0	8
5	10.5	5.0	4.0	2	5.0	10
6	14.0	7.5	6.0	2	6.0	12
7	17.5	10.0	8.0	2	7.0	14
8	–	12.5	10.0	2	8.0	16
9	–	15.0	12.0	2	9.0	18
10	–	17.5	14.0	2	10.0	20
11	–	20.0	16.0	2	11.0	22
12	–	22.5	18.0	2	12.0	24
13	–	25.0	20.0	2	13.0	26
14	–	27.5	22.0	2	14.0	28
15	–	30.0	24.0	2	15.0	30
16	–	32.5	26.0	2	16.0	32

Oxygen uptake (VO₂) and metabolic equivalents (METs)

The rate of oxygen uptake by the body relates to the ability to achieve a given work-load. At rest, the VO_2 is about 3.5 ml/kg per minute, which is described as 1 MET (1 metabolic equivalent). Average peak VO_2 in cardiac patients is about 21 ml/kg per minute (6 METs); those who can achieve 10 METs have a prognosis with medical therapy as good as those with operative intervention, and those who can achieve 13 METs have an excellent prognosis regardless of other exercise responses. Since exercise protocols differ, effort capacity should be expressed in METs.

There are various parameters that can be observed and assessed during an exercise test. These may be:

- *Symptomatic*: onset of symptoms and relationship to exercise
- *Haemodynamic*: changes in blood pressure and heart rate
- *Electrocardiographic*: changes in the ST segment and cardiac rhythm

A standard resting ECG should be obtained before the test and current medication needs to be recorded. During the test, the patient should be encouraged to exercise for as long as possible, but signs of fatigue, pain and dyspnoea should be noted, especially in the stoic patient. The systolic blood pressure should be recorded at the termination of each stage by palpation of the brachial artery. The diastolic blood pressure is difficult to measure and does not add to the value of the test.

Automatic ECG recorders will usually record a full 10-second ECG at predetermined time intervals (three leads recorded simultaneously for 2.5 seconds), and the test is continued until completion or another endpoint has been reached (Table 5.4). At the end of testing, the level of the test achieved (with timing and MET equivalent) should be recorded, with the reason for stopping. All symptoms and blood pressure readings should be recorded. Maximal ST depression should be noted, although it is best to report only on planar or down-sloping ST segments as indicative of possible myocardial ischaemia.

Indications for stress testing

Assessing patients with chest pain

A major indication for exercise stress testing is in the diagnosis of chest pain. Unfortunately, ST changes are not always present during exercise in patients with

Table 5.4 Endpoints of the exercise stress test

Absolute	Relative
Patient's request	Chest pain without ECG changes
Fall in blood pressure or heart rate	Less serious symptoms (anxiety, dizziness, cramp)
Sustained dysrhythmias	
Progressive angina	Attainment of predicted maximal heart rate
Severe dyspnoea, fatigue or faintness	Marked ST depression (>5 mm)
Equipment failure	Increasing ectopic activity or heart block
	Marked hypertension (SP > 220 mmHg; DP > 110 mmHg)

angiographically-defined coronary artery disease, especially if lesions are limited to the circumflex and distal right coronary arteries. False negative tests may also be obtained if the patient is taking beta-blockers, which limit cardiac work, or if exercise has been submaximal. False positive results may be obtained in up to 10% of men and 25% of women who have normal resting ECGs. Diagnostic stress testing is, therefore, of limited value in women (Sullivan et al, 1994). There have been many explanations for these findings, including ST changes due to hyperventilation or increased sympathetic tone. In some young women, multiple resting ST/T wave changes are found on the resting ECG, which worsen (often dramatically) on exercise.

Another peculiar syndrome describes angina in patients with angiographically normal coronary arteries (Syndrome X). Invasive studies often show abnormal myocardial contractility, and the condition probably reflects an early form of cardiomyopathy.

Assessing prognosis

Exercise testing has become routine in most hospitals to determine prognosis in patients with ischaemic heart disease. The greater the degree of ST segment shift on exercise, the greater the chance of significant multivessel disease. The exercise time is very important and is often used for risk stratification and to determine mortality (Table 5.5).

The prognosis of patients following myocardial infarction is mostly dependent on left ventricular function, which may be reflected by workload and blood pressure response to formal exercise, as well as circulation to the unaffected myocardium. Whilst ST changes may reflect poor coronary perfusion (Akhras et al, 1982), it is the exercise time and blood pressure response that matter most. Inability to perform the test and/or a rise of less than 30 mmHg in the systolic blood pressure seem to identify the high-risk patients and are predictive of future cardiac events (Campbell et al, 1988). Symptom-limited exercise stress testing may be safely carried out before discharge in selected patients. These are patients under 65 years of age, without dysrhythmias, recurrent ischaemic pain or cardiac failure. Information on functional capacity is not only useful for prognostic reasons, but may also help in advising future activities and the appropriateness of rehabilitation. For logistic reasons, exercise testing often has to be carried out following discharge from hospital. Those patients who were unable to have a predischarge

Table 5.5 Mortality for patients with coronary heart disease assessed by the Bruce Exercise Test (Coronary Artery Surgery Study, 1983)

Risk group	Test result	Mortality	
		12 months (%)	24 months (%)
Low	Stage III	1	5
Moderate	Stage II	2	11
High	Stage I	5	19

stress test should have the test performed prior to their first outpatient appointment. In general, those with normal exercise tests have a good prognosis, as opposed to those with poor exercise tests. Patients without cardiac pain after myocardial infarction, and without ST changes during exercise stress testing, do not need coronary angiography (Cross et al, 1993). Those with abnormal tests should be examined further by echocardiography, radionuclide studies or arteriography. Since thrombolysis has become routine, there is some concern that dynamic stress testing may have limited value in assessing the prognosis in post-infarct patients (Stevenson et al, 1993). By recanalising the infarct-related artery, thrombolytic treatment exposes the patient to the risk of reocclusion. This risk will not be revealed by conventional stress testing, which has been designed to detect reversible ischaemia and left ventricular performance. It may be that other non-invasive techniques (such as nuclear studies) will become the investigation of choice in post-infarct patients.

Assessing other exercise-related symptoms

The aetiology of atypical anginal pain, dyspnoea, palpitations and dizziness may all be clarified by an exercise test. Functional capacity can be gauged by an objective assessment of the severity of symptoms and the degree of limitation imposed by cardiac or other disease. Occasionally, intermittent dysrhythmias may be recorded, and an exercise test should form part of the evaluation of patients with suspected cardiac rhythm abnormalities (Podrid and Graboys, 1984).

In patients with cardiac failure, an exercise capacity of <6METs associates with decreased survival, and a capacity below 4METs provides a strong reason for considering heart transplantation.

NUCLEAR SCANS AND NUCLEAR ANGIOGRAPHY

In recent years, there has been a rapid development of radioisotope techniques for the assessment of myocardial disease. Nuclear scans can be used to assess:

- Myocardial perfusion
- Ventricular function
- Myocardial viability
- Prognosis

Myocardial perfusion has mainly been assessed using thallium and technetium, which are injected intravenously and taken up by the heart, which is then visualised in planar or tomographic modes by a gamma camera. Radiolabelled agents identify and delineate areas of myocardial hypoperfusion, either by being preferentially taken up by damaged or necrosed myocardium (hot spot detection) or by demonstrating areas of hypoperfusion (cold spot detection). Technetium-99m-labelled pyrophosphate is most commonly used for the former and thallium-201 for the latter.

- *The thallium scan.* Thallium-201 is a potassium analogue, which concentrates in normal myocardial cells and can be used to demonstrate myocardial ischaemia and infarction. Abnormal tissue does not take up the tracer and, therefore, appears as a cold spot on the scan.
- *The technetium-99m pyrophosphate scan.* In contrast to thallium scanning, technetium-labelled pyrophosphate is taken up by damaged myocardial cells and is imaged as a hot spot. This may be useful in the diagnosis of recent myocardial infarction, when traditional investigations (enzymes, ECG, etc.) have not been of help. This investigation is popular in the USA but is not often carried out in the UK.

These multiple planar techniques have been superseded by SPECT (single photon emission computed tomography) imaging, a three-dimensional imaging technique that allows accurate localisation of perfusion defects. This is particularly of value in identifying the coronary vessel involved. Technetium-labelled methoxy-iso-butyl isonitrile (99mTc-MIBI) is the usual agent employed, although technetium-labelled tetrofosmin is now being used to produce superior imaging.

Nuclear stress testing

Where routine perfusion scanning has not produced enough information, scanning may be repeated using either pharmacological or exercise (dynamic) stress testing. In the USA, nuclear stress testing has almost replaced ECG treadmill stress tests.

For dynamic testing, the patient exercises on a bicycle until he becomes symptomatic. Thallium is then injected and the image is obtained in separate views with a gamma camera. Cold spots may disappear as the myocardium reperfuses, and fixed cold spots indicate old infarct. Patients with significant triple vessel disease often take up thallium very poorly, with a very slow wash-out.

In those unable to exercise, dipyridamole or adenosine is injected to promote coronary blood flow, and then thallium scanning can be used to detect differential flow through normal and stenosed arteries. Alternatively, dobutamine may be given to precipitate myocardial ischaemia without exercise, and simultaneous echocardiography and SPECT scanning can be extremely effective in detecting coronary vessel stenosis.

Radionuclide ventriculography

Radionuclide ventriculography is helpful in defining those patients with poor left ventricular function whose prognosis may be improved with surgery. More recently, the importance of right ventricular dysfunction in low output states has been recognised, particularly following inferior and right ventricular infarction. Nuclear scanning may be invaluable for examining these difficult areas of the heart. Ischaemic dysfunction that may only develop during exercise can also be easily visualised by nuclear angiography and is usually seen as a fall in cardiac output, with the development of regional contraction abnormalities (Dymond et al, 1984).

There are two main techniques of radionuclide ventriculography: first-pass scanning and multigated acquisition (MUGA) scanning.

1. *First-pass scanning.* A radiotracer (usually technetium-99m) is injected as a bolus into a peripheral vein and its radioactivity counted on its first passage through the heart. The chambers can be visually separated by its time of passage through the right and left heart, so that images of the right and left heart can be constructed. Wall motion of the anterolateral and inferior aspects of the left ventricle can also be demonstrated.

2. *The MUGA scan.* Technetium is used to label the patient's red cells, which are then reinjected. A period of equilibration is then allowed; radioactivity is then measured within the heart as it beats and recorded frame by frame by the gamma-camera, which is activated by the ECG (one frame per cycle). This enables regional wall motion to be visualised (for defining dyskinetic segments and ventricular aneurysms) and can provide information on ventricular volumes, ejection fraction and cardiac output.

In patients recovering from myocardial infarction, radionuclide ventriculography is an excellent way to identify poor left ventricular anatomy and function, which is important prognostically.

Nuclear imaging in acute myocardial infarction

In most cases of myocardial infarction, there is adequate diagnostic evidence of myocardial infarction from the history, ECG and cardiac enzymes. In more difficult cases, nuclear imaging may then complement other investigations, for example in the:

- Diagnosis and localisation of a myocardial infarction in the presence of left bundle branch block or subendocardial necrosis
- Diagnosis of right ventricular infarction
- Detection of new areas of infarction close to old areas of fibrosis
- Diagnosis of perioperative myocardial infarction

Thallium-201 cold spot scans are nearly always positive in the first 6 hours following myocardial infarction but are less reliable thereafter. Unfortunately, reversible defects may be found in patients with coronary artery spasm or crescendo angina, and fixed defects may be found if there is myocardial infiltration or old infarction. Technetium-99m scanning is of particular value in right ventricular infarction (Rodrigues et al, 1986) and, in combination with thallium scanning, may be used to separate areas of recent and previous myocardial infarction. Exercise stress testing with thallium is about twice as good at detecting residual ischaemia following myocardial infarction, in comparison to traditional ECG treadmill testing. It, therefore, provides a more accurate way of assessing prognosis in postinfarct patients.

SPECT scanning may be used to detect 111-In radiolabelled monoclonal Fab fragments of specific antibody to cardiac myosin. When myocardial cell membranes rupture soon after infarction, they expose structural myosin, to which these monoclonal antibodies attach. This technique allows very early confirmation of myocardial infarction but is very expensive. SPECT scanning facilities are currently limited in the UK.

Magnetic resonance imaging (MRI) is a safe, non-invasive imaging technique that utilises a strong magnetic field to generate a three-dimensional image of the body, including the heart (Hartnell, 1991). Myocardial perfusion studies (using specific contrast agents) can differentiate between infarcted and ischaemic myocardium and can be used in quantification of infarct size. MRI is also useful for assessing left ventricular function (using ECG-gated cine-MRI), assessing the severity of valvular lesions and demonstrating the complications of acute myocardial infarction, including left ventricular aneurysm, intraventricular clot and ventriculoseptal defects. Rapid sequence cine-MRI is being used to assess graft patency following bypass surgery, and flow contrast techniques allow the estimation of coronary blood flow through vein grafts.

Detecting myocardial viability

Many patients with poor left ventricular function can benefit from revascularisation procedures if their cardiac muscle is shown not to be irreversibly damaged (so-called 'stunned' or 'hibernating' myocardium). *Positron emission tomography (PET)* may provide information on myocardial viability by detecting the uptake of fluorodeoxyglucose (FDG). Normally functioning myocardium takes up this glucose analogue, and PET scanning can differentiate between normal myocardium (preserved contractility and positive FDG uptake), infarcted myocardium (impaired contractility and no FDG uptake) and hibernating myocardium (impaired contractility and positive FDG uptake).

CARDIAC CATHETERISATION AND CORONARY ANGIOGRAPHY

In addition to coronary angiography, cardiac catheterisation may need to be carried out:

- To record intracardiac pressures and demonstrate pressure gradients
- To measure cardiac output and detect shunting (by measuring blood gases) at different levels
- To identify anatomical and functional anomalies, such as ventricular aneurysms and valvular disease.

Coronary angiography

Selective coronary angiography was introduced in 1959 and may be considered as the gold standard for defining the coronary circulation. The images are usually recorded on high speed cine-film to provide a dynamic record of ventricular wall movement, blood flow and intravascular anatomy. The extent and severity of the lesions, with assessment of left ventricular function, can be used to determine the patient's prognosis. The investigation is expensive and requires a minimum of five people (a doctor, two nurses, a radiographer and a technician). The procedure takes about half an hour and is performed under local anaesthesia. There is a small morbidity and mortality rate (due to myocardial infarction and dysrhythmias), but this is so low these days as to allow day-case investigation in low-risk cases.

Angiography is usually recommended:

- For patients with stable angina whose symptoms are significantly affecting their life-style, to decide whether surgery is indicated
- For patients with unstable angina following stabilisation
- Following acute myocardial infarction. Between 10 and 15% of patients who leave hospital will die in the first year, and they need identification. Up to 10% of patients are found to have left main stem stenosis, and 30% have triple artery disease. The remainder do not have severe coronary artery disease and do not need surgery to improve their symptoms or prognosis. Fortunately, we do not have to perform coronary angiography in all patients following acute myocardial infarction, and high- and low-risk groups can be identified non-invasively (Campbell et al, 1988; Cross et al, 1993).

The need for angiography is usually not urgent, and it is probably better to await resolution of the atheromatous plaques and endogenous remodelling of the coronary vasculature (Davies et al, 1990).

HAEMODYNAMIC MONITORING

The ability to recognise and assess serious circulatory changes in patients recovering from acute myocardial infarction is of major importance, both diagnostically and for assessing therapy and prognosis. Whilst clinical examination of the patient remains of major importance, it may be difficult to assess many patients without invasive monitoring. For example, infarction of the right ventricle may complicate one third of inferior myocardial infarctions and is associated with a low left atrial pressure, despite elevation of the jugular venous pressure. In patients with long-standing cardiac failure, selective peripheral vasoconstriction may maintain blood pressure, whilst masking a low cardiac output. This group of patients may also develop thickening of the pulmonary vessel walls, allowing a substantial rise in pulmonary capillary pressures before the clinical signs of pulmonary congestion develop. So, while the patient may be judged to have mild left ventricular failure on clinical grounds, haemodynamically there may be pulmonary hypertension, with a substantial reduction in cardiac output.

The term 'haemodynamic monitoring' describes a method of monitoring the blood pressure, volume and circulation, usually by indwelling catheters inserted into the heart or major blood vessels. The catheters are connected by fluid-filled tubing to pressure transducers and recording systems. The most frequently measured parameters on coronary care are the pulse, arterial blood pressure, central venous pressure (CVP), intracardiac pressures and cardiac output. In recent years, many techniques have become available that permit easy bedside analysis of the patient's haemodynamic status and cardiac function. The precise method of obtaining and recording these haemodynamic data varies from hospital to hospital and is usually dependent upon the expertise of the staff and available equipment. Typical indications for invasive monitoring are shown in Table 5.6.

Table 5.6 Indications for invasive haemodynamic monitoring

Cardiogenic shock
Moderate or severe heart failure
Unexplained hypotension
Suspicion or presence of:
- Pulmonary embolism
- Right ventricular infarction
- Severe hypertension
- Aortic dissection
- Mechanical heart defects (e.g. ruptured septum or mitral valve)

Once the catheter has been inserted, it is usually the responsibility of the nursing staff to ensure the patient's comfort and safety and the maintenance of the system, and to obtain and record data. Since the patient's treatment will often rely heavily on the results of monitoring, it is essential that such data are accurate. The nurse should be aware of problems inherent in data acquisition, including common technical and physiological variables that may affect the data. In addition, the nurse should be aware of the effect that specific nursing interventions (e.g. feeding, bathing and positioning) may have on haemodynamic measurements.

Pressure transducer systems

Pressure transducers are electromechanical devices that detect energy changes (e.g. those in pressure and temperature) and convert them to electrical signals. In most forms of haemodynamic monitoring, they detect intravascular pressure changes and convert them into electrical charges for amplification and digital readout. Usually, pressure changes are transmitted via fluid-filled tubing connected to a supple diaphragm located in a transducer dome. Changes in the intravascular pressure are transmitted from the in-dwelling cannula to fluid that passes through the transducer dome. Pressure waves are directly transmitted to a diaphragm within the dome, which is connected to a strain gauge. The more the diaphragm is moved by the pressure waves, the greater is the electrical charge generated and the higher the pressure reading on the monitor.

Measuring the central venous pressure (CVP)

Central venous pressure monitoring is used to measure pressure of blood in the right atrium or superior vena cava. On the ward, measurement is usually intermittent via water manometers, whilst on intensive care units, continuous monitoring via a pressure transducer with oscilloscopic display is more usual.

The central venous pressure reflects right ventricular end diastolic pressure (filling pressure or preload) and is determined by blood volume, vascular tone and cardiac performance. Elevation of the CVP is common following acute myocardial infarction, usually reflecting raised right-sided pressures secondary to left ventricular failure. Other causes are right ventricular infarction, tricuspid incompetence and cardiac tamponade. Low CVP readings are usually due to hypovolaemia, when infusion of fluid may improve cardiac performance.

CVP catheters are inserted percutaneously, usually into the subclavian or jugular veins, and are advanced to lie in the superior vena cava or right atrium. During central venous catheterisation, it is important that the patient is placed in the Trendelenburg position (i.e. head down). This distends the central veins, which not only reduces the risk of air embolism, but also makes cannulation easier. The right side of the patient is chosen preferentially to prevent damage to the thoracic duct. Placement of the catheter is confirmed by chest X-ray, which also will exclude the presence of a pneumothorax.

The pressure is normally measured using manometry, although because of the sluggish response, a pressure transducer may be preferred, particularly if continuous display of the CVP is required.

Manometry

The manometer (Figure 5.8) should be placed with the baseline at the level of the right atrium. The baseline may be at zero on the scale, but it is preferable to set it at a higher value (e.g. 10 cm), so that negative pressures may be recorded. A spirit level should be used to ensure that the zero reference point on both the patient and the manometer coincide. The line should be well flushed, by opening up the intravenous fluid line. Free passage of fluid through the system should occur when the infusion rate is turned up, and blood should be freely aspirated if required. Respiratory oscillations should be visible.

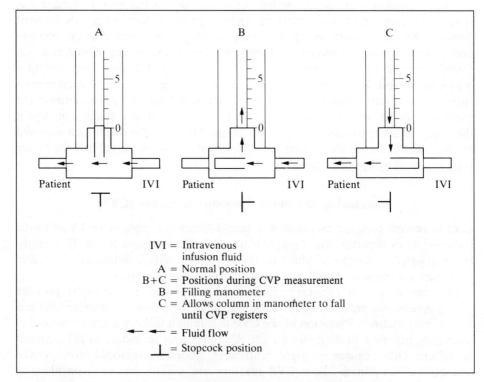

Fig. 5.8   Central venous pressure (CVP) monitoring, showing stopcock positioning

The manometer column should be filled by turning the stopcock from the normal position A to position B (Figure 5.8). The stopcock is then turned to position C, and the fluid is allowed to run down and equilibrate through the CVP line. Normally, the fluid falls freely, although it fluctuates with venous pulsation and respiration. Once the column has settled, the CVP should be measured at the end of expiration and expressed in cmH_2O (normal = 0–10 cmH_2O).

Following CVP measurement, the stopcock should be returned to position A and the infusion rate adjusted as required.

Electrical pressure transducers

This method is most frequently used when measurements are made via the right atrial port of a four-channel Swan–Ganz catheter. The reading recorded by the transducer is displayed in mmHg (normal = 0–8 mmHg).

Correlation of CVP in mmHg and cmH_2O is shown in Table 5.7.

Positioning the patient is extremely important during measurement of the CVP. Ideally, the patient should be lying flat, without a pillow, but if the patient's condition does not permit this, he can be positioned at 45° or less. During normal respiration, the intrathoracic pressure falls on inspiration. Measuring haemodynamic pressures at end expiration is considered to be the most valid, because the intrathoracic pressure is closest to zero at this point.

Intra-arterial blood pressure monitoring

In clinically unstable patients, measurement of the blood pressure with the traditional sphygmomanometer and stethoscope is often difficult, particularly if the patients are hypotensive. In shock, readings taken in this way may differ from the actual arterial blood pressure by over 30 mmHg. The insertion of an arterial pressure line is useful for directly and continuously measuring systolic, diastolic and mean arterial blood pressures, as well as for giving easy access for repeated blood gas sampling. Sites commonly employed are the radial, brachial and dorsalis pedis arteries. However, the closer the cannula is to the heart, the more accurate the waveform and the pressure reading.

Table 5.7 Conversion of mmHg to cmH_2O (approximate)

(mmHg × 1.36 = cmH_2O)	
1 = 1	11 = 15
2 = 3	12 = 16
3 = 4	13 = 18
4 = 5	14 = 19
5 = 7	15 = 20
6 = 8	16 = 22
7 = 10	17 = 23
8 = 11	18 = 24
9 = 12	19 = 26
10 = 14	20 = 27
(cmH_2O/1.36 = mmHg)	

Cannulation is performed under local anaesthetic, using a 20-gauge Teflon catheter, which is attached to a T-connector and a pressurised heparin/saline flushing system. This runs continuously at 3–5 ml/hr to minimise clotting, vasospasm and intimal damage. A transducer converts the pressures into a digital readout and displays the arterial waveform. The readings displayed are systolic blood pressure, diastolic blood pressure and mean blood pressure. The mean arterial pressure (MAP) is, however, not the sum of the systolic and the diastolic pressure divided by two; it is a measurement that integrates the area under the arterial waveform curve to obtain a true mean.

Complications of intra-arterial monitoring are not common but include:

- Arterial occlusion
- Arterial spasm
- Haemorrhage
- Air embolism
- Sepsis
- Ecchymoses

When the line is removed, pressure over the insertion site should be maintained for at least 5 minutes, or longer if thrombolytic agents or anticoagulants have been used.

Pulmonary artery and pulmonary artery wedge pressures

The value of CVP measurement is limited, because it basically reflects the functional state of the right ventricle, which does not always parallel that of the left ventricle. Information about left ventricular function is often essential for complete evaluation.

Monitoring pulmonary artery (PA) and pulmonary artery wedge (PAW) pressures may be useful following myocardial infarction, since they provide data to guide and evaluate therapy. One of the most important advances in haemodynamic monitoring has been the development of pulmonary artery flotation (Swan–Ganz) catheters (Swan et al, 1970). The Swan–Ganz catheter has been used to subclassify patients following acute myocardial infarction by measurement of cardiac index and wedge pressures (Forrester et al, 1976). This enables prediction of short-term prognosis and the selection of appropriate therapy (Table 5.8).

The Swan–Ganz catheter (Figure 5.9) is about 80–110 cm in length, marked at 10 cm intervals, and is available in three sizes: 5 FG (for children), 6 FG and 7 FG (for adults). The basic model has two lumina. The larger lumen terminates at the tip of the catheter and is used for recording intracardiac pressures, infusion of fluids and sampling of mixed venous blood. A smaller lumen serves to inflate the latex balloon that not only helps the catheter to float through the right heart, but also allows repeated, reversible, pulmonary artery occlusion for recording wedge pressures. In the more complicated models, there is a third lumen, terminating 30 cm proximal to the catheter tip, which enables simultaneous measurement of right atrial (RA) pressures, and a fourth channel that leads to a thermistor located close to the tip. These latter two channels are used together for calculation of right ventricular cardiac output by thermodilution. Other types of catheter are available

Table 5.8 Classification, therapy and mortality of patients following acute myocardial infarction

Class	Cardiac Output	Index*	Wedge pressure (mmHg)	Therapy	Mortality (%)
No cardiac failure	Normal	>2.2	<18	Bed rest	3
Pulmonary congestion	Normal	>2.2	>18	Lower wedge pressure with: diuretics (blood pressure normal) vasodilators (blood pressure raised)	9
Peripheral hypoperfusion	Low	<2.2	<18	Plasma expanders	23
Pulmonary congestion and peripheral hypoperfusion	Low	<2.2	>18	Reduce wedge pressure with diuretics/ vasodilators If hypotensive, use inotropic agents	51

*Cardiac index (l/min per m^2) = cardiac output (litres) per minute per body surface area (m^2) (From Forrester et al, 1976. Reproduced by kind permission of the *New England Journal of Medicine*)

for pulmonary angiography and pacing, and all can be floated into the pulmonary artery by observing pressure tracings made during passage through the right heart, without requiring fluoroscopy. The catheter is normally inserted at the bedside under local anaesthesia via a peripheral vein (usually the subclavian or antecubital).

Uses of catheters

Measurement of PAW and PA pressures

PAWP is the pressure recorded when the Swan–Ganz catheter has been floated through the right heart and wedged into a peripheral pulmonary artery. The pulmonary arteries are end arteries, and the pulmonary veins contain no valves. The catheter, therefore, registers the pressure transmitted retrogradely from the left atrium. The PAWP closely relates to the left atrial pressure and provides an indirect method of assessing left atrial pressure. Normal intracardiac pressures recorded by the Swan–Ganz catheter are shown in Table 5.9.

Table 5.9 Intracardiac pressures measured by the Swan–Ganz catheter

	Pressure (mmHg)
Right atrium	0–8
Pulmonary artery: systolic	15–30
diastolic	5–12
Pulmonary artery wedge pressure	5–12

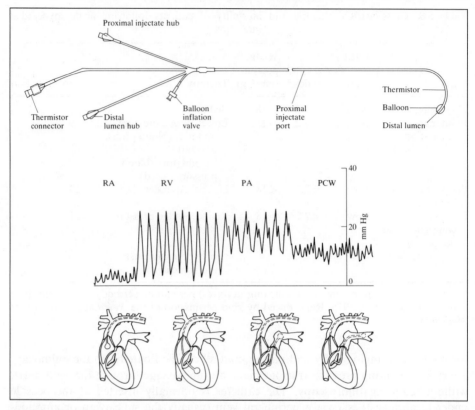

Fig. 5.9 The Swan–Ganz thermodilution catheter and typical pressures recorded during its passage through the heart (From Stokes and Jowett, 1985. Reproduced by kind permission of Churchill Livingstone)

Cardiac output

The measurement of cardiac output provides useful information about cardiac performance and response to therapy. Cardiac output may be measured at the bedside using the four-channel Swan–Ganz catheter by injecting 10 ml of 5% dextrose at 4°C or room temperature into the right atrium via the 30 cm port. A temperature drop of the blood is recorded by the thermistor at the tip of the catheter, which lies in the pulmonary artery. From the recorded changes in temperature, a bedside computer can calculate the cardiac output. A mean of three serial readings is usually taken for the value of cardiac output.

Blood gas analysis

Blood gas analysis can be made on mixed venous blood, slowly aspirated via the tip port. Another type of pulmonary artery flotation catheter has become available (Opticath by Oximetrix of California), which has a separate channel containing two fibreoptic bundles for light transmission. By connecting these to an oximeter, continuous measurement of the Po_2 is possible.

Complications

Complications arising from the use of Swan–Ganz catheters are infrequent but include the following:

1. *Dysrhythmias.* These include heart block and ventricular tachycardia (Sprung et al, 1981). They are caused by mechanical irritation of the endocardium or valves and are usually noted at the time of catheter insertion, manipulation or removal. Continuous ECG monitoring is, therefore, desirable, with special attention paid to the rhythm during catheter manipulation.

2. *Infection.* As with any centrally-placed line, scrupulous asepsis is mandatory, not only during catheter insertion, but also when manipulating the catheter and during infusion of fluids. If the catheter is not secured to the skin, the non-sterile portion can migrate inwards and cause infection. A permanently-indwelling introducer, with a flexible polythene sleeve, may be used to protect the proximal 30 cm of the catheter and allow manipulation if the catheter needs repositioning.

3. *Pulmonary infarction.* This may be caused by frequent, prolonged or over-inflation of the balloon, or by thrombus formation around the catheter tip (Renke et al, 1975). With time, the catheter tends to migrate through the heart and to wedge spontaneously. If unnoticed, pulmonary infarction can result. Pressures should be displayed continuously on an oscilloscope, so that any pressure damping (indicating thrombus formation) or spontaneous wedging may be immediately recognised.

4. *Perforation of the pulmonary artery.* Too rapid an inflation of the balloon not only increases the risk of balloon rupture, but may also rupture the pulmonary capillary (Lemen et al, 1975). This is rare, but patients with pulmonary hypertension are at risk. Balloon inflation should, therefore, always be slow.

5. *Balloon rupture and air embolism.* Balloon rupture should be suspected when there is no resistance to attempted inflation and failure to wedge. It becomes more common the longer the catheter is left in place.

STATIC MONITORING

The continuous monitoring of cardiac rhythm is one of the most important aspects of cardiological investigation and forms a vital part of assessment of patients in coronary care and other high-dependency units. The major impact of the coronary care unit on the mortality from acute myocardial infarction has resulted from the detection and treatment of related dysrhythmias (Wagner, 1984; Brownlee, 1985). Static monitoring has provided the capability to anticipate the occurrence of potentially fatal dysrhythmias, with the opportunity for prompt treatment of other changes in rhythm likely to have adverse haemodynamic consequences.

These advances have become possible by the widespread availability of electronic oscilloscopes (monitors) that can continuously detect and display the electrical activity of the heart. As may be anticipated, the results of such monitoring vary, according to whether all potentially serious dysrhythmias are recognised. Much 'manual' recording is limited by fatigue, boredom or distraction, but the recent introduction of computer-linked monitors can lead to detection of almost all serious dysrhythmias.

Nurses from all wards and specialties are more frequently caring for patients attached to such monitors and must, therefore, be familiar with electrode placement and monitor operation, as well as being able to recognise and distinguish normal and abnormal rhythms.

Electrodes

Electrodes are small sensors that can be fixed to the skin to allow the electrical activity of the heart to be detected and transmitted to the monitor for amplification and display. Great advances have been made in the design of these electrodes, and modern disposable, pregelled, self-adhesive electrodes usually obtain excellent skin contact with minimal or no skin preparation. There are several steps that may be taken if the signal is poor:

1. The skin should be shaved, particularly if the patient is very hairy. Not only will skin contact be enhanced, but the patient will also be grateful during electrode removal.

2. Rubbing the skin with dry gauze or a wooden spatula will remove loose, dry skin (the stratum corneum) and aid electrode contact.

3. Wiping the skin with alcohol will remove excess tissue debris, body oil and sweat. If the patient is perspiring heavily, a small amount of tincture of benzoin can be applied and allowed to dry before electrode placement. Special electrodes have been manufactured for those patients who are perspiring heavily.

4. The expiry date of the electrode should be checked, and it should be confirmed that there is a gel-filled sponge on the electrode. Old electrodes may have lost their sponge or have dried out. When in use, the gel soaks into the skin, and a period of up to 15 minutes may elapse before good contact is made. Electrode jelly massaged into the skin before application will reduce this time. The electrodes should be applied 'centre first', so that the adhesive holds the gelled area tightly to the skin.

The electrode site should be examined daily for allergic skin reactions, but otherwise there is no need to change the electrodes routinely, unless the signal becomes poor. Non-allergenic electrodes may be used if the patient is sensitive to the adhesive, and any inflammation may be treated with a small quantity of 1% hydrocortisone cream.

The admitting nurse must select the appropriate lead placement for the individual patient before electrode application. The monitor wires either clip or snap onto the chest wires, although it is preferable to do this before the electrodes are placed on the chest, so that the patient is not hurt if pressure is required to push them on.

The monitor cable

The signals detected by the electrodes are transmitted to the oscilloscope by a monitor cable. At the distal end, this comprises thin wires of about 12 inches in length, which connect directly to the surface electrodes. These may be of different colours or labelled 'right', 'left' and 'ground' (or 'earth'). These correspond to the right arm electrode (RA), the left arm electrode (LA) and the right leg electrode (RL), respectively. Some cables may allow for a further two surface electrodes to be attached, so that leads aVR, aVL and aVF may also be recorded. The contacts with the electrodes should be clean and compatible with the surface electrodes being used. The wires should be inspected for breaks in the insulation and any bends or knots. It is useful to form a 'stress loop' with this part of the cable to prevent traction on the electrodes and monitor connections, with consequent electrode separation and movement artefact. A lead-fault indicator signal may be present on the monitor, which alerts the nurse to problems in signal transmission.

The thin chest leads connect to a junction box that attaches to the proximal end of the lead cable, which is thicker and plugs directly into the monitor. This part of the monitor cable should be flexible and long enough to allow the patient to walk around the bed area and use the commode.

The bedside monitor

A bedside monitor is an oscilloscope connected to the patient by the monitor cable, which displays the patient's ECG tracing on a continuous basis. Where there is a central monitoring system with a central console, the ECG pattern is duplicated for all monitored beds and occasionally for telemetry units too.

The heart rate is usually calculated by a computer that senses the interval between the tallest component of the complexes (usually the R waves). False heart rates may be registered if, for example, the T wave is of amplitude equal to that of the R wave, since this will be read as another QRS complex. The amplitude of these complexes may be adjusted by using the gain control, or if this is insufficient, another lead can be selected by the lead selector control. This control allows the ECG complexes to be recorded in different selected patterns without moving the chest electrodes. A three-electrode system allows the standard limb leads I, II and III to be selected. Five-electrode systems allow leads aVR, aVL and aVF to be obtained as well. An alarm system is set to sound when predetermined parameters are met or exceeded. For example, the rate alarm may be set at 10–15 beats above and below the rates estimated as acceptable for each individual patient.

Many bedside units have a secondary trace under the actual 'real-time' trace. This may run continually but be delayed so that the trace can be frozen to capture rhythm disturbances by use of the 'run/hold' switch. Depending on the degree of sophistication, the memory loop will hold from a few seconds of the preceding ECG to several minutes. It may allow specific rhythm retrieval and a 'hard copy' rhythm strip to be obtained for more detailed examination or to provide a permanent copy for the patient's records.

An initial rhythm strip is usually taken as a baseline, which should be interpreted and documented in the patient's notes. Some coronary care units repeat this procedure at fixed intervals (e.g. 2–4 hourly), as well as whenever there is a change in rhythm or QRS morphology.

The ECG tracing should be observed for the quality of the recording. Monitoring is usually at 25 mm/second. If the machine is set at 50 mm/second, the rate appears to be slowed and intervals prolonged. The tracing should be clear and well defined and should travel across the screen on the same level. The exact configuration of the QRS complexes is not important, unless complexes are changing from beat to beat; it is the rhythm, rather than the shape, that is usually of greatest importance. The minimum brightness should be selected on the contrast control to prevent a 'halo' effect around the tracing.

Monitoring

Standard electrocardiographic limb leads are recorded from the right arm, left arm and left leg to produce limb leads I, II and III. In order to help with patient mobility and reduce movement interference, monitoring on coronary care is usually via three chest electrodes. These are normally placed in the two infraclavicular spaces (right, negative; left, positive) and at the right sternal edge (earth), which are areas free from underlying muscular masses, thus minimising muscle potential artefact. In this configuration, a tracing similar to standard limb lead I is obtained. Additionally, a clear site is left for application of chest electrodes for full 12-lead ECG recording, defibrillation and external cardiac massage should they be required.

The ECG tracing should be observed for the following features:

- Rate
- Rhythm
- PR interval
- Ectopic beats

Dysrhythmias may be recognised in any lead, but as a general rule monitoring the three-lead equivalent of chest lead V1 is the best. This is because it clearly demonstrates the P wave and usually allows clear differentiation between ventricular ectopic beats and those arising from the supraventricular region but being conducted aberrantly. Aberration should be expected when the ectopic beat is preceded by a P wave different from that of a normal sinus beat or is of a right bundle branch block (RSR') pattern in V1. This lead is also useful for diagnosing bundle branch block and for differentiating between left and right ventricular ectopic beats. In right bundle branch block, the left ventricle is depolarised before the right, and the net electrical movement is towards the V1 electrode, producing a predominant positive complex. This will also be seen in an ectopic beat arising in the left ventricle. In left bundle branch block and right ventricular ectopics, the reverse is seen, with a predominantly negative V1 complex being recorded.

Although the V1 lead has all these undoubted advantages, it would seem to require fixation of four limb leads as well as a chest lead. Fortunately, a modified version of chest lead V1 has been described by Marriott (1983), designated MCL-1 (Modified Chest Lead 1), shown in Figure 5.10. The positive (+) electrode is placed in the normal V1 intercostal space (4th right), whilst the negative (−) and the earth (G) electrodes are located near the left shoulder and right shoulder respectively.

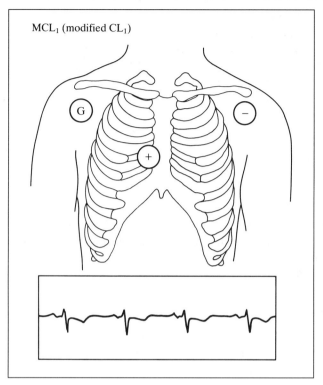

Fig. 5.10   Modified chest lead 1 (MCL-1)
+ = positive electrode; − = negative electrode; G = ground electrode (From Jowett et al, 1985. Reproduced by kind permission of Churchill Livingstone)

It must be noted that although routine monitoring by a familiar lead such as MCL-1 has obvious advantages, special leads are occasionally necessary to determine the origin of ectopic beats. A modified chest lead equivalent to V6 (MCL-6) is of particular value in differentiating between ventricular ectopy and aberration.

Computerised monitoring

Although visual observation of the oscilloscope by a trained observer is used on many units and on general medical wards, many dysrhythmias are missed. Over half of ventricular ectopic beats are not noticed, as well as between 5 and 10% of multifocal ectopics. The use of computers for the detection of dysrhythmias in acute care units and for the review of rhythms over an extended period is therefore preferred (Knoebel and Lovelace, 1983). The simplest example of this is the rate detector alarm, which will sound if preset heart rate limits are not met or are exceeded. Microchip technology has led to the development of an enormous number of computer-linked monitors that are able to recognise many dysrhythmias and sound alarms appropriately. Analysis can be performed at various levels of sophistication, from simple dysrhythmia recognition to full reporting of standard 12-lead ECGs. Using a storage mode, display of premature ventricular beat counts and trend analysis is possible for a 24-hour period. The complexity of the ECG signal and the frequent interference introduced by artefact have retarded the anticipated advances in this field. As a result, complex rhythm analysis is not usually feasible, and most systems are limited to determination of rate with recognition of pauses, premature ventricular complexes (PVCs) and tachycardias of both ventricular and supraventricular origin.

Problems with monitoring

Monitoring faults are not uncommon. These include the following.

Problems with the trace

If the trace does not appear, all connections should be checked, and the brightness switch should be turned up. The trace position switch may have been set such that the trace is off the screen; it should be adjusted if required. The 'run/hold' switch should also be activated.

Incorrect heart rate display

The heart rate is normally shown on the rate meter, which counts successive R waves and calculates the heart rate per minute. However, the system is not infallible. If the R waves are too small or vary in height, they will not be counted. It is also important to ensure that the T wave is not too large, or else it may be counted and analysed as an extra QRS complex. As a result, a doubled heart rate will be displayed.

Wandering baseline

Respiration or changes in the patient's position in bed may affect the height of the complexes, or give rise to a wandering baseline. If this is a recurrent problem, the chest electrodes should be moved or a different lead selected by the lead selector control.

Artefacts and interference

The most frequent problem of static monitoring is false alarms due to movement artefact or loose and poorly connected electrodes. Very small or 'fuzzy' complexes may result on the screen, as may the appearances of asystole. Sixty-cycle interference may be present if the bed or other nearby equipment is not earthed. Similarly, electrical equipment close to the monitor, such as X-ray machines, vacuum pumps, fluorescent lights or electric razors, may cause interference.

Low-voltage ECGs

Low-voltage complexes (<6mm) may occur in the frontal leads (peripheral low voltage) or in both the frontal and horizontal planes (total low voltage). Causes may be cardiac (pericardial effusion, cardiomyopathy or diffuse ischaemic heart disease) or non-cardiac (obesity, emphysema or hypothyroidism) or both. It may be necessary to resite the electrodes.

Nurses should take time to inform the patient and his relatives that although the heart is being monitored, it does not necessarily mean that the patient is critically ill. The patient must always be checked each time an alarm sounds to determine its validity, particularly on cubicled units. The patient and any visitors should receive an explanation if the alarm sounds.

AMBULATORY MONITORING

Abnormalities of cardiac rhythm are common and may affect individuals with or without cardiac disease. Such abnormalities may be detected by static monitoring, but if the dysrhythmia is infrequent or transient, extended monitoring techniques are required.

The standard 12-lead ECG provides little information about cardiac rhythm. The average ECG records about 50 complexes, typically taken with the patient lying down and at rest. Static monitoring techniques also have their limitations and are unsuitable for detection of short rhythm disturbances, especially if induced by exertion or other factors in the daily life of the patient (Jowett and Thompson, 1985; Jowett et al, 1985). Documentation of abnormal electrical activity may, therefore, require prolonged continuous recording during exercise.

Ambulatory ECG monitoring was initially designed to document transient disturbances in heart rhythm and conduction, with the aim of establishing a relationship between symptoms and accompanying disturbances in cardiac rhythm. The role of ambulatory monitoring has now expanded to assessing antidysrhythmic therapy, detecting ischaemia and determining prognosis (Mickley, 1994).

The standard ambulatory monitor

Norman 'Jeff' Holter, an American, first put forward ideas for a portable ECG recorder in the late 1940s, and hence these recording machines are often known as 'Holter recorders', whatever their origin. From the initial bulky, short-duration recorders, these monitors have been refined to light, small, strong machines capable of recording the heart rhythm continuously for up to 48 hours, several channels of ECG data being recorded simultaneously.

The complete unit consists of a small tape recorder carried in a harness that is worn by the patient. The recording electrodes are applied to the chest, usually in modified V1 and V5 positions. The second channel allows QRS vector (axis) changes to be detected if, for example, there is an intraventricular conduction defect or transient ventricular pre-excitation.

Faithful reproduction of the ST segment has been difficult in the past, but this has now been much improved. Monitoring ST segment shift provides an increasing indication for the use of these monitors to document symptomatic and silent myocardial ischaemia. Secondary channels may also be used to monitor blood pressure and respiratory patterns.

Usually, an ordinary tape cassette is inserted into the machine, although solid state technology has replaced this in some machines. The patient is told to carry on normal daily activities, and a detailed diary for the day's activities (e.g. sleeping, working and watching television) should be kept, with clear descriptions and timing of any symptoms, especially faintness, palpitations and dizziness. Some machines have an 'event marker', a button that may be pressed to mark the tape at the onset of symptoms, so that the cardiac rhythm at that exact time is recorded. The diary of timed symptoms and the referral note are of major value during tape analysis and interpretation.

The typical 24-hour recording provides about 100 000 complexes for analysis, but, fortunately, high speed electrocardioscanners (Figure 5.11) are able to replay the tapes in as little as 6 minutes, although selection of rhythm strips and print out make full processing a little longer. Presentation of the contents depends upon the clinical circumstances. A full disclosure presentation can print all the complexes in miniature, which is particularly useful for identifying periods of interest. If the patient has experienced symptoms, these periods may be selectively recalled, with a normal-sized ECG printout, including the periods before and after the event. Precise timing is noted on the strips, to allow comparison with the patient's diary, in order to correlate symptoms and dysrhythmias.

Other recording methods

Holter monitoring is limited both by storage capacity and by the fact that events must take place during the period of study. Patients frequently complain that 'It

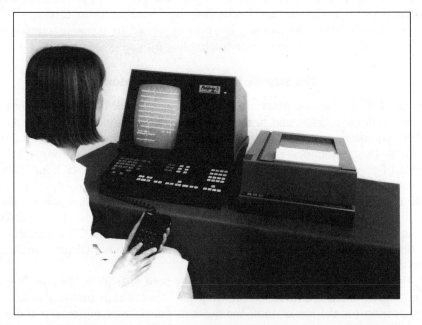

Fig. 5.11 High-speed electrocardioscanner (Reproduced by kind permission of Reynolds Medical Limited)

never happens when I'm attached to the recorder'. Fortunately, several modified recording devices have been developed that aid dysrhythmia detection.

Event recorders

Event recorders are able to record for about 30 minutes total duration but, instead of running continuously, can be manually activated at the onset of symptoms or will activate automatically should any sudden change in rate or rhythm (according to preset criteria) occur. Unfortunately, these will not always show the exact onset of the dysrhythmia, which is often important in demonstrating the origin of the dysrhythmia and prescribing appropriate therapy.

Transtelephonic recorders

These are small, hand-held, solid state recorders, with electrodes affixed to the back. During an attack, the patient presses the unit firmly to the chest and a short rhythm sample is recorded. This may be transmitted as a modulated audio signal to the hospital (usually to the coronary care unit), where the signal is decoded and printed out on a conventional ECG rhythm strip. The recorder can then be reset and used again. It is, therefore, very useful for infrequent, short-lived and recurrent symptoms.

Telemetric units

Telemetry is often used within hospitals for extended peri-infarction cardiac monitoring. The patient is fitted with standard chest electrodes attached to a small transmitter, carried in a chest harness or pyjama pocket. The cardiac rhythm is transmitted continuously to a receiver (normally situated on the coronary care unit), where it is displayed, observed and analysed in the same way as for patients on static monitors. The advantage of this system is that patients may be mobilised in the early period following myocardial infarction, whilst still having the benefits of dysrhythmia monitoring. The transmission range of these units is usually short and thus relatively free from extrinsic radio-interference. Longer-range units have been developed for use by cardiac arrest teams, who may be further away from the receiver units, and by ambulance and paramedic teams outside the hospital. In both cases, the cardiac rhythm may be monitored and advice on drug therapy be given by more experienced physicians 'back at base'.

Normal limits and recording artefacts

The use of ambulatory monitoring has disclosed many dysrhythmias in apparently normal individuals (Bjerregaard, 1983); these are not necessarily pathological, but we do not currently have consistent ways of separating normality from abnormality. Most of the general population have isolated ventricular ectopic beats, two-thirds have sinus bradycardia and about one fifth have very brief episodes of atrial fibrillation. About 0.2% of apparently healthy adults have ventricular bigeminy. Pauses of 2–3 seconds are very common in athletes, who have high vagal tone.

The interpretation of the pathological significance of rhythm abnormalities is very much dependent on the circumstances. The view may be entirely different in unselected adults compared to patients recovering from myocardial infarction. In general, rhythm disturbances are more important and tolerated less well in the elderly than in younger adults.

Whichever recording system is used, artefactual interference is often encountered. Frequent causes include poor electrode contact, body movement and poor tape quality (due to tape stretch or inadequate erasure). Men with nylon shirts, or women with nylon underwear, may generate static electricity, which can distort recordings. Such garments should not be worn during ambulatory recording. Recording artefacts are normally obvious during rhythm analysis, although many complexes may closely resemble rhythm abnormalities. Hence, careful examination of related rhythm strips is often required to demonstrate that the recording is artefactual.

The value of ambulatory monitoring

There are several major uses of ambulatory monitoring techniques:

1. *Diagnosing the aetiology of symptoms.* Confirmation of a dysrhythmia-induced symptom requires the coincidence of the symptom and a dysrhythmia. Asymptomatic recordings do not usually help, although evidence of asymptomatic abnormalities, such as short runs of ventricular tachycardia or ischaemic episodes, may help further management.

Approximately 60–70% of Holter recordings will show no abnormality, and a further 20–30% will be normal despite the presence of symptoms during the recording period. A positive diagnosis is only made in 10% of cases where symptoms coincide with a dysrhythmia (Clarke et al, 1980).

2. *Assessment of the incidence and frequency of previously identified ischaemia or dysrhythmias.* Rate-dependent conduction disturbances or dysrhythmias caused by metabolic or ischaemic changes are often demonstrated this way. An increasing use is for the detection of silent myocardial ischaemia.

3. *Immediate analysis of a dysrhythmia.* By use of transtelephonic or telemetric units, immediate rhythm analysis is available. This mode of monitoring is widely used for pacemaker function reports. Inpatient telemetry also allows extended ambulatory monitoring of patients with recent myocardial infarction.

4. *Assessment of antidysrhythmic therapy.* Comparison of tapes before and after drug administration can help in assessing the efficacy of any chosen drug and give warning of potential toxicity. Serial 24-hour tapes may reveal the variability in the incidence of dysrhythmias on different days in the same patient. An important implication of this is that a chosen antidysrhythmic drug may only be said to be effective if the number of episodes are reduced by 80% (Petch, 1985).

5. *Assessment of patients following cardiac arrest or cardiac surgery.* Continuous monitoring following cardiac arrest may demonstrate frequent ventricular extrasystoles or short runs of ventricular tachycardia. In some patients, these observations provide a valuable guide for long-term prognosis and therapy. Holter monitoring may also reveal advanced degrees of sino-atrial or atrioventricular block, which may have been the underlying cause of the cardiac arrest.

6. *Pacemaker assessment*. Special recorders are applied to detect pacing stimuli and are very useful in assessing dual chamber pacing systems. They may also be of value in assessing implanted defibrillators.

7. *Detecting myocardial ischaemia*. Unlike rhythm monitoring, which can use any lead system, faithful reproduction of the ST segment often requires multilead systems and even then may produce false positive and false negative results, as with formalised exercise stress testing. Nonetheless, much research is being carried out with this technique to assess the total ischaemic burden on the heart (i.e. episodes of painful and painless ischaemia). It appears that silent ischaemia carries the same adverse prognosis as that indicated during symptomatic exercise testing (Dagenais et al, 1988).

8. *Newer applications*. The role of ambulatory monitoring for recording late potentials, as in normal signal-averaged ECGs, is being explored, as is QT interval variability (dynamic QT analysis), which may relate to susceptibility to dysrhythmias and prognosis of ischaemic heart disease.

Heart rate variability (beat-to-beat variation) is an index of overall autonomic control on the heart and is a powerful predictor of prognosis following acute myocardial infarction. New systems can measure heart rate variability, but we do not currently know how it may be influenced.

References

Akhras F, Upward J, Scott R and Jackson G (1982) Early exercise testing and coronary angiography after uncomplicated myocardial infarction. *British Medical Journal,* **284:** 1293–1294.

Bjerregaard P (1983) Mean 24 hour heart rate, minimum heart rate and pauses in healthy subjects 40–79 years of age. *European Heart Journal,* **4:** 44–51.

British Cardiac Society (1987) Cardiology in the district hospital. *British Heart Journal,* **58:** 537–546.

British Cardiac Society (1993) Guidelines on exercise testing when there is not a doctor present. *British Heart Journal,* **70:** 488.

Brownlee W T (1985) Acute arrhythmias. *British Journal of Hospital Medicine,* **33:** 138–145.

Bruce R A, Blackman J R, Jones J W and Strait G (1963) Exercise tests in adult normal subjects and cardiac patients. *Pediatrics,* **32:** 742–756.

Campbell S, Hern R A, Quigley P, Vincent R, Jewitt D and Chamberlain D (1988) Identification of patients at low risk of dying after acute myocardial infarction by simple clinical and sub-maximal exercise test criteria. *European Heart Journal,* **9:** 938–947.

Clarke P I, Glasser S P and Spoto E (1980) Arrhythmias detected by ambulatory monitoring: lack of correlation with symptoms of dizziness and syncope. *Chest,* **77:** 722–725.

Coronary Artery Surgery Study (CASS) Principal Investigators and Associates (1983) A randomised trial of coronary artery bypass surgery: survival data. *Circulation,* **68:** 939–950.

Cross S J, Lee H S, Kenmure A, Walton S and Jennings K (1993) First myocardial infarction in patients under 60 years old: the role of exercise tests and symptoms in deciding who to catheterise. *British Heart Journal,* **70:** 428–432.

Dagenais G R, Rouleau, J R, Hochart P, Magrina J, Cantin B and Dumesnil J G (1988) Survival with painless strongly positive exercise electrocardiograms. *American Journal of Cardiology,* **62:** 892–895.

Davies S W, Marchant B, Lyons J P, Timmis A D, Rothman M T and Layton C A (1990) Coronary lesion morphology in acute myocardial infarction: demonstration of early remodelling after streptokinase treatment. *Journal of the American College of Cardiology*, **16**: 1079–1086.

Dymond D S, Foster C, Grenier R P, Carpenter J and Schmidt D H (1984) Peak exercise and immediate post exercise imaging for the detection of left ventricular functional abnormalities in coronary artery disease. *American Journal of Cardiology*, **53**: 1532–1537.

Epstein S E (1978) Value and limitation of electrocardiographic response to exercise in the assessment of patients with coronary heart disease. *American Journal of Cardiology*, **42**: 667–674.

Fletcher G F, Froelicher V F, Hartley L H, Haskell W L and Pollock M L (1990) Exercise standards. A statement for health professionals from the American Heart Association. *Circulation*, **82**: 2286–2320.

Forrester J S, Diamond G, Chatterjee K and Swan H J C (1976) Medical therapy of acute myocardial infarction by application of hemodynamic subsets. *New England Journal of Medicine*, **295**: 1356–1362.

Hartnell G G (1991) Cardiac magnetic resonance imaging. *Clinical MRI*, **1**: 43–64.

Houston A B (1993) Doppler ultrasound and the apparently normal heart. *British Heart Journal*, **69**: 99–100.

Irving J B, Bruce R A and de Rouen T (1977) Variations in and significance of systolic pressure during maximal exercise (treadmill) testing. *American Journal of Cardiology*, **39**: 841–848.

Jowett N I and Thompson D R (1985) Electrocardiographic monitoring. II. Ambulatory monitoring. *Intensive Care Nursing*, **1**: 123–129.

Jowett N I, Thompson D R and Bailey S W (1985) Electrocardiographic monitoring. I. Static monitoring. *Intensive Care Nursing*, **1**: 71–76.

Knoebel S B and Lovelace D E (1983) Symposium on arrhythmias. I. Computers and clinical arrhythmias. *Cardiology Clinics*, **1**: 121–137.

Lemen R, Jones J G and Cowan G (1975) A mechanism of pulmonary artery perforation by Swan–Ganz catheters. *New England Journal of Medicine*, **242**: 211–212.

Marriott H J L (1983) *Practical Electrocardiography*. Baltimore: Williams and Wilkins.

Mickley H (1994) Ambulatory ST segment monitoring after myocardial infarction. *British Heart Journal*, **71**: 113–114.

Naughton J, Balke B and Nagle F (1964) Refinements in methods of evaluation and physical conditioning before and after myocardial infarction. *American Journal of Cardiology*, **14**: 837–843.

Oakley C M (1984) Mitral valve prolapse: harbinger of death or variant of normal. *British Medical Journal*, **288**: 1853–1854.

Petch M C (1985) Lessons from ambulatory electrocardiography. *British Medical Journal*, **291**: 617–618.

Podrid P J and Graboys T B (1984) Exercise stress testing in the management of cardiac rhythm disorders. *Medical Clinics of North America*, **68**: 1139–1152.

Renke R T, Higgins C B and Atkin J W (1975) Pulmonary infarction complicating the use of Swan–Ganz catheters. *British Journal of Radiology*, **48**: 885–888.

Rodrigues E A, Dewhurst N G, Smart L M, Hannan W J and Muir A L (1986) Diagnosis and prognosis of right ventricular infarction. *British Heart Journal*, **56**: 19–26.

St John Sutton M (1994) Should ACE inhibitors be used routinely after infarction? Perspectives from the SAVE trial. *British Heart Journal*, **71**: 115–118.

Sprung C L, Jacobs L J, Caralis P V and Karpf M (1981) Ventricular arrhythmias during Swan–Ganz catheterisation of the critically ill patient. *Chest*, **79**: 413–415.

Stevenson R, Umachandran V, Ranjadayalan K, Wilkinson P, Marchant B and Timmis A D (1993) Reassessment of treadmill stress testing for risk stratification in patients with acute myocardial infarction treated by thrombolysis. *British Heart Journal*, **70**: 415–420.

Stokes P H and Jowett N I (1985) Haemodynamic monitoring with the Swan–Ganz catheter. *Intensive Care Nursing*, **1**: 9–17.

Sullivan A K, Holdright D R, Wright C A, Sparrow J L, Cunningham D and Fox K M (1994) Chest pain in women: clinical, investigative and prognostic features. *British Medical Journal*, **308:** 883–886.

Swan H J C, Ganz W, Forrester J S, Marcus H, Diamond G and Chonette D (1970) Catheterisation of the heart in man with the use of a flow-directed balloon catheter. *New England Journal of Medicine*, **283:** 447–451.

Wagner C S (1984) Arrhythmias in acute myocardial infarction. *Medical Clinics of North America*, **68:** 1001–1008.

6

Management of Acute
Myocardial Infarction

In Western countries, myocardial infarction is responsible for between one third and half of all deaths and half to three-quarters of all cardiac deaths. In the UK, this means about 270 000 patients with myocardial infarction and over 180 000 deaths per annum. Over 60% of these fatalities occur within 2 hours of the onset of symptoms, most before the arrival of help, let alone admission to hospital. The development of prehospital care must be a major target for the 1990s.

Once in hospital, patients are best managed on acute cardiac units rather than on general medical wards. The chances of resuscitation are two to three times higher on specialist units, and many patients admitted to medical wards do not seem to be considered soon enough for active intervention (including thrombolytic therapy) or for secondary preventative measures prior to discharge (Lawson–Matthew et al, 1994). Inpatient mortality fell by about 10% following the introduction of coronary care units in the 1960s, and inhospital mortality is still falling, being about 10–15% in patients under the age of 70 years. Whilst the initial fall in cardiac mortality was due to the prompt recognition and treatment of potentially fatal dysrhythmias, the more recent improvement has been due to better and faster admission procedures, infarct limitation strategies (including thrombolysis and surgery) and enhanced therapy for cardiogenic shock and heart failure.

Initial management of acute myocardial infarction is aimed at relieving the symptoms (predominantly pain), with haemodynamic stabilisation. The next priority is to limit the infarct size, and, finally, prompt recognition and treatment of any ensuing complications.

LIMITING THE EXTENT OF INFARCTION

Therapeutic intervention in the course of acute myocardial infarction aims to prevent or limit the extent of myocardial necrosis and preserve normal myocardial performance. This demands early reperfusion of the myocardium at risk. The important zone of potentially salvageable myocardium lies between the irreversibly-damaged central core and normal myocardial tissues at the periphery. The size of this 'border zone' will be influenced by the severity and location of the coronary artery occlusion, the patency of other coronary arteries and the presence of collateral vessels.

Re-establishing coronary perfusion is the principal way of improving oxygenation of the injured myocardium. The majority of patients with acute myocardial infarction have evidence of fresh coronary arterial thrombus in association with a fissured atheromatous plaque. Whilst it has been recognised for over 50 years that the extent of myocardial infarction is related to the duration of coronary occlusion (Blumgart et al, 1941), the clinical importance of opening the infarct-related artery (the 'open artery' theory) to increase or re-establish normal myocardial perfusion has only recently been realised and has since become a major goal (Braunwald, 1993). Early reperfusion limits infarct size, preserves global and regional left ventricular function and increases survival (Van der Laarse et al, 1986). Thrombolytic agents will induce early coronary recanalisation and patency, and where these fail, coronary angioplasty or bypass surgery can be used acutely to re-establish myocardial blood flow. The GUSTO Angiographic Investigators (1993) have shown that the earlier and more completely that coronary patency is achieved, the better the prognosis. It is going to be very important in coming years that non-invasive techniques are developed to indicate the failure of early thrombolytic therapy, so that retreatment or emergency revascularisation procedures may be carried out.

Supplemental oxygen therapy is usual in most coronary care units. Most patients with acute myocardial infarction have arterial hypoxaemia, and there is some evidence from ST segment mapping that oxygen therapy can reduce myocardial ischaemia. Oxygen might induce vasoconstriction, and it is postulated that, by constricting normal coronary arteries, blood is diverted to the affected coronary artery. Certainly, the oxygen gradient between the normal myocardium and border zone myocardium may be increased, helping myocardial oxygenation.

Coronary arterial spasm in the presence of a fixed atheromatous lesion may complicate over one third of cases of myocardial infarction. The use of nifedipine and nitrates may help to overcome this and re-establish coronary blood flow.

Cardiac drugs may be used to limit myocardial work and oxygen consumption:

- The *beta-adrenergic blocking agents* are often used to reduce heart rate and contractility, limit myocardial damage and perhaps inhibit dysrhythmias (including ventricular fibrillation). Early administration of beta-blockers has been reported to decrease the final infarct size by 15–20% (Herlitz and Hjalmarson, 1986)
- *Nitrates* may be useful in decreasing preload and thus reducing myocardial work and augmenting endocardial perfusion. In addition, they diminish left ventricular volume, thus reducing compression on the collateral coronary arteries, which may enhance collateral circulation
- The beneficial use of *aspirin* in unstable angina and acute myocardial infarction has been confirmed (Anti-platelet Trialists' Collaboration, 1994), and it is probably a combination of reduction of inflammation and prevention of coronary platelet emboli that helps to limit the extent of myocardial necrosis following acute myocardial infarction

PREHOSPITAL MANAGEMENT

The first evidence of myocardial infarction may be sudden death. Up to one half of all coronary deaths occur in the first hour following the onset of symptoms of myocardial ischaemia (Table 6.1), and most are due to ventricular fibrillation. As this acute rhythm disturbance can be treated effectively, the first priority is to get the patient to a defibrillator (or vice versa). Not all sudden cardiac deaths are necessarily due to coronary thrombosis, and acute ischaemia (e.g. owing to coronary arterial spasm or platelet emboli) of a critical area of myocardium may be responsible, as may myocarditis, aortic stenosis or aortic dissection. Warning symptoms are common (Table 6.2), although their significance frequently goes unrecognised by the patient or by those from whom he may seek advice. In the majority of those who do experience a warning symptom, it is usually chest pain, although this is not always typically anginal in nature. Chest pain is the sole prodromal symptom in 75% of patients and is usually recurrent. Pain may be felt in the arms (especially in the distribution of the ulnar nerve) or in the back, and is frequently attributed to indigestion.

Only 40% of acute coronary deaths occur in hospital; another 40% occur in the home and the remainder in public places, such as at work (6%) or in the street (Goldman and Cook, 1984). Most of these deaths occur before the call for help is made (Fitzpatrick et al, 1992). Studies in Seattle, USA, have shown that

Table 6.1 Time between onset of coronary symptoms and death

Time (hr)	Male (%)	Female (%)
<0.5	35	44
0.5–1	5	5
1–2	5	2
2–3	6	7
4–24	15	12
>24	34	30

Table 6.2 Premonitory symptoms in 100 sequential cases of myocardial infarction at Leicester General Hospital

Symptoms*	Percentage
Angina	
New	11
Old	17
Chest pain	26
Emotional stress	19
Dyspnoea	13
Lethargy	10
Palpitations	4
None	46

*Note that some symptoms were multiple

bystander-initiated resuscitation combined with paramedical services can halve the number of these deaths, and over half the patients who are resuscitated survive to live a normal life (Crampton et al, 1975). Reports from other parts of the US are not quite so impressive (Gray et al, 1991), but it is clear that public education can lead to lives being saved.

'Coronary ambulances' (Pantridge and Adgey, 1969) are often employed to carry trained staff with equipment for resuscitation, haemodynamic stabilisation and rhythm monitoring to the patient with minimal delay. The main advantage in summoning an ambulance directly is that a defibrillator will be brought to the patient immediately. Initially, these ambulances were manned by medical practitioners and specialist nursing staff, but now paramedical personnel have been trained and provide primary emergency care in many areas (Briggs et al, 1976). ECG transmission by cellular phone to the cardiac unit allows the ambulance personnel to receive guidance if they are in doubt (Califf and Harrelson–Woodlief, 1990). The most important part of coronary ambulance training is the application of early cardiac defibrillation, which has had a major impact on the reduction of out-of-hospital coronary mortality. The effectiveness of such a system has been shown in many cities around the world, including Brighton, Belfast, Seattle and Melbourne. In these areas, prehospital care may have decreased the overall observed coronary mortality rate by as much as 14% (Crampton et al, 1975; Goldman and Cook, 1984). However, these services cannot function satisfactorily unless there has been community education in the recognition of the possible presenting symptomatology of myocardial infarction, with basic training in cardiopulmonary resuscitation, allowing emergency services to reach the patient (Thompson et al, 1979).

Apart from the role of effective resuscitation, there are other first-line measures that these ambulance services can provide. The insertion of intravenous cannulae and the administration of analgesics and oxygen are helpful, and there is much current interest in the role of out-of-hospital thrombolysis. The GREAT and EMIP studies have demonstrated that resuscitation with thrombolysis can be given with success in the community, particularly to patients at a distance from hospital (GREAT Study Group, 1992; EMIP, 1993).

Delays in the treatment of coronary thrombosis

There are several (usually unavoidable) delays between the onset of symptoms and admission to the coronary care unit (Birkhead, 1992). These may occur:

- Between the onset of symptoms and the call for help
- Between the call for assistance and the arrival of medical help
- During transport to hospital
- Within the hospital

It is well recognised that many patients postpone seeking medical attention after the onset of symptoms, and this has been our experience (Table 6.3). Why patients delay seeking help is unknown, and these patterns of behaviour may not be modifiable by education. Where they occur, prodromal symptoms are experienced by 50% of patients up to 1 week before myocardial infarction, and many can predate

Table 6.3   Time between onset of coronary symptoms and call for medical help in 200 patients
admitted to coronary care* with and without previous myocardial infarction (MI)

Time (hr)	Previous MI	No previous MI
<0.5	28	20
0.5–1	18	15
1–3	42	27
3–24	5	9
>24	7	29
Total	100	100

*Leicester General Hospital

symptoms to up to a month before the attack. The advice of the patient's family is usually sought before any contact is made with a medical practitioner, and further time is wasted in waiting for the emergency physician to visit, formulate a diagnosis, arrange hospital admission and organise transport. The British Heart Foundation Working Group (1989) has urged general practitioners to organise a rapid response mechanism for acute cardiac patients, in conjunction with paramedical ambulance teams. In Nottingham (Rowley et al, 1992), the heart attack register suggests that calling the ambulance directly can significantly reduce the waiting time (247 minutes vs 100 minutes). The journey to hospital is usually brief, but delay can occur during admission procedures and in radiography and casualty departments. Unless these delays can be minimised, the role of acute coronary care is limited, and one wonders whether patients would not be better off initially being stabilised and treated at home, without being rushed around at a time when they are probably at greatest danger.

THE HOSPITAL VS HOME CONTROVERSY

In the 1970s, conflicting advice about the best place to manage acute myocardial infarction led to great uncertainty within the medical profession, especially among general practitioners, with whom the decision often lies. Studies at that time (Mather et al, 1971; Dellipiani et al, 1977; Hill et al, 1978) suggested that if there was going to be a prolonged delay in arranging hospital admission, or if the patient had presented some time after the onset of chest pain, there was no difference between the mortality of patients treated at home or in hospital. Since these studies, thrombolysis has become routine in the treatment of myocardial infarction, and current practice demands that most patients need rapid transmission to hospital to allow early and safe thrombolysis (Fox, 1990). Management at home should only be considered if myocardial infarction is confirmed and has occurred more than 24 hours before assessment and providing there are no complications. Home management does, of course, mean that the general practitioner is often committed to frequent visits in the first 48–72 hours, which is not always possible in busy practices.

The alternative view may be taken that since it is the speed in giving thrombolysis that is important ('call-to-needle' time), the general practitioner should be instituting immediate treatment, including thrombolytic therapy, at home (the 'stay and stabilise' policy). The logistics of this are complicated, and unless general practitioners have been specially trained and supported (Waine et al, 1993), or alternatively there is provision of a well-equipped, well-trained mobile emergency unit, as in the EMIP study (1993), most would feel that ensuring rapid transmission of the patient is what is required. In today's mediocolegal and economic climate, this is probably best served by a rapid response ambulance and direct admission to a coronary care unit (the 'scoop and run' policy). General practitioners should be prepared to make a diagnosis on the basis of information over the telephone, and unless they can reach the patient within 15 minutes, they should send an ambulance rather than attend the patient first (Rowley et al, 1992).

IMMEDIATE MANAGEMENT IN HOSPITAL

Direct admission to coronary care or rapid assessment and admission policies must exist if cardiac mortality and morbidity are to be minimised. Unless admissions are organised, delays of up to 6 hours from the onset of symptoms to the arrival in the coronary care unit are not infrequent, and it is obvious that, by this time, the immediate danger period is over and the role of thrombolysis limited. Significant reduction in admission time can be made if there is a direct telephone line to the coronary care unit, which bypasses the hospital switchboard (Burns et al, 1989; Wallbridge et al, 1992). These direct lines may be used by both general practitioners and the ambulance service and, despite worries, do not usually lead to congestion of the unit or a significant number of inappropriate admissions. Our experience (Table 6.4) shows that the majority of cases are correctly directed to the cardiac care unit (80%), although only half of these will actually have sustained acute myocardial infarction. The original concept of coronary care units being only for cases of suspected or established myocardial infarction has, anyway, been superseded, and the unit should be available for any condition that merits cardiovascular monitoring facilities, including acute left ventricular failure, dysrhythmias, aortic dissection or major pulmonary emboli.

Table 6.4 Analysis of a year's admissions to the coronary care unit at Leicester General Hospital (1985) (966 patients)

Diagnosis	Male	Female	Totals	
			Number	Percentage
Myocardial infarction	267	93	360	37.3
Other cardiac	259	143	402	41.6
Non-cardiac	129	75	204	21.1

Where there is no direct admission policy, a 'fast-track' admission system may be used to diminish the components of in-hospital delay. In this fast-track/triage system, patients are selected for treatment by the cardiac care team on predefined clinical and electrocardiographic criteria, and routine evaluation by the admitting medical team is bypassed (Pell et al, 1992). Immediately on arrival at hospital (or preferably whilst in the ambulance), the presentation should be recognised as an acute cardiac problem. The receiving doctor should take no more than a few minutes to confirm or reject the diagnosis of acute myocardial infarction, obtain a 12-lead electrocardiogram and ensure that there are no contraindications to thrombolysis. Patients may then be classified as:

- *Fast track*: myocardial infarction, qualifying ECG (ST elevation or bundle branch block) and no contraindications for thrombolysis
- *Slow track*: probable myocardial infarction with dubious ECG changes or relative contraindications to thrombolysis
- *No track*: myocardial infarction unlikely or thrombolysis is contraindicated

'Fast-track' patients should be able to receive thrombolytic treatment within 15 minutes of admission. Such a system should not require any additional staff or resources and may halve the in-hospital delay to the institution of thrombolysis.

The original approach of watchful waiting over coronary patients has given way to active intervention, with the development of therapies intended to re-establish coronary perfusion and limit or reduce the extent of the myocardial damage, with prompt resuscitation if required. Of equal importance is the appreciation of the psychological stress placed upon the patient who has been rushed into hospital, usually via an emergency ambulance, to be delivered to the high-technology world of the coronary care unit. Verbal and tactile communication is important, and the patient's confidence must be obtained and further developed by careful explanation at all stages.

There are several interventions that need immediate consideration following admission to the coronary care unit. Many of these will happen simultaneously, and the usual medical sequence of history, examination, investigation and treatment is not usually the most effective way of patient assessment. If fast tracking/triage has not already been carried out, a rapid clinical appraisal is the first step to assess the likelihood of myocardial infarction and the possible need for resuscitation. An early confirmation of qualifying criteria for thrombolysis is vital, so that early treatment can be instituted and any immediate complication anticipated.

History and examination of the patient

Taking a history from patients on a coronary care unit is often easy; somebody, somewhere must have thought the history was suggestive of myocardial infarction. The initial enquiry should be brief, and serve to answer two questions:

- Does the patient need thrombolysis?
- Are there any contraindications to receiving thrombolysis?

Taking a more complete clinical history will still be needed, but this can usually wait until treatment is commenced. Obtaining essential information in the acute phase of the illness, when the patient is in pain and feeling faint or nauseated, is not ideal, and the complete story often becomes more clear when the patient has been settled with analgesia and antiemetics.

All drug therapy being taken on admission needs recording and reviewing. Many medications can be stopped and should only be reinstituted if specifically required. This will prevent adverse drug actions or interactions. Beta-adrenergic blocking agents should be continued unless there are contraindications, such as excessive bradycardia, hypotension or heart failure. Sudden withdrawal of these agents may be accompanied by further chest pain, dysrhythmias or extension of the myocardial infarction.

The physical appearance and clinical findings in patients suffering from acute myocardial infarction are extremely variable and alter with time and the presence of any coexistent complications. It is not uncommon to find no physical abnormalities at all. The general appearance of the coronary patient is dependent upon the physical and psychological impact that the illness has upon the particular individual. Hence, although some patients will appear quiet and anxious, others may appear excessively agitated and restless. The situation will be ameliorated or aggravated if the patient has had a previous hospital admission or myocardial infarction, depending upon his clinical and social course in hospital.

Autonomic imbalance or impaired left ventricular function may result in nausea, vomiting, sweating, peripheral vasoconstriction and varying degrees of dyspnoea. The typical patient will, therefore, be cool, clammy, in pain and frightened.

Pulse and blood pressure

Variation in pulse rate and blood pressure usually depend on the amount of pain, the size of the infarct and the degree of left ventricular dysfunction but may be influenced by overactivity of the autonomic nervous system. Inferior and true posterior myocardial infarctions are usually associated with parasympathetic overactivity (bradycardia, hypotension and atrioventricular heart block), whilst anterior and lateral infarction myocardial infarctions are associated with sympathetic stimulation (tachycardia and hypertension).

In some patients, profound hypotension may follow the administration of nitrates. A small dose of atropine should be considered if there is significant bradycardia or hypotension.

Pulse irregularities may indicate the presence of a dysrhythmia or conduction defect, which usually requires electrocardiographic monitoring for full elucidation.

The jugular venous pressure

The jugular venous pressure (JVP) is usually normal unless there is pre-existing congestive heart failure or pulmonary disease or there has been right ventricular infarction. The pressure waveform, however, may be useful in detecting dysrhythmias. For example, cannon waves may be seen in complete heart block and irregular 'a' waves in ventricular tachycardia.

The heart sounds

The first heart sound is often diminished and muffled as a result of left ventricular dysfunction, and reversed splitting of the second sound is common, probably reflecting conduction delay or mechanical abnormalities within the ischaemic left ventricle. Fourth heart sounds are nearly always present (Hill et al, 1969), so that their absence makes myocardial infarction an unlikely diagnosis. Third heart sounds are less common and usually reflect left ventricular failure. As such, the presence of this added sound is associated with poor prognosis. Detecting these low-pitched sounds is often difficult in patients who are obese or have hyper-inflated chests, such as those with emphysema. Auscultation over the carotid or subclavian vessels may then amplify these sounds.

Cardiac murmurs

The murmur of mitral incompetence is present in about 50% of patients in the early stages of myocardial infarction and is due either to papillary muscle dysfunction or to dilatation of the mitral ring in association with left ventricular failure (Heikkila, 1967). Other murmurs may indicate pre-existing valvular disease, which may or may not have predisposed the individual to myocardial infarction. For example, aortic valve disease may cause myocardial infarction in the presence of little or no coronary atherosclerosis.

Intravenous access and blood samples

Insertion of an intravenous line will allow administration of an analgesic and an antiemetic by injection. Intramuscular routes are inadequate, since drug absorption from vasoconstricted muscle capillary beds in the 'shut down' patient is erratic. In addition, this route is contraindicated if thrombolysis is being considered. The routine use of an intravenous port has simplified prolonged venous catheterisation. A Venflon-type catheter can be used, which is inserted under sterile conditions into a peripheral (forearm) vein and flushed with sterile normal saline. The use of topical antiseptics such as Betadine does not reduce the risk of cannula-related infection, and cleaning the skin with an alcohol swab (Steret) is sufficient (Thompson et al, 1989). This has the added advantage of removing skin oils and allowing the cannula to be fixed more securely to the skin with adhesive tape. The cannula needs to be flushed every 8–12 hours with normal saline and before and after every intravenous drug. The use of a heparin solution does not prolong cannula patency or reduce infection (Jowett et al, 1986).

Baseline blood tests can be taken at the same time as cannula insertion, but care should be taken if blood samples are withdrawn through the cannula; too small a cannula or too rapid an aspiration can cause haemolysis of the blood sample, with misleading results. Blood should be sent for analysis of the following.

Full blood count

This will detect anaemia or polycythaemia. The white cell count (WBC) and erythrocyte sedimentation rate (ESR) are initially normal but rise in response to muscle necrosis. The leucocytosis peaks at about $15\,000$ cells/mm^3 after 2–4 days, and higher levels suggest complications, such as infection or pericarditis. The ESR often remains elevated for 2–3 weeks.

Urea and electrolytes

Levels of these are needed to assess renal function and potassium levels, which are particularly important in patients taking digoxin or diuretics.

Cardiac enzymes

Following myocardial infarction, the levels of some of the myocardial enzymes will rise, and estimation of their serum levels is often of diagnostic importance. Cardiac enzymes not only help to confirm the diagnosis of myocardial infarction (even in the absence of electrocardiographic evidence), but also the degree of their elevation may give some indication of the size of the myocardial infarction; enzyme release is thought to reflect irreversible cell damage. The most commonly

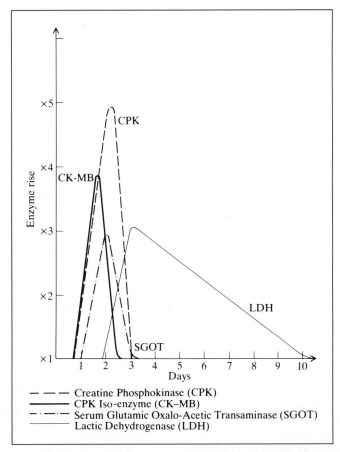

Fig. 6.1   Serum enzyme elevation in acute myocardial infarction

measured cardiac enzymes are *creatine kinase* (CK), *lactate dehydrogenase* (LDH) and *serum glutamic oxaloacetic transaminase* (SGOT or AST). The timing of enzyme release and concentration peaks in relation to chest pain are also of importance (Figure 6.1).

It should be noted that thrombolysis causes an earlier enzyme release due to 'wash out' of enzymes from recanalised vessels, displacing the concentration curves to the left. The above enzymes are not cardiospecific and may be released from other tissues in response to different stimuli or illnesses (Table 6.5). Isoenzymes of LDH and CK may be used to increase specificity, and, recently, assays of a highly specific cardiac enzyme, Troponin T, have become possible, although these are not yet available in most district general hospitals. The routine measurement of cardiospecific enzymes could improve the speed and accuracy of diagnosis of myocardial infarction (Roberts, 1984).

Creatine kinase (CK)

CK is found in high concentrations in both skeletal and cardiac muscle, as well as the brain. Its estimation is the most sensitive single enzyme assay for detecting acute infarction (positive in over 90% of cases). Serum levels rise within 4–8 hours of myocardial infarction, peak at 24 hours and return to normal after about 3–5 days. Elevated levels can also be seen following muscle damage (including intramuscular injections) and extreme muscular exercise. Bedside estimation of CK levels by trained nurses is possible (Downie et al, 1993) and may be of value in confirmation of the diagnosis in patients with non-diagnostic ECGs or left bundle branch block.

CK is composed of two subunits, M (muscle) and B (brain), which can be linked together as MM, BB or MB. The last is of greatest diagnostic importance, since it is almost exclusively found in the human heart. This does not mean that CK-MB

Table 6.5 Other possible causes of enzyme elevation

SGOT	Pulmonary embolism
	Hepatic congestion
	Liver disease
	Shock
	Trauma (including surgery or cardioversion)
	Gall-bladder disease
	Drugs (steroids, cholestatic agents and the oral contraceptive pill)
LDH	Heart failure
	Liver disease
	Renal failure
	Myocarditis
	Pulmonary embolism
	Muscle disease or injury (including severe exercise and intramuscular injections)
CK	Muscle disease or injury (surgery, intramuscular injections or after defibrillation)
	Stroke
	Haemorrhage
	Following sustained tachycardias

is only liberated following myocardial infarction; cardiac damage and consequent enzyme release can occur following defibrillation or cardiac surgery. The isoenzyme may also be elevated in cases of hypothermia and with some muscle diseases.

After acute myocardial infarction, CK-MB levels rise rapidly to reach a peak at 24 hours and disappear again by about 72 hours. A CK-MB release of more than 15% of the total CK is suggestive of myocardial infarction.

Lactate dehydrogenase (LDH)

LDH is found widely throughout the body tissues, especially the liver, as well as skeletal and cardiac muscle. It is elevated in over 85% of cases of myocardial infarction, with elevated levels starting within 24–48 hours, peaking at 3–6 days and returning to normal over 1–2 weeks. False elevation of levels occurs commonly in haemolysed blood samples.

Normal LDH is composed of five chemically distinct isoenzymes. There are high concentrations of LDH_1 in cardiac tissue, so that release leads to a change in the concentration ratio of LDH_1 to total LDH.

Glutamic oxaloacetic transaminase (SGOT or AST)

The heart is the major source of SGOT, and elevation of this enzyme is found in over 70% of cases of myocardial infarction. Levels start to rise in the serum after 8–12 hours, peaking towards the end of the second day and remaining elevated for about 5 days.

Troponin T (TnT)

Troponin T is a structurally-bound protein found in both skeletal and cardiac muscle, but the amino acid sequence in each is different. Antisera to cardiospecific troponin T has been raised and can be used to detect release of this cardiospecific enzyme. Levels climb early (1–10 hours; median 4 hours), and its elevation is highly sensitive for diagnosing.myocardial infarction (Hillis et al, 1993). In addition, measuring serial troponin T levels may give some indication of whether the infarct-related artery has been opened (Figure 6.2), allowing further strategies to be implemented to relieve the coronary obstruction (Miyata et al, 1993).

Myoglobin

Myoglobin is not specific to heart muscle but is suitable for rapid immunoturbidimetric assay. It is released early following myocardial infarction, peaking at 4–12 hours. It has been found to be more sensitive than either CK or even CK-MB, and results can be obtained in less than 2 minutes (Mair et al, 1992). Bedside estimation in the emergency room or on the coronary care unit may allow certain patients to have a diagnosis of myocardial infarction excluded very early following admission to hospital.

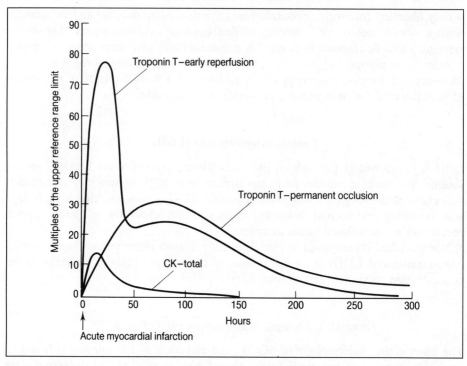

Fig. 6.2 Pattern of troponin T release with early reperfusion of the myocardium following coronary thrombosis

Random serum lipid levels

Early assessment of random serum lipid concentrations will give an indication of pre-existing hyperlipidaemia (Ryder et al, 1984). If not carried out on admission, formal assessment will not be possible until about 3 months, since cholesterol concentrations are suppressed following acute myocardial infarction.

Blood glucose level

The venous blood glucose concentration is of prognostic importance (Burden et al, 1978). Those with an admission blood sugar of less than 7 mmol/l usually have uncomplicated courses, whereas those with concentrations over 9 mmol/l are much more likely to develop complications. Hyperglycaemia may be precipitated by the stress of the illness or may even predate it. About 5–6% of coronary admissions are previously undiagnosed diabetics (Oswald et al, 1984).

Aspirin and nitrates

Soluble aspirin should be given at the earliest opportunity. Aspirin enhances the benefits of thrombolysis and has been shown to reduce early and late morbidity (ISIS-2, 1988). The initial dose should be at least 150 mg, which should be chewed and held in the mouth rather than being swallowed. This enhances absorption and prevents the dose being regurgitated.

Coronary arterial spasm is a common associate of acute coronary thrombosis, and nitrates may not only have a synergistic effect with thrombolysis in reestablishing vessel patency, but also open up collateral blood vessels and reverse inappropriate coronary artery vasoconstriction. The findings of ISIS-4 (1995) have thrown some doubt on the role of nitrates in acute myocardial infarction, but most would still recommend acute administration at the earliest opportunity (e.g. sublingual or buccal nitrate or 2 puffs of GTN spray), particularly for those with ST segment elevation on the ECG. Hypotension may follow administration of nitrates, and caution is required if the patient is already hypotensive or is already taking nitrate therapy. Intravenous nitrates may be of value in heart failure or recurrent pain.

Analgesia

The provision of early and adequate pain relief is of major importance and should be given by nursing staff on their own initiative. Intravenous opiates are the drugs of choice and are usually very well tolerated following myocardial infarction. They relieve the pain and anxiety that may stimulate catecholamine release, the latter leading to a lowered threshold for dysrhythmias, an increase in myocardial work and provocation of coronary arterial spasm (Lown et al, 1977). Intravenous beta-blockers, thrombolysis and nitrates all reduce pain and reduce the need for analgesic drugs, probably by limiting ischaemic damage (Herlitz et al, 1988).

The most common side-effects of opiate therapy are nausea and vomiting, which can be reduced by simultaneous administration of an antiemetic such as metoclopramide (Maxolon). Cyclizine (Valoid) causes vasoconstriction, and prochlorperazine can only be given by mouth or intramuscularly; these drugs should not be used. Comparison of the various opiate preparations suggests that diamorphine provides the earliest complete analgesic action, with no more side-effects than other similar preparations (Scott and Orr, 1969). An initial intravenous dose of 2.5–5.0 mg should be given at 1 mg per minute, followed by further 2.5 mg doses until pain is relieved. Opiates must be used with care in patients with chronic bronchitis or cor pulmonale. Respiratory side-effects may occur within minutes of administration of the drug and last up to 6 hours. Respiration is depressed by direct action upon the respiratory centre, leading to a fall in respiratory rate and tidal volume, which is why opiates should be administered in small, frequent doses rather than a single large dose. Nalorphine is a useful antagonist to have at hand if in doubt. A less well considered complication of opiate therapy is that of reduced gastric and intestinal motility. Apart from leading to constipation, the oral absorption of important drugs (such as diuretics and antidysrhythmic agents) may be impaired. Persistent anxiety may require treatment with diazepam (Valium), which is an effective anxiolytic agent and, as a beneficial side-effect, probably improves left ventricular function by reducing systemic and left ventricular filling pressures.

Oxygen

Patients with acute myocardial infarction, particularly those with left ventricular failure and cardiogenic shock (*British Medical Journal*, 1976), are often hypoxaemic. The reason for the hypoxaemia is unknown, but it probably results from a combination of pulmonary congestion, pulmonary ventilation/perfusion defects and a slowing of peripheral circulation. Many studies (e.g. McNicol and Kirby, 1972) have suggested that there are benefits of oxygen therapy despite the possible rise in mean peripheral resistance. Since hypoxaemia may increase the size of the myocardial infarction (Radvany et al, 1975), improving oxygen delivery to the ischaemic peri-infarction area may help to reduce the final infarct size (Maroko et al, 1975). It is common practice for low-flow oxygen to be administered to most patients for 24–48 hours (100% oxygen at 2–4 l/min). Nasal cannulae are preferred to face masks, which spend most of their time oxygenating the skin of the forehead. Care is required in patients with coexistent chronic airways disease, in whom the concentration of inspired oxygen should be altered according to arterial blood gas estimation (Table 6.6). Pulse oximetery is a useful adjunct to assess adequate arterial oxygenation but should not be used as the sole means of assessing adequacy of ventilation (Davidson and Hosie, 1993). In patients with severe heart failure and cardiogenic shock, positive end expiratory pressure ventilation (PEEP) has been used to increase oxygen transport to ischaemic tissues, but its use is limited by the accompanying dramatic fall in cardiac output as a consequence of reduced venous return, inhibited by raised intrathoracic pressures.

Arterial hypoxaemia may last for up to 3 weeks following uncomplicated myocardial infarction, and longer if there has been significant heart failure or shock.

Chest radiography

An portable anteroposterior chest film is usually taken on admission to the unit. This initial film serves to exclude other causes of chest pain, such as aortic aneurysm, pneumonia and pneumothorax. It may also give some guide to pulmonary congestion, although assessment of pulmonary hypertension is not always easy. A normal film usually excludes significant heart failure, but an abnormal film does not mean that pulmonary pressures are still raised; radiographic findings may take up to 4 days to resolve following haemodynamic stabilisation (Kostuk et al, 1973). Conversely, there may be a 12-hour lag between haemodynamic dysfunction and the radiographic appearances of cardiac failure. There may also be a degree of non-cardiac pulmonary oedema in some patients, caused by reduced plasma oncotic pressure (serum albumin levels fall in acute myocardial infarction) and aggregation of leucocytes.

Table 6.6 Oxygen masks, flow rates and approximate concentrations of delivered oxygen

Mask oxygen flow (litres/min)	Edinburgh (%)	MC (%)	Nasal cannulae (%)	Hudson (%)
1	25–30	–	25–30	–
2	30–35	30–50	30–35	25–38
4	35–40	40–70	32–40	35–45
6	–	55–75	–	50–60
8	–	60–75	–	55–65
10	–	65–80	–	60–75

Electrocardiographic monitoring

Careful monitoring of cardiac rhythm and the prompt treatment of dysrhythmias have sharply reduced hospital deaths from myocardial infarction (Norris, 1982). Following admission, the patient should be connected to a suitable cardiac monitor (Jowett et al, 1985). If the patient is being transferred via the accident and emergency department, a portable monitor must accompany the patient to the coronary care unit. Chest electrodes should be kept away from areas used for cardiac auscultation or defibrillation by placing the 'negative' electrode below the right clavicle (or on the right arm), the 'earth' below the left lateral clavicle (or on the left arm) and the 'positive' electrode in the 4th intercostal space immediately to the right of the sternum (V1 position; see Chapter 5).

THE ECG IN ACUTE MYOCARDIAL INFARCTION

A standard 12-lead ECG should be carried out as soon as possible to confirm the diagnosis and assess the suitability for thrombolysis. The left ventricular subendocardium infarcts within 30 minutes of thrombotic occlusion of a coronary vessel, but extension to the full thickness of the ventricular wall usually takes several hours. The ECG can change within seconds of coronary occlusion, and over 80% of patients with acute myocardial infarction have an abnormal ECG on presentation. Despite some limitations, the ECG remains probably the best way of diagnosing acute myocardial infarction (Timmis, 1990).

There is no single ECG change produced by myocardial ischaemia and infarction; the findings are dependent on the duration of the ischaemic insult and the part of the heart affected. The initial ECG is sometimes normal, and even pre-existing abnormalities are not helpful if they do not change with time. In the early stages, the ECG may change rapidly. ST elevation may fluctuate, T waves may invert and ST depression can occur. Pathological Q waves may also appear within 2 hours of the onset of chest pain (Adams et al, 1993). Daily, and often subtle, electrocardiographic changes may be of major value in the diagnosis of myocardial infarction, especially when viewed with knowledge of the clinical history and changes in serum enzyme levels.

In typical transmural myocardial infarction, there is an evolving sequence of ST–T changes with Q wave formation (Figure 6.3). If the ischaemic insult has been insufficient to cause actual infarction, either ST depression or ST elevation (Prinzmetal changes) may be seen. Infarction limited to the inner part of the ventricular wall (subendocardial infarction) interferes with repolarisation (although not depolarisation), leading to ST depression and deep symmetrical T wave inversion (Figure 6.4).

Acute transmural myocardial infarction

The hallmark of transmural myocardial infarction is the Q wave. By definition, this is the initial negative (downward) deflection of the QRS complex. Normally, there are small ('septal') Q waves in the left ventricular leads, caused by depolarisation of the septum from left to right. Q waves greater than 0.04 second (one small square on standard ECG recording paper) in duration and greater than 2 mm in

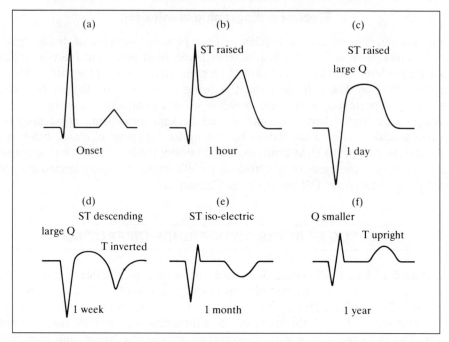

Fig. 6.3 Evolution of ECG changes following acute transmural myocardial infarction:
(a) ECG may be normal or show non-specific changes
(b) development of Q wave and concave ST segment elevation
(c) fully developed Q wave and convex ST elevation
(d) ST segment descends and T wave inverts
(e) ST segment now isoelectric; T wave often still inverted
(f) Q wave permanent but smaller. In 10% of patients the ECG is normal

depth are pathological and imply infarction. The ventricles are depolarised from the inside outwards, and hence if an electrode were placed inside the heart, it would record a large negative deflection, the impulse travelling from within out. Myocardial necrosis produces an electrical 'window' in the ventricle, so that an overlying recording skin electrode will record a cavity potential, as if the electrode were inside the heart, i.e. show a large Q wave.

The Q wave in standard lead III should only be considered abnormal if it exceeds 0.03 second and if it is accompanied by Q waves in leads II and aVF. The 'normal' Q wave in lead III usually diminishes or disappears on deep inspiration, but a pathological Q wave will remain. Q waves may be produced by any process that forms a myocardial window and, as described above, are usually due to myocardial necrosis or fibrosis. However, other conditions may lead to damage or replacement of myocardial tissue, including myocarditis, cardiomyopathies, amyloidosis and cardiac tumours.

Determining the site of infarction

Infarction Q waves will appear within the first 24–48 hours in those leads facing the area of necrosis. Determination of the site of the infarction may be made by correlating the ECG findings with knowledge of the coronary circulation. However, normal coronary vasculature varies widely from person to person, so it is only possible to make generalisations.

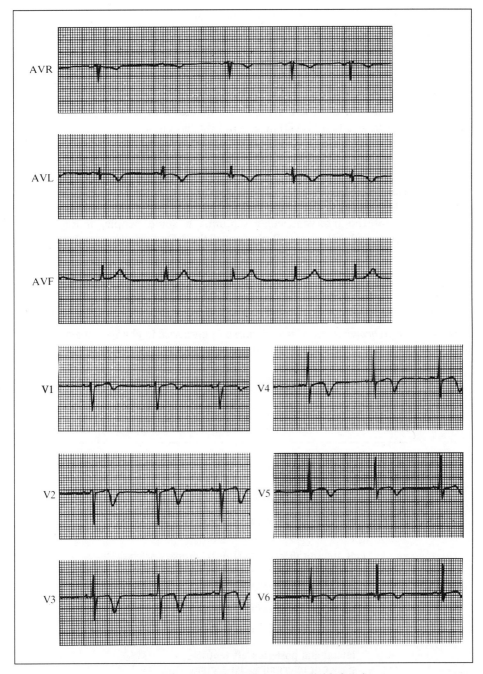

Fig. 6.4   ECG: subendocardial myocardial infarction

The three major coronary vessels (Table 6.7) are:
- The right coronary artery (RCA)
- The left anterior descending artery (LAD)
- The left circumflex artery (LCx)

The RCA supplies the right atrium, the right ventricle and the inferior left ventricle. Blood is also conveyed to the sinus-node, the AV node and the posterior portion of the ventricular septum. Hence, occlusion of the RCA can produce infarction of the inferior and posterior left ventricle and, sometimes, the right atrium and ventricle. Ischaemia or oedema of the sinus and AV nodes may produce bradycardia and heart block (Figure 6.5).

The left coronary artery ('left main stem') divides into its two main branches: the left anterior descending (LAD) artery and the left circumflex (LCx) artery. The former supplies the anterior left ventricular wall, the apex and the interventricular septum. There are septal perforating branches, which additionally supply blood to the bundle of His and bundle branches. Occlusion of the LAD leads to infarction of the anterior left ventricular wall, the cardiac apex and the interventricular septum. The LCx supplies the remainder of the left ventricle and, sometimes, the posterior part of the interventricular septum. In some people, it additionally supplies the sinus and AV nodes. Occlusion of the LCx leads to lateral infarction, sometimes associated with conduction problems.

Common ECG patterns of infarction

The following ECG patterns of infarction may be seen in the standard 12-lead ECG.
- *Anterior myocardial infarction* (Figure 6.6) gives rise to changes in leads V1–V4 (anteroseptal infarction), standard leads I and aVL and V4–V6 (anterolateral infarction)
- *Inferior myocardial infarction* produces changes in the inferior leads II, III and aVF (Figure 6.7)

Table 6.7   Major coronary arteries and structures supplied by each

Right coronary artery (RCA):
    right atrium
    right ventricle
    inferior left ventricle
    sinus node
    atrioventricular node
    posterior interventricular septum

Left anterior descending (LAD) coronary artery:
    anterior wall of left ventricle
    anterior interventricular septum
    apex of left ventricle
    bundle of His and bundle branches

Left circumflex (LCx) coronary artery:
    left atrium
    lateral and posterior left ventricle
    posterior interventricular septum

- *High lateral myocardial infarction* may be seen only in leads I and aVL
- *Apical infarction* can be seen in leads V5 and V6
- *Posterior myocardial infarction* does not produce Q waves in the standard 12-lead ECG, since no lead directly overlies the area of necrosis. Instead, the diagnosis must be implied on the basis of reciprocal R waves in leads opposite the area, usually chest leads V1–V3 (Figure 6.5)

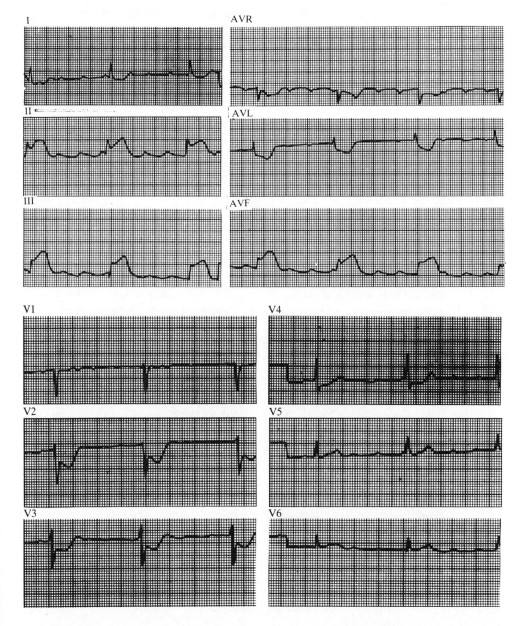

Fig. 6.5 ECG: complete heart block following occlusion of the right coronary artery

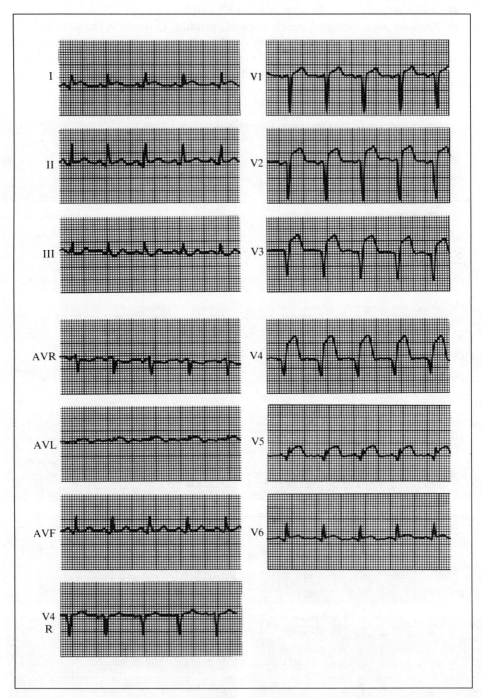

Fig. 6.6   ECG: acute anterior myocardial infarction

Of course, the areas of myocardial infarction do not have strict boundaries and may be affected by anatomical differences in collateral coronary circulation. Hence, changes do not always appear in the classical leads. Further leads may be required to locate infarcts at unusual sites. For example, V7 and V8 (placed further round the chest) are useful for diagnosing lateral infarcts, and leads in the 2nd and 3rd intercostal spaces may locate high lateral infarcts.

With the passage of time following myocardial infarction, the Q waves may regress or even disappear. This may be because the scar contracts away from the surface electrode or because small intraventricular conduction pathways are established in relation to the infarct (Goldberger, 1979).

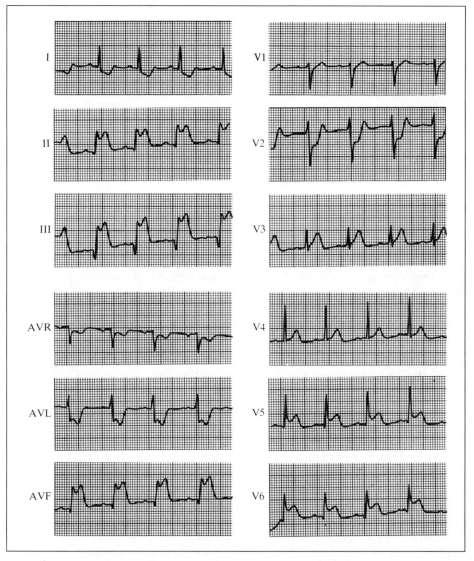

Fig. 6.7   ECG: acute inferolateral myocardial infarction

ST segment and T wave changes

The earliest ECG sign of acute transmural myocardial ischaemia is elevation of the ST segment, the so-called 'current of injury'. This is sometimes accompanied by very tall, hyperacute T waves. The ST segments are usually convex upwards, although they are occasionally concave or flattened. These acute ST–T wave changes resolve within hours or days, to leave inverted T waves. ST segment depression is often seen in leads facing away from the affected area, reflecting 'reciprocal' electrical changes. However, it is possible that these changes may indicate ischaemic myocardial tissue away from the infarction site and could give a clue to the presence of atherosclerotic disease in other coronary vessels. It is likely that this group of patients has a worse long-term prognosis (Krone et al, 1993).

The ST–T wave changes usually resolve over the following weeks, although T wave inversion may last for an indefinite time. Persistent ST elevation in the chest leads often indicates formation of a ventricular aneurysm.

Patients with acute myocardial infarction presenting with ST depression alone do not appear to benefit from thrombolysis and may have a worse prognosis (Gheorghiade et al, 1993).

Right ventricular and atrial infarction

Isolated or additional infarction of the atria or right ventricle is probably more common than realised (Wartman and Hellerstein, 1948) and is often difficult to recognise clinically. About one third to one half of patients with inferior infarction sustain some damage to the right ventricle, and isolated right ventricular infarction is found in between 5 and 10% of autopsies (Rodrigues et al, 1986). Right ventricular infarction generally appears as an inferior infarct with changes in standard leads II, III and aVF (Cohn et al, 1974). Lead V4R, however, and also sometimes V5R and V6R, may show ST–T wave changes, with ST elevation of greater than 1 mm. Although this change in lead V4R is a useful diagnostic pointer (Klein et al, 1983), false positive recordings may occur in inferior myocardial infarction, left bundle branch block and pericarditis. Atrial infarction is found in about 10% of cases of myocardial infarction and occurs more commonly in the right atrium. The ECG often shows altered P wave morphology and deviation of the PR segment. Atrial dysrhythmias are a common complication, particularly atrial fibrillation (Liu et al, 1961).

Subendocardial myocardial infarction

The subendocardial portion of the ventricular myocardium is especially prone to ischaemia because its blood supply is impeded by the high intraventricular pressure. In myocardial infarction limited to the subendocardium, Q waves do not usually develop on the ECG, since the damage is not transmural; Q wave development usually requires more than 50% of the wall thickness to be involved. Subendocardial infarction, therefore, is inferred from ST–T wave changes, usually demonstrated as permanent ST depression with deep, symmetrical T wave inversion (see Figure 6.4).

ECG changes that mimic myocardial infarction (pseudo-infarction)

There are many circumstances in which ECG appearances may be confused with those of myocardial infarction. It is important to recognise these, since confusion may lead to the inappropriate administration of thrombolytic drugs.

1. *Normal ECG variants.* High ST take-off is often seen in young adults, especially in the septal leads, and ST changes can also be produced by changes in posture or by hyperventilation. T wave inversion may be normal in leads V1 and V2 (and V3 in negroes).

Poor R wave progression across the chest leads, or QS complexes, occasionally occur in V1 and V2 as a normal variant in tall, thin individuals or those with chest wall deformities (e.g. pectus excavatum), because of positional changes of the electrodes relative to the heart.

2. *Myocarditis and pericarditis.* Reference has already been made to non-pathological Q wave changes in myocarditis or with myocardial infiltrates, which may be misdiagnosed as myocardial infarction. Concave ST elevation with widespread T wave inversion occurs with pericarditis, but in contrast to myocardial infarction, reciprocal ST depression does not occur.

3. *Metabolic influences.* Transient Q wave formation may follow metabolic insult (especially hyperkalaemia or hypoglycaemia), and ST/T wave changes are characteristic of hypo- and hyperkalaemia.

4. *Left ventricular hypertrophy.* Left ventricular hypertrophy secondary to hypertension or aortic stenosis may produce poor R wave progression in leads V1–V3. These may be confused with pathological Q waves, particularly if there are coexistent ST/T wave changes of left ventricular strain.

5. *Pulmonary embolism.* QR waves in leads V1–V3 are seen in right ventricular hypertrophy or strain. The classic S1/Q3/T3 pattern described in acute pulmonary embolism is associated with non-infarction Q waves in standard leads III and aVF. Widespread T wave inversion and tachycardia are more usually seen.

6. *Miscellaneous conditions.* Very deep inverted T waves are sometimes found after intracerebral bleeds, probably due to altered autonomic tone, and may be confused with the changes of subendocardial infarction. Similar T wave changes are often seen after tachydysrhythmias or Stokes–Adams attacks.

TREATMENT OF CORONARY THROMBOSIS

The increasing use of coronary angiography has demonstrated that most cases of myocardial infarction are associated with the presence of fresh thrombus in the affected coronary artery, usually at the site of a ruptured atheromatous plaque (Davies and Thomas, 1985; *Lancet*, 1985). Coronary artery thrombus has been found in many patients suffering sudden cardiac death and as many as 95% of patients dying from acute transmural myocardial infarction (Davies et al, 1976).

Thrombotic occlusion may occur without resulting in infarction, and subendo-cardial infarction can follow acute coronary insufficiency without evidence of thrombosis. Nevertheless, in the majority of cases of transmural myocardial infarc-tion, complete absence of blood flow in the diseased coronary artery is typical, although spontaneous thrombolysis may take place to a varying degree in about 30% of patients within the first 12–24 hours (DeWood et al, 1980). Present evidence suggests that there is a dynamic interaction involving coronary artery spasm, platelet aggregation and a fissured atheromatous plaque (Gold and Leinbach, 1980; Davies and Thomas, 1985). Occlusive thrombi probably originate at the site of an intimal tear, and it is likely that small coronary emboli are shed before the artery becomes occluded, causing multiple, small, distal occlusions in the area supplied by the coronary vessel ('micro-infarcts'). The tear may either heal and regress or initiate thrombosis, leading to complete occlusion. Hence, there may be varying consequences, ranging from micro-infarcts to full transmural infarction (Stehbens, 1985).

Coronary thrombolysis has become one of the most significant advances in the treatment of acute myocardial infarction this century. Ironically, the observation in the 1930s that streptokinase (a breakdown product of some Streptococcus strains) could lyse clotted blood came long before coronary care units, bedside monitors, defibrillators and loop diuretics existed. It was another 25 years before attempts to recanalise the coronary arteries with streptokinase were reported in the treatment of acute myocardial infarction (Fletcher et al, 1958; Dewar et al, 1963). Although there are many drugs that may be used to break up thrombi, most clini-cal trials so far have reported the use of streptokinase. Intracoronary administra-tion of streptokinase in acute myocardial infarction has been studied in the USA since 1978, but it was the exceptionally important GISSI study (1987) that showed that early peripheral administration of streptokinase significantly reduced mortal-ity without the need for coronary catheterisation.

Before therapeutic intervention is carried out with thrombolytic agents, there are certain considerations including:

- Who should be treated
- When and how to administer the drug
- The choice of thrombolytic agent
- What to do after thrombolysis

Who should be treated

Early work suggested that fewer than 50% of cases of myocardial infarction may be suitable for thrombolysis (Jagger et al, 1987; Murray et al, 1987), but this may have been because trial protocols were more rigid than the criteria applied in everyday clinical practice (De Bono, 1987). Such strict criteria may exclude many patients from receiving the benefits of thrombolysis, and indivi-dual units have usually developed their own indications. The overview from the Fibrinolytic Therapy Trialists' Collaborative Group (1994) has helped consider-ably in clarifying the situation, and our current guidelines for thrombolysis are shown in Table 6.8.

Table 6.8   Guidelines for thrombolysis in acute myocardial infarction

1. *Pain*
   - Chest pain consistent with acute myocardial infarction

2. *ECG changes*
   - ST elevation of >0.1 mV (1 mm) in at least two contiguous leads
   - New, or presumed new, bundle branch block

   (NB Posterior infarction may present with ST depression with prominent R wave in leads V1–V2)

3. *Time since onset of symptoms*
   - 0–6 hours: greatest benefit
   - 6–12 hours: probable benefit
   - >12 hours: diminishing benefit unless continuing or stuttering pain

4. *Age*
   - Age is not an important consideration
   - Biological age is probably more important
   - Clear-cut benefits are seen in patients less than 75 years old
   - Very elderly patients have few clear-cut benefits

The main contraindications to administration of thrombolytic drugs are:

- A high risk of bleeding (recent surgery or trauma, stroke or active peptic ulceration)
- Uncontrolled hypertension (BP more than 200/120)
- Proliferative diabetic retinopathy

Relative contraindications include:

- Cerebrovascular surgery
- Previous stroke
- Ongoing anticoagulant therapy
- Aortic aneurysm
- A need for pacing

Complications

The major risks of thrombolysis are intracranial haemorrhage, systemic haemorrhage, immunological complications, hypotension and cardiac rupture.

Intracranial haemorrhage complicates between 0.2 and 1% of cases and may be disastrous. This appears to be a greater risk in elderly patients treated with tissue plasminogen activator (TPA).

Systemic haemorrhage is very common and may be severe in about 5% of cases (Timmis et al, 1982). Venepuncture following thrombolysis must be carried out with care to prevent bleeding and bruising. Pacemakers and Swan–Ganz catheters may be better inserted via the antecubital fossa or femoral vein to prevent possible occult bleeding following central catheterisation. Haemorrhagic complications may be treated by direct pressure on the source of bleeding, tranexamic acid (1 g by slow iv injection) or fresh frozen plasma.

Fever and allergic reactions are frequent with streptokinase and anistreplase and may be reduced by pretreatment with hydrocortisone and chlorpheniramine.

Anaphylaxis is a rare complication, although the accompanying hypotension may be mistaken for cardiogenic shock. Hypotension is a very frequent accompaniment of thrombolytic therapy with streptokinase and APSAC. This is often easily managed in most patients, but may require substituting tissue plasminogen activator.

Dysrhythmias may accompany recanalisation and reperfusion of the ischaemic myocardium. These 'reperfusion dysrhythmias' are usually without clinical significance. Idioventricular rhythm is the most frequent abnormality, although some cases will develop ventricular tachycardia or fibrillation. Intravenous beta-blockers may help to protect the myocardium during thrombolysis and could reduce the incidence of reperfusion dysrhythmias and cardiac rupture, another recognised complication of late thrombolysis.

When and how to administer the drug

For myocardial salvage to be effective, thrombolysis must be attempted as early as possible, although some thrombolytic trials suggest that intervention may have some effect for up to 24 hours (GISSI Study Group, 1987; ISIS-2, 1988). Experimental work suggests that irreversible cardiac damage occurs within 3–4 hours of coronary artery occlusion, but in clinical myocardial infarction, left ventricular viability may be preserved by such factors as the presence of a pre-existing collateral circulation and residual antegrade coronary blood flow (Rude et al, 1981; Rogers et al, 1984). Additionally, it is likely that acute coronary occlusion is not always a sudden, but a stuttering, event, often marked by episodic chest pain. Currently, the data from all available trials suggest that the usual time limit for thrombolysis should be 12 hours after the onset of symptoms (Cobbe, 1994). Unfortunately, admission to hospital after the start of symptoms may vary widely and has been reported to be between 13 and 505 minutes (mean 80 minutes) in the UK, often with a further delay of 70 minutes between arrival at hospital and transfer to the coronary care unit (*Lancet*, 1987). The current median interval between onset of pain and the start of treatment in British hospitals lies between 3 and $4\frac{1}{2}$ hours (Birkhead, 1992; Wallbridge et al, 1992). Prehospital thrombolysis is feasible, either by the general practitioner (GREAT, 1992) or by emergency response vehicles with trained personnel (EMIP, 1993), but current resources cannot support the widespread clinical application of these strategies. Most doctors feel that rapid admission to coronary care is more important (Petch, 1991; Weston and Fox, 1991), where re-evaluation of emergency services and hospital triage is merited. Since specific therapy for acute myocardial infarction now exists, it is the organisation of care that now needs to be improved (Julian et al, 1988).

The route of administration of thrombolytic agents has also been subject to study and controversy (Marder and Francis, 1984). In angiographic centres, fibrinolytic agents are often infused directly into the occluded artery. This involves an angiographic catheter being introduced into the aortic root via the femoral artery. Nitrates or nifedipine are given to alleviate any coronary artery spasm, before streptokinase is infused directly over the thrombus. Clearly, this method of treatment could never be given to the majority of patients presenting with acute myocardial infarction, and systemic administration of thrombolytics has, therefore, emerged as the preferred route. Systemic administration of the drug is faster and enables the distal surface of the thrombus to be reached by retrograde coronary flow through collateral blood vessels.

The choice of thrombolytic agent

There are three main thrombolytic agents in common usage.

Streptokinase

Streptokinase is a metabolic product of the group C beta-haemolytic Streptococcus, which causes activation of plasminogen, leading to lysis of the fibrin within the thrombus. Streptokinase is antigenic and may produce allergic side-effects, such as fever, rash and even anaphylactic shock. It is now clear that very high antistreptolysin titres begin to develop from the third day following its use and persist for years. These may well neutralise the lytic effect if the patient is treated with streptokinase again (Buchalter et al, 1992). This also applies to recent streptoccal infections.

Dose   1.5 million units intravenously over 1 hour.

Current cost per dose   £80.

Tissue plasminogen activator (TPA)

Tissue plasminogen activator (TPA) is a naturally occurring protein with greater clot specificity than streptokinase and hence is less likely to activate systemic fibrinolysis. Cloning of the TPA gene has provided large quantities of the drug for clinical use, but it remains very expensive.

Dose   100 mg.

- *Normal regime*: 10 mg by intravenous bolus, 50 mg over 1 hour and the remainder over 2 hours.
- *Accelerated regime*: 15 mg bolus, 50 mg over 30 minutes and the remainder over 60 minutes
- *Bolus regime* (experimental): two 50 mg boluses 30 minutes apart

Current cost per dose   £816.

Anisoylated plasminogen-streptokinase activator complex (APSAC or anistreplase)

The advantage of this agent is that it may be given as a bolus rather than by infusion and hence could be given by a general practitioner before the patient is admitted to hospital. As with streptokinase, administration of this drug produces an acute allergenic and longer-term antibody response, which may neutralise further administration with this or streptokinase. Some centres feel that patients who have ever had streptokinase or APSAC should not be rechallenged and that TPA should be used instead (White, 1991).

Dose   30 units over 3–5 minutes intravenously.

Current cost per dose   £495.

One of the largest therapeutic trials ever, ISIS-3, randomised these three major thrombolytic drugs blindly against each other in 41 299 patients with suspected acute myocardial infarction (ISIS-3, 1992). There was no difference in mortality between the treatment groups, but there were fewer cerebral bleeds with strepto-kinase, and, overall, this appears to be the safest drug. However, the GUSTO trial (1993) found that TPA given by an initial faster infusion rate (so-called 'accelerated' or 'front-loaded' TPA) might save an extra life for every 100 patients treated with TPA, and TPA was found to be more beneficial in younger patients treated within 4 hours of their infarct, especially if the infarct was large and ante-riorly situated. It is likely that this superior result is produced by a more rapid and complete restoration of coronary blood flow (GUSTO Angiographic Investigators, 1993). For the best results, the infarct related artery must:

- Be opened early
- Be opened completely
- Have maintained patency

Reocclusion is associated with a two-fold increase in mortality, in comparison to those who do not maintain patency. Unfortunately, only one third of patients will have symptomatic reocclusion, making identification difficult.

There are newer, third-generation thrombolytic agents being developed, which it is hoped will be less antigenic, not so expensive and more effective. Staphylokinase (STAR) is showing great promise. This agent is produced by *Staphylococcus aureus* and has already been shown to be effective in man (Collen and Van de Werf, 1993). Modified TPA, prourokinase and plasminogen activators coupled to monoclonal antibodies are under development to enhance clot specificity, and specific antithrombin drugs, such as hirudin and hirolog, are being tested currently.

What to do after thrombolysis

Successful reperfusion of the myocardium is usually accompanied by relief of chest pain and a rapid return to normal of elevated ST segments on the ECG. The left ventricular ejection fraction increases (Valentine et al, 1986), and the improvement in left ventricular function is particularly marked in patients with anterior myocar-dial infarction and those with their first infarct (Res et al, 1986). Continuing chest pain or persistent ST elevation on the ECG may indicate failure of thrombolysis. Resistance to streptokinase may be present and can be confirmed if the fibrinogen level is more than 2 mmol/l 1 hour or more after thrombolysis. Retreatment with TPA may then be justified.

Because the circumstances that caused coronary thrombosis usually still prevail after successful thrombolysis, reaccumulation of thrombus may occur, with esti-mates of up to 40% within the first week, although these will not always be so severe. Symptomatic reocclusion of the infarct-related artery occurs in about 5–8% of patients, mostly within the first 3 days. These patients have a more compli-cated clinical course and a higher mortality if further attempts to achieve patency are not made or fail (Ohman et al, 1990).

Strategies aimed at preventing reocclusion and opening the artery as completely as possible seem to be important. Patients should receive antiplatelet therapy (aspirin or dipyridamole) to counter platelet aggregation, and whilst anticoagulation was thought to be important to prevent recurrent thrombosis, ISIS-3 did not seem to show any major benefit from giving heparin, although the 6-month follow-up of patients in the GISSI-3 trial (1992) found that those treated with streptokinase plus heparin had a better survival after the first 12 hours. These results seem to confuse rather than clarify the situation, and many centres still believe heparin to be important, particularly following treatment with clot-specific agents (De Bono, 1987). The concept of post-thrombotic vulnerability to reocclusion after TPA is supported by several other studies, including TAMI-3 (Topol et al, 1989) and the European Co-operative study (De Bono et al, 1992). Our current practice is to use an intravenous heparin bolus of 5000 U, followed by 1000 U/hr for 24 hours after thrombolysis with TPA. It is essential to ensure that the heparin is achieving therapeutic concentrations by monitoring the APTT (activated partial thromboplastin time) or heparin levels.

Residual atheromatous stenoses may be found by angiography in 80–90% of cases following thrombolysis (Serruys et al, 1983). Whilst it may be thought that tackling this abnormality by coronary angioplasty (PTCA – percutaneous transluminal coronary angioplasty) is logical, active intervention does not seem to confer any additional advantage over conservative management (TIMI Study Group, 1989; Arnold et al, 1992). However, primary coronary angioplasty used as an alternative to thrombolysis may be beneficial as an initial intervention (Gibbons et al, 1993; Grines et al, 1993; Zijlstra et al, 1993). Not all studies agree on this strategy (Ribeiro et al, 1993), and using PTCA as a primary intervention is, anyway, not feasible for most patients in the UK.

Inappropriate administration of thrombolytic therapy

Whilst thrombolysis has become standard care for myocardial infarction, the appropriate selection of patients is sometimes difficult, which is why different centres have developed different criteria. Although there is little doubt about the benefits of thrombolysis, apprehension over its complications may limit its use. Understanding the clinical risks of therapy may be critical in appropriate patient selection. In many cases, those who appear to be at greatest risk seem to have the most to gain from thrombolysis.

The risk of bleeding and stroke are well appreciated, and reports of the disastrous consequences in patients with aortic dissection and pericarditis reinforce this issue (Blankenship and Almquist, 1989). Serious consequences of misdiagnosis were observed in the ASSET trial, where patients with non-coronary chest pain who underwent thrombolysis had a mortality of 9.5%, against a mortality of 1.2% in those treated with placebo (Wilcox et al, 1988).

Given the high incidence and multiple aetiologies of chest pain, one needs to guard against inappropriate administration of thrombolytic agents. For example, misdiagnosis rates of 41% have been reported if ECG criteria are not used (TEAHAT Study Group, 1990). For patients with a normal or near-normal ECG, inappropriate thrombolysis may be avoided if the ECG is repeated regularly for a few hours, and treatment is only given if definite abnormalities develop that indicate the administration of a fibrinolytic agent (Fibrinolytic Therapy Trialists' Collaborative Group, 1994). The TAMI (Thrombolysis and Angioplasty in Myocardial Infarction) trial investigators have shown that, by following specific criteria (similar to those shown in Table 6.8 above), appropriate patient selection was associated with a low rate of inappropriate administration, and all those who were inappropriately treated survived (Chapman et al, 1993). Thus, in most clinical settings, it is desirable to have a simple algorithm with specific criteria for the safe administration of thrombolytic therapy, and perhaps we should remember to 'first – do no harm' (Califf et al, 1992).

Thrombolysis and complete heart block

The highest incidence of complete heart block occurs outside hospital following acute inferior myocardial infarction. Provided there are no contraindications, thrombolysis should be given immediately, as for other cases of myocardial infarction, along with atropine. In the majority of cases, AV conduction improves, and many cases of complete heart block may be tolerated without the need to insert a temporary pacemaker (Jowett et al, 1989). Anterior myocardial infarction complicated by complete heart block warrants temporary pacing, but thrombolysis should be given first, preferably using TPA.

Intravenous beta-blockade

Intravenous beta-blockade reduces pain, recurrent ischaemia and mortality in patients with acute myocardial infarction (Yusuf et al, 1985). The TIMI II-B study has confirmed the additional benefits of beta-blockade when given in conjunction with thrombolysis. Despite these benefits, intravenous beta-blockade is not often given acutely in the UK, and it is not clear why. Metoprolol and atenolol are safe to use, provided there is no bradycardia, hypotension or heart failure.

Angiotensin converting enzyme (ACE-) inhibitors

The place of ACE-inhibitors in patients with congestive cardiac failure has been unequivocally demonstrated (Packer, 1992). Their routine use in unselected patients following acute myocardial infarction has been addressed by two major studies: GISSI-3 (1994) and ISIS-4 (1995). Broadly speaking, the studies show a small benefit with early administration, but, practically, the use of ACE-inhibitors probably only needs consideration in patients with overt cardiac failure or significant left ventricular damage (an ejection fraction under 40%). The SAVE (Pfeffer et al, 1992) and AIRE (AIRE Investigators, 1993) studies both looked at this type of patient following recent myocardial infarction, and the results are clear: ACE-inhibition should be commenced within 1 week of myocardial infarction to reduce mortality and serious cardiovascular events (St John Sutton, 1994).

Magnesium

Despite early reports of the large benefits of intravenous magnesium sulphate (Woods et al, 1992), the ISIS-4 study showed a non-significant mortality excess in patients treated this way. Routine use is not recommended, but there may be a role in patients with hypokalaemia: low serum potassium is often associated with low serum magnesium.

Anticoagulants

The use of anticoagulants in acute myocardial infarction is controversial, but should be of benefit in:

Preventing deep vein thrombosis and pulmonary emboli
● Preventing left ventricular thrombi and peripheral embolisation
● Possible limitation of infarct size

Low-dose subcutaneous heparin therapy is probably sufficient for most patients as prophylaxis for venous thromboembolism (THRIFT Consensus Group, 1992). Our recommended practice is for 5000 iu heparin to be given 8 hourly to all patients, from admission until the patient is ambulant. Low-dose therapy is effective only as a prophylactic measure and has no effect on established thrombus.

Routine use of heparin following thrombolysis does not improve outcome (ISIS-4, 1995), but it is still recommended in conjunction with clot-specific thrombolytic agents, such as TPA. Full-dose anticoagulant therapy (heparin followed by warfarin, or high-dose calcium heparin) is given to those considered to be at increased risk of thromboembolic complications, including those with:

Active thromboembolic phenomena
Prolonged cardiac failure
Atrial fibrillation
Left ventricular aneurysm
Cardiogenic shock
Severe obesity
An inability to ambulate
Extensive anterior myocardial infarction

The duration of therapy is not clear, but 3 months should be adequate in most cases (Genton and Turpie, 1983).

The incidence of peripheral embolisation following extensive myocardial infarction is well appreciated. Formal anticoagulation with high-dose subcutaneous calcium heparin or warfarin will reduce the occurrence of mural thrombi (SCATI Study Group, 1989).

Long-term anticoagulation has been used for secondary prevention following acute myocardial infarction. The WARIS trial (Jafri et al, 1992) found that long-term warfarin therapy reduced the number of deaths and strokes. Routine anticoagulant treatment of all post-infarction patients is, however, not practicable, in terms of numbers alone, but perhaps should be considered in 'high-risk' patients.

IMPORTANT PHYSICAL FINDINGS IN THE
POST-INFARCTION PATIENT

A low-grade fever is often recorded in the first 3 days after myocardial infarction and is more common with large areas of myocardial damage. Other causes, such as deep vein thrombosis and infection, should be excluded, especially if the pyrexia exceeds 38°C. Chest and urinary tract infections are common, and bacteraemia may be caused by intravenous cannulae, pacing wires or urinary catheters. Occasionally, drugs may be the cause of late or unusual fevers.

Respiratory system

Pulmonary embolism

Thromboembolic phenomena have become less frequent since the introduction of prophylactic low-dose heparin therapy and early mobilisation. The diagnosis of pulmonary embolism must be considered in any patient with chest pain associated with dyspnoea, tachycardia and fever. Physical examination is often unhelpful, unless there is pulmonary infarction. It is probably better to treat on suspicion rather than to rely on hard diagnostic criteria.

Chest infections

Chest infections are common, especially in the elderly, the obese and smokers. Pulmonary congestion and left ventricular failure predispose to infection, and opiate therapy is associated with small areas of atelectasis and ventilation/perfusion abnormalities in the lungs. Aspiration pneumonia may follow cardiopulmonary resuscitation.

Pneumothorax

This complication may follow central venous catheterisation, temporary cardiac pacing or cardiopulmonary resuscitation. Usually, pneumothoraces do not need treating, but they should be anticipated following trauma, and drainage should be carried out if required.

Gastrointestinal tract

Gastric dilatation may sometimes result from nasal administration of oxygen, leading to discomfort, nausea or vomiting.

Constipation and occasional paralytic ileus may result from bed-rest and atropine or opiate therapy. Straining at stool must be avoided to prevent excessive vagal stimulation by the Valsalva manoeuvre.

Gastro-oesophageal reflux is a common coexistent cause of precordial chest pain, and even endoscopic evidence of oesophagitis does not exclude the diagnosis of concomitant myocardial infarction. Stress ulceration of the oesophagus, stomach or duodenum may occur, sometimes presenting as gastrointestinal haemorrhage. This latter complication may be occult, may present with tachycardia, hypotension and shock in a previously stable patient and may be misdiagnosed as cardiac failure or cardiogenic shock.

Urinary tract

Urinary problems may result from drug therapy or bladder catheterisation. Atropine and opiates may precipitate urinary retention, especially in the elderly male, which is often exaggerated by a sudden diuretic response to frusemide or bumetanide. Catheterisation may be necessary, although it is not without risk of introducing infection and vagal stimulation.

Acute renal failure may result from prolonged hypotension or renal arterial embolisation from left ventricular mural thrombi.

Nervous system

Alterations in mental state are common on intensive care units, where there may be anxiety or even hostility arising as a response to psychological stress. Decreased cerebral perfusion may give rise to psychiatric symptoms and is predisposed to by pre-existing cerebrovascular disease. Hypoxaemia and deteriorating left ventricular function will exaggerate these effects. Narcotics and anxiolytic drugs may alter perception, and intravenous lignocaine can produce hallucinations and seizures. Mural thrombi may give rise to cerebral embolisation and stroke, and cerebral haemorrhage is a recognised complication of thrombolytic therapy, particularly in the elderly.

The metabolic system

Diabetes or gout may be precipitated by myocardial infarction or drugs (e.g. thiazide diuretics). The blood glucose concentration should be checked routinely on admission and monitored if elevated. Although hyperglycaemia is common in coronary care admissions, so-called 'stress' hyperglycaemia of greater than 10 mmol/l on admission to the unit probably represents pre-existing diabetes mellitus (Husband et al, 1983). The peri-infarction mortality in diabetics is higher than in non-diabetics, but thrombolysis has had a major impact on this and should not be denied because of the fear of retinal haemorrhage (Lynch et al, 1993). High admission blood sugars are frequent in those developing cardiogenic shock and those who will need temporary cardiac pacing (Jowett et al, 1989).

Shock from any cause, notably severe myocardial infarction or cardiac arrest, causes metabolic acidosis, because of hypoxia in the tissues leading to the accumulation of organic acids, particularly lactic acid (Table 6.9). Accumulation of high blood concentrations of lactic acid are serious, and the clinical picture of lactic acidosis is usually dominated by shock, with Kussmaul respiration, in the presence of high blood concentrations of hydrogen ions (a low pH). Lactic acidosis needs to be recognised and treated vigorously with oxygen and inotropic support. Sodium bicarbonate may be used to correct the acidaemia, and is best given in small hypertonic concentrations (e.g. 50–100 ml of 8.4% solution). Great care is needed in patients with myocardial infarction because of sodium and fluid overload.

Table 6.9   Some causes of lactic acidosis

Due to impaired tissue oxygenation	Other causes
Myocardial infarction	Diabetes mellitus
Left ventricular failure	Renal failure
Pulmonary embolism	Liver disease
Shock	Drugs:
Sepsis	Biguanides
Pancreatitis	Alcohol
	Cyanide (sodium nitroprusside)
	Aspirin

Hypertension

Many patients with myocardial infarction are found to be hypertensive on admission to coronary care. This may represent pre-existing hypertension or may be a response to the stress of myocardial infarction, with sympathetic overactivity. Coronary mortality is higher in hypertensive patients, and a systolic blood pressure of more than 160 mmHg persisting for more than 3 hours after admission predisposes to cardiac rupture. If the blood pressure does not settle after relief of pain and anxiety, active treatment should be commenced. This should be considered as urgent when ischaemic pain continues or there is heart failure. Short-acting beta-adrenergic blocking agents (such as metoprolol) are useful for the management of sympathetic overactivity in the early stages of infarction, but caution is required: tachycardia and hypertension may represent a cardiovascular response to left ventricular failure, rather than being indicative of pure sympathetic overactivity. Incipient left ventricular failure is more likely in the presence of tachypnoea, a wide pulse pressure and a loud first heart sound (Gunnar et al, 1979), and vasodilator therapy is a better therapeutic choice.

POST-INFARCT CARE

Most units have a policy for a gradual return to physical activity (e.g. Table 6.10).

The usual period spent by patients on the unit is about 24–48 hours, although longer admissions will be needed for those patients with extensive myocardial infarction, severe heart failure or recurrent serious dysrhythmias. About half of the coronary admissions will have an uncomplicated course and probably need little intensive care (Mulley et al, 1980). Very early discharge (day 3) may be possible for a few uncomplicated infarcts who have no evidence of residual ischaemia (Topol et al, 1988), but most will go home between 5 and 10 days post infarct. Just after the Second World War, the minimum period of bed-rest was 4 weeks, with some patients spending months in bed. Even now, there is a wide variation in the time people stay in hospital, the average time in the UK being 7 days, whilst in Germany, it is 3 weeks.

Table 6.10 Typical physical activity plan following acute myocardial infarction

Time	Activity
Day 1	Bed-chair rest
Day 2	Sit out of bed or chair; discharge from CCU
Day 3	Walk around ward and to toilet
Day 4	Try stairs
Days 5–7	Discharge home
Days 7–14	Exercise within home and garden
Days 14–28	Gradual increased walking outside home
	Enrol in rehabilitation programme
Days 28–35	Exercise stress test*
Week 4–6	Outpatient review
	Return to work
	Recommence driving (in line with DVLA regulations)

*Predischarge exercise stress testing may be preferable if resources allow.

The patient and family will need support and advice on life-style and secondary prevention measures. Ideally, an assessment of prognosis should be made prior to discharge, preferably aided by exercise stress testing and perhaps 3-hour Holter monitoring. Blood cholesterol must be assessed and hyperlipidaemia treated vigorously. Long-term aspirin and beta-blocker therapy improve survival.

References

Adams J, Trent R and Rawles J M, on behalf of the GREAT Group (1993) Earliest electrocardiographic evidence of myocardial infarction: implications for thrombolytic treatment. *British Medical Journal*, **307**: 409–413.

AIRE (Acute Infarction Ramipril Efficacy) Investigators (1993) Effect of Ramipril on mortality and morbidity of survivors of acute myocardial infarction with clinical evidence of heart failure. *Lancet*, **342**: 821–828.

Anti-platelet Trialists' Collaboration (1994) Overview I: Prevention of death, myocardial infarction and stroke by prolonged anti-platelet therapy in various categories of patients. *British Medical Journal*, **308**: 81–106.

Arnold A E R, Simoons M L and Van de Werf F (1992) Recombinant TPA and immediate angioplasty in acute myocardial infarction. *Circulation*, **86**: 111–120.

Birkhead J S (1992) Time delays in provision of thrombolytic treatment in six district hospitals. *British Medical Journal*, **305**: 445–448.

Blankenship J C and Almquist A K (1989) Cardiovascular complications of thrombolytic therapy in patients with a mistaken diagnosis of acute myocardial infarction. *Journal of the American College of Cardiology*, **14**: 1579–1582.

Blumgart H L, Gilligan R and Schlesinger M J (1941) Experimental studies on the effect of temporary occlusion of coronary arteries. II. The production of myocardial infarction. *American Heart Journal*, **22**: 374–389.

De Bono D (1987) Coronary thrombolysis. *British Heart Journal*, **57**: 301–305.

De Bono D P, Simoons M L, Tijssen J, Arnold A E R and Betriu A, for the European Co-operative Study Group Trial (1992) Effect of early intravenous heparin on coronary patency, infarct size and bleeding complications after alteplase thrombolysis. *British Heart Journal*, **67**: 122–128.

Braunwald E (1993) The open artery theory is alive and well – again. *New England Journal of Medicine*, **329**: 1650–1652.

Briggs R S, Brown P M, Crabb M E, Cox T J, Ead H W, Hawkes R A, Jequier P W, Southall D

P, Grainger R, Williams J H and Chamberlain D A (1976) The Brighton resuscitation ambulances: a continuing experiment in pre-hospital care by ambulance staff. *British Medical Journal*, **2**: 1161–1165.

British Heart Foundation Working Group (1989) Role of the general practitioner in managing patients with myocardial infarction: impact of thrombolytic treatment. *British Medical Journal*, **298**: 555–557.

British Medical Journal (1976) Oxygen in myocardial infarction (editorial). *British Medical Journal*, **i**: 731.

Buchalter M B, Suntharalingam G, Jennings I, Hart C, Luddington R J, Chakraverty R, Jacobson S K, Weissberg P L and Baglin T P (1992) Streptokinase resistance: when might streptokinase administration be ineffective? *British Heart Journal*, **68**: 449–453.

Burden A C, Kupfer R, Davies M K and Pohl J E F (1978) Blood sugar and prognosis of myocardial infarction. *Lancet*, **i**: 820–821.

Burns J M, Hogg K J, Rae A P, Hillis W S and Dunn F G (1989) Impact of a policy of direct admission to a coronary care unit on use of thrombolytic therapy. *British Heart Journal*, **61**: 322–325.

Califf R M and Harrelson-Woodlief S L (1990) At home thrombolysis. *Journal of the American College of Cardiology*, **15**: 937–939.

Califf R M, Fortin D F, Tenaglia A N and Sane D C (1992) Clinical risks of thrombolytic therapy. *American Journal of Cardiology*, **69**: 12A–20A.

Chapman G D, Ohman E M, Topol E J, Candela R J, Kereiakes D J, Samaha J, Berrios E, Pieper K S, Young S Y and Califf R M (1993) Minimising the risk of inappropriately administering thrombolytic therapy (TAMI study group). *American Journal of Cardiology*, **71**: 783–787.

Cobbe S M (1994) Thrombolysis in myocardial infarction. *British Medical Journal*, **308**: 216–217.

Cohn J N, Guiha N H, Broden M I and Limas C J (1974) Right ventricular infarction – clinical and haemodynamic features. *American Journal of Cardiology*, **33**: 209–214.

Collen D and Van de Werf F (1993) Coronary thrombolysis with recombinant staphylokinase in patients with evolving myocardial infarction. *Circulation*, **87**: 1850–1853.

Crampton R S, Aldrich R F, Gascho J A, Miles J R and Stillerman R (1975) Reduction of pre-hospital, ambulance and community coronary death rates by the community-wide emergency cardiac care system. *American Journal of Medicine*, **58**: 151–165.

Davidson J A H and Hosie H E (1993) Limitations of pulse oximetry: respiratory insufficiency – a failure of detection. *British Medical Journal*, **307**: 372–373.

Davies M J and Thomas A C (1985) Plaque fissuring – the cause of acute myocardial infarction, sudden death and crescendo angina. *British Heart Journal*, **53**: 363–373.

Davies M J, Woolf N and Robertson W B (1976) Pathology of acute myocardial infarction with particular reference to occlusive coronary thrombi. *British Heart Journal*, **38**: 659–664.

Dellipiani A W, Colling W A, Donaldson R J and McCormack P (1977) Teesside coronary survey: fatality and comparative severity of patients treated at home, in the hospital ward and the coronary care unit after myocardial infarction. *British Heart Journal*, **39**: 1172–1178.

Dewar H A, Stephenson P, Horler A R, Cassells-Smith A J and Ellis P A (1963) Fibrinolytic therapy of coronary thrombosis. *British Medical Journal*, **1**: 915–920.

DeWood M A, Spores J, Notske R, Mouser L T, Burroughs R, Golden M S and Lang H T (1980) Prevalence of total coronary occlusion during the early hours of transmural myocardial infarction. *New England Journal of Medicine*, **303**: 897–902.

Downie A C, Frost P G, Fielden P, Joshi D and Dancy C M (1993) Bedside measurement of creatine kinase to guide thrombolysis on the coronary care unit. *Lancet*, **341**: 452–454.

EMIP (European Myocardial Infarction Project Group) (1993) Pre-hospital thrombolytic therapy in patients with suspected acute myocardial infarction. *New England Journal of Medicine*, **329**: 383–389.

Fibrinolytic Therapy Trialists' Collaborative Group (1994) Indications for fibrinolytic therapy in suspected acute myocardial infarction: collaborative overview of early and major morbidity results from all randomised trials of more than 1000 patients. *Lancet*, **343**: 311–322.

Fitzpatrick B, Watt G and Tunstall-Pedoe H (1992) Potential impact of emergency intervention on sudden deaths from coronary heart disease in Glasgow. *British Heart Journal*, **67**: 250–254.

Fletcher A P, Alkjaersig N, Smyrniotis F E and Sherry S (1958) The treatment of patients suffering from early myocardial infarction with massive and prolonged streptokinase therapy. *Transcripts of the Association of American Physicians*, **71**: 287–295.

Fox K A A (1990) Thrombolysis and the general practitioner. *British Medical Journal*, **299**: 867–868.

Genton M D and Turpie A G G (1983) Anticoagulant therapy following acute myocardial infarction. *Modern Concepts in Cardiovascular Disease*, **52**: 49–51.

Gheorghiade M, Shivkumar K and Schultz L (1993) Prognostic significance of ECG persistent ST depression in patients with their first myocardial infarction in the placebo arm of the Beta-Blocker Heart Attack Trial. *American Heart Journal*, **126**: 271–278.

Gibbons R J, Holmes D R and Reeder G S (1993) Immediate angioplasty compared with the administration of a thrombolytic agent followed by conservative treatment for acute myocardial infarction. *New England Journal of Medicine*, **328**: 685–691.

GISSI Study Group (1987) Long-term effects of intravenous thrombolysis in acute myocardial infarction: final report of the GISSI study. *Lancet*, **ii**: 871–874.

GISSI-3 (Gruppo Italiano per lo Studio della Sopravvivenza nell'Infarto Miocardico) (1992) Study protocol on the effects of lisinopril, of nitrates and of their association in patients with acute myocardial infarction. *American Journal of Cardiology*, **70**: 62C–69C.

GISSI-3 (1994) Effect of lisinopril and transdermal glyceryl trinitrate singly and together on 6 week mortality and ventricular function after acute myocardial infarction. *Lancet*, **343**: 1115–1122.

Gold H K and Leinbach R C (1980) Coronary obstruction in anterior myocardial infarction: thrombus or spasm? *American Journal of Cardiology*, **45**: 483.

Goldberger A L (1979) *Myocardial Infarction: Electrocardiographic Differential Diagnosis*. St Louis: C V Mosby.

Goldman L and Cook E F (1984) The decline in ischaemic heart disease mortality rates. *Annals of Internal Medicine*, **101**: 825–836.

Gray W A, Capone R J and Most A S (1991) Unsuccessful medical resuscitation – are continuous efforts in the emergency department justified? *New England Journal of Medicine*, **325**: 1393–1398.

GREAT Study Group (1992) Feasibility, safety and efficacy of domiciliary thrombolysis by General Practitioners: the Grampian Regional Early Anistreplase Trial. *British Medical Journal*, **305**: 548–553.

Grines C L, Browne K F and Marco J (1993) A comparison of immediate angioplasty with thrombolytic therapy for acute myocardial infarction. *New England Journal of Medicine*, **328**: 673–679.

Gunnar R M, Loeb H S, Scanlon P J, Moran J F, Johnson S A and Pifarre R (1979) Management of acute myocardial infarction and accelerating angina. *Progress in Cardiovascular Diseases*, **22**: 1–30.

GUSTO Angiographic Investigators (1993) The effects of TPA, streptokinase or both on coronary artery patency, ventricular function and survival after acute myocardial infarction. *New England Journal of Medicine*, **329**: 1615–1622.

GUSTO (Global Utilisation of Streptokinase and Tissue plasminogen activator for Occluded coronary arteries) Investigators (1993) An international randomised trial comparing 4 strategies for acute myocardial infarction. *New England Journal of Medicine*, **329**: 673–682.

Heikkila J (1967) Mitral incompetence complicating acute myocardial infarction. *British Heart Journal*, **29**: 162–169.

Herlitz J and Hjalmarson A (1986) The role of beta-blockade in the limitation of infarct development. *European Heart Journal*, **7**: 916–924.

Herlitz J, Hjalmarson A and Waagstein F (1988) Treatment of pain in acute myocardial infarction. *British Heart Journal*, **61**: 9–13.

Hill J C, O'Rourke R A, Lewis R P and McGranahan G M (1969) The diagnosis value of the atrial gallup in acute myocardial infarction. *American Heart Journal*, **78:** 194–201.

Hill J D, Hampton J R and Mitchell J R A (1978) A randomised trial of home versus hospital management for acute myocardial infarction. *Lancet*, **i:** 837–841.

Hillis W S, Birnie D and Docherty A (1993) Troponin T and myocardial damage. *British Journal of Cardiology*, **1:** 16–21.

Husband D J, Alberti K G and Julian D G (1983) 'Stress' hyperglycaemia during acute myocardial infarction: an indicator of pre-existing diabetes? *Lancet*, **ii:** 179–181.

ISIS-2 Collaborative Group (1988) Randomised trial of intravenous streptokinase, oral aspirin, both or neither amongst 17,187 cases of suspected acute myocardial infarction. *Lancet*, **ii:** 349–360.

ISIS-3 (Third International Study of Infarct Survival) Collaborative Group (1992) A randomised comparison of streptokinase ·vs tissue plasminogen activator vs anistreplase and of aspirin plus heparin vs aspirin alone among 41,299 cases of suspected myocardial infarction. *Lancet*, **339:** 753–770.

ISIS-4 Collaborative Group (1995) A randomised trial assessing early oral captopril, oral mononitrate and intravenous magnesium sulphate in 58,050 patients with suspected acute myocardial infarction. *Lancet*, **345:** 669–685.

Jafri S M, Gheorghiade M and Goldstein S (1992) Oral anti-coagulation for secondary prevention after myocardial infarction with special reference to the Warfarin Re-infarction Study (WARIS). *Progress in Cardiovascular Disease*, **34:** 317–324.

Jagger J D, Murray R G, Davies M K, Littler W A and Flint E J (1987) Elegibility for thrombolytic therapy in acute myocardial infarction. *Lancet*, **i:** 34–35.

Jowett N I, Thompson D R and Bailey S W (1985) Electrocardiographic monitoring. I. Static monitoring. *Intensive Care Nursing*, **2:** 71–76.

Jowett N I, Stephens J M, Thompson D R and Sutton T W (1986) Do indwelling cannulae on coronary care need a heparin flush? *Intensive Care Nursing*, **2:** 16–19.

Jowett N I, Thompson D R and Pohl J E F (1989) Temporary transvenous cardiac pacing: 6 years experience in one coronary care unit. *Postgraduate Medical Journal*, **65:** 211–215.

Julian D G, Pentecost B L and Chamberlain D A (1988) A milestone for myocardial infarction. *British Medical Journal*, **297:** 497–498.

Klein H O, Tordjman T, Ninio R, Sareli P, Oren V, Lang R, Gesen J, Pauzner C, Di Segni E, David D and Kaplinski E (1983) The early recognition of right ventricular infarction: diagnostic accuracy of the V4R lead. *Circulation*, **67:** 558–565.

Kostuk W, Barr J W, Simon A L and Ross J (1973) Correlation between the chest film and hemodynamics in acute myocardial infarction. *Circulation*, **48:** 624–632.

Krone R J, Greenberg H and Dwyer E M (1993) Long-term prognostic significance of ST segment depression during acute myocardial infarction. *Journal of the American College of Cardiology*, **22:** 361–367.

Lancet (1985) Treatment of coronary thrombosis. *Lancet*, **i:** 375–376.

Lancet (1987) Thrombolytic therapy for acute myocardial infarction. *Lancet*, **ii:** 138–140.

Lawson-Matthew P J, Wilson A T, Woodmansey P A and Channer K S (1994) Unsatisfactory management of patients with acute myocardial infarction admitted to general medical wards. *Journal of the Royal College of Physicians of London*, **28:** 49–51.

Liu C K, Greenspan G and Piccirillo R T (1961) Atrial infarction of the heart. *Circulation*, **23:** 331.

Lown B, Verrier R L and Rabinowitz S H (1977) Neural and psychological mechanisms and the problem of sudden cardiac death. *American Journal of Cardiology*, **39:** 890–902.

Lynch M, Gammage M D, Lamb P, Nattrass M and Pentecost B L (1993) Acute myocardial infarction in diabetic patients in the thrombolytic era. *Diabetic Medicine;* **11:** 162–165.

McNichol M W and Kirby B J (1972) Oxygen therapy in myocardial infarction. In *Textbook of Coronary Care*, Melzer L E and Dunning A J (eds). Amsterdam: Excerpta Medica.

Mair J, Artnre-Dworzak E, Lechleitner P et al (1992) Early diagnosis of acute myocardial infarction by the newly developed rapid immuno-turbidimetric assay for myoglobin. *British Heart Journal*, **68:** 462–468.

Marder V J and Francis C W (1984) Thrombolytic therapy for acute transmural myocardial infarction: intracoronary versus intravenous. *American Journal of Medicine*, **77:** 921–927.

Maroko P R, Radvany P and Braunwald E (1975) Reduction in infarct size by oxygen inhalation following acute coronary occlusion. *Circulation*, **52:** 360–368.

Mather H G, Pearson N G and Read K L (1971) Acute myocardial infarction – home and hospital treatment. *British Medical Journal*, **3:** 334–338.

Miyata M, Abe S, Yamashita T et al (1993) Non-invasive detection of reperfusion using cardiac Troponin T one hour after the initiation of reperfusion therapy. *Circulation*, **88**(2): Abstract 0806.

Mulley A G, Thibault G E, Hughes R A, Barnett G O, Reder V A and Sherman E L (1980) The course of patients with suspected myocardial infarction. The identification of low risk patients for early transfer from intensive care. *New England Journal of Medicine*, **302:** 943–948.

Murray N, Lyons J, Layton C and Balcon R (1987) What proportion of patients with myocardial infarction are suitable for thrombolysis? *British Heart Journal*, **57:** 144–147.

Norris R M (1982) *Myocardial Infarction*. Edinburgh: Churchill Livingstone.

Ohman E M, Califf R M, Topol E J, Candela R, Abbottsmith C and Ellis S (1990) Consequences of re-occlusion after successful reperfusion therapy in acute myocardial infarction. *Circulation*, **82:** 781–791.

Oswald G A, Corcoran S and Yudkin J S (1984) Prevalence and risks of hyperglycaemia and undiagnosed diabetes in patients with acute myocardial infarction. *Lancet*, **i:** 1265–1267.

Packer M (1992) Pathophysiology of chronic heart failure and treatment of heart failure. *Lancet*, **340:** 88–95.

Pantridge J F and Adgey A A J (1969) Pre-hospital coronary care: the mobile coronary care unit. *American Journal of Cardiology*, **24:** 666–673.

Pell A C H, Miller H C, Robertson C E and Fox K A A (1992) Effect of "fast-track" admission for acute myocardial infarction on delay to thrombolysis. *British Medical Journal*, **304:** 83–87.

Petch M C (1991) Coronary thrombolytic therapy at home. *British Medical Journal*, **302:** 1287–1288.

Pfeffer M A, Braunwald E, Moyle L A, Basta L et al (1992) Effect of captopril on mortality and morbidity in patients with left ventricular dysfunction after myocardial infarction: results of the survival and ventricular enlargement trial (SAVE). *New England Journal of Medicine*, **327:** 669–677.

Radvany P, Maroko P R and Braunwald E (1975) Effects of hypoxaemia on the extent of myocardial necrosis after experimental coronary occlusion. *American Journal of Cardiology*, **35:** 795–800.

Res J C, Simoons M L, Van der Waal E E, Van Eenige J, Vermeer F, Verheugt F W, Wijns W, Braat S, Remme W J and Serruys P W (1986) Long-term improvement in global left ventricular function after early thrombolytic treatment in acute myocardial infarction. *British Heart Journal*, **56:** 414–421.

Ribeiro E E, Silva L A and Carneiro R (1993) Randomised trial of direct coronary angioplasty versus intravenous streptokinase in acute myocardial infarction. *Journal of the American College of Cardiology*, **22:** 376–380.

Roberts R (1984) The two out of three criteria for the diagnosis of infarction: is it passé? *Chest*, **86:** 511–513.

Rodrigues E A, Dewhurst N G, Smart L M, Hannan W J and Muir A L (1986) Diagnosis and prognosis of right ventricular infarction. *British Heart Journal*, **56:** 19–26.

Rogers W J, Hood W P, Mantle J A, Baxley W A, Kirklin J K, Zorn G L and Nath H P (1984) Return of left ventricular function after reperfusion in patients with myocardial infarction: importance of sub-total stenosis and intact collaterals. *Circulation*, **69:** 338–349.

Rowley J M, Mounser P, Skene A M and Hampton J R (1992) Management of myocardial infarction: implications for current policy derived from the Nottingham Heart Attack Register. *British Heart Journal*, **67:** 255–262.

Rude R E, Muller J E and Braunwald E (1981) Efforts to limit the size of myocardial infarcts. *Annals of Internal Medicine*, **95:** 736–761.

Ryder R E J, Hayes T M, Mulligan I P, Kingswood J and Williams S (1984) How soon after myocardial infarction should plasma lipids be assessed? *British Medical Journal*, **289:** 1651–1653.

SCATI Study Group (1989) Randomised controlled trial of subcutaneous calcium heparin in acute myocardial infarction. *Lancet*, **ii:** 182–186.

Scott M E and Orr R (1969) Effects of diamorphine, methadone, morphine and pentazocine in patients with suspected acute myocardial infarction. *Lancet*, **i:** 1065–1067.

Serruys P W, Wijns W, Van Den Brand M, Ribeiro V, Fiorretti P, Simoon M, Kooijman C J, Reiber J H and Hugenholtz P G (1983) Is transluminal coronary angioplasty mandatory after successful thrombolysis? Quantitative coronary angiographic study. *British Heart Journal*, **50:** 257–265.

Stehbens W E (1985) Relationship of coronary artery thrombosis to myocardial infarction. *Lancet*, **ii:** 639–642.

St John Sutton M (1994) Should ACE inhibitors be used routinely after infarction? Perspectives from the SAVE trial. *British Heart Journal*, **71:** 115–118.

TEAHAT Study Group (1990) Very early thrombolysis in suspected myocardial infarction. *American Journal of Cardiology*, **65:** 401–407.

Thompson D R, Jowett N I, Folwell A M and Sutton T W (1989) A trial of providone–iodine antiseptic solution for the prevention of cannula-related thrombophlebitis. *Journal of Intravenous Nursing*, **12:** 99–102.

Thompson R C, Hallstrom A P and Cobb L A (1979) Bystander-initiated CPR in the management of ventricular fibrillation. *Annals of Internal Medicine*, **90:** 737–740.

THRIFT (Thrombo-embolic Risk Factors) Consensus Group (1992) Risk of and prophylaxis for venous thrombo-embolism in hospital patients. *British Medical Journal*, **305:** 567–574.

TIMI Study Group (1989) Comparison of invasive and conservative strategies after treatment with intra-venous TPA in acute myocardial infarction. *New England Journal of Medicine*, **320:** 618–627.

Timmis A D (1990) Early diagnosis of acute myocardial infarction. *British Medical Journal*, **301:** 941–942.

Timmis G C, Gangadharan V, Hauser A M, Rames R G, Westveer D C and Gordon S (1982) Intracoronary streptokinase in clinical practice. *American Heart Journal*, **104:** 925–938.

Topol E J, Burek K and O'Neil (1988) A randomised controlled trial of hospital discharge 3 days after myocardial infarction in the era of reperfusion. *New England Journal of Medicine*, **318:** 1083–1088.

Topol E J, George B S, Kereiakes D J and the TAMI group (1989) A randomised controlled trial of intravenous TPA and early intravenous heparin in acute myocardial infarction. *Circulation*, **79:** 281–286.

Valentine R P, Pitts D E, Brooks-Brunn L, Woods J, Nyhuis A, Van Hove E and Schmidt P E (1986) Effect of thrombolysis on left ventricular function during acute myocardial infarction. *American Journal of Cardiology*, **58:** 896–899.

Van der Laarse A, Vermeer F, Hermens W T, Willems G M, de Neef K, Simoons M L, Serruys P W, Res J, Verheugt F W and Krauss X H (1986) Effects of early intra-coronary streptokinase in infarct size estimated from cumulative enzyme release and on enzyme release state: a randomised trial of 533 patients with acute myocardial infarction. *American Heart Journal*, **112,** 672–681.

Waine C, Hannaford P and Kay C (1993) Early thrombolysis therapy: some issues facing general practitioners. *British Heart Journal*, **70:** 218.

Wallbridge D R, Tweddel A C, Martin W and Cobbe S M (1992) The potential impact of patient self referral on mortality in acute myocardial infarction. *Quarterly Journal of Medicine*, **85:** 901–909.

Wartman W B and Hellerstein H K (1948) The incidence of heart disease in 2000 consecutive autopsies. *Annals of Internal Medicine*, **28:** 41.

Weston C and Fox K A A (1991) Pre-hospital thrombolysis: current status and future prospects. *Journal of the Royal College of Physicians of London*, **25:** 312–320.

White H (1991) Thrombolytic treatment for recurrent myocardial infarction. *British Medical Journal*, **392:** 428–429.

Wilcox R G, Olsson C G, Skene A M, von der Lippe G and Hampton J R (1988) Trial of TPA for mortality reduction in acute myocardial infarction (ASSET). *Lancet*, **ii:** 525–530.

Woods K L, Fletcher S, Roffe C and Haider Y (1992) Intravenous magnesium sulphate in suspected acute myocardial infarction: results of the second Leicester intravenous magnesium trial (LIMIT-2). *Lancet*, **339:** 1553–1558.

Yusuf S, Peto R, Lewis J, Collins R and Sleight P (1985) Beta-blockade during and after myocardial infarction: an overview of randomised trials. *Progress in Cardiovascular Diseases*, **27:** 335–371.

Zijlstra F, De Boer M J and Hoorntje J C A (1993) A comparison of immediate coronary angioplasty with intravenous streptokinase in acute myocardial infarction. *New England Journal of Medicine*, **328:** 680–684.

7

Nursing Management of Acute Myocardial Infarction

Nursing management of acute myocardial infarction is designed to help the patient overcome various physical and psychological insults. Therapeutic goals are broadly designed to promote healing of the damaged myocardium, prevent complications (such as dysrhythmias, heart failure and shock) and facilitate the patient's rapid return to normal health and life-style (Webster and Thompson, 1992).

Meeting the basic needs of the patient, such as comfort, rest, sleep and elimination, forms an essential component of nursing intervention. Some of these needs will require immediate attention, whereas others will be dealt with in later days. The nurse should be aware of what will be required and should be able to anticipate problems, rather than waiting for them to occur.

Patients in hospital, especially those on high-dependency units, are bound to be under a great deal of stress and anxiety, both during their hospital stay and (usually) after discharge. There will be uncertainty about their surroundings, fear of what has happened to them and worry about lack of control over what may occur in the following days. The situation may be exacerbated by lack of information, pain, discomfort or inability to obtain adequate rest.

The acute illness brings changes for the patient and family in terms of usual patterns of living, which, although hopefully only short term, may persist after discharge from hospital. Acute myocardial infarction, in particular, poses major threats to the patient, usually because of the suddenness of the illness (often with no warning) and because of the connotations that heart disease carries. Fear of sudden death is the immediate worry, usually followed by a realisation that the patient may become disabled for the rest of his days. Apart from these changes in self-image, there are also feelings of loss in terms of status within the family unit, working environment and social circle. The secure knowledge of a regular financial income, the ability to care for the family and continuing full physical fitness are no longer present.

The responses that individual patients make to these threats include emotional crisis, defence mechanisms and coping behaviours. The patient's personal beliefs, attitudes, responsibilities, values and experiences will all influence how he or she perceives and responds to the infarct. In the unfamiliar and frightening environment of the coronary care unit, the nurse needs to establish a close rapport with the patient and family in order to be effective in reducing anxiety and fear, promoting the resolution of losses, encouraging adjustment to change and planning together for complete recovery and successful rehabilitation. This will include detailed explanations about the significance of the illness, the nature of coronary heart disease and the goals of treatment, including the part that the coronary care unit plays. The personnel involved in the provision of care will need introducing, and the roles of these people and the surrounding equipment should be fully explained. The encouragement of independence and the fostering of a realistic, but optimistic, outlook are of great importance. Such interventions should involve the nurse in providing care in an individualised and flexible fashion, rather than the traditional rigid task-orientated system. The coronary care unit is an ideal setting for the nurse, patient and family to meet and discuss progress and future management. Care plans should be based upon an assessment completed within the initial hours of admission, so that priorities of care can then be established early and modified as the patient improves.

It can thus be seen that nursing intervention involves many challenges in the management of acute myocardial infarction, and a considerate and sensitive approach to the patient and his family is required to permit full evaluation of present and potential problems and to establish an overall plan of care, which hopefully, will overcome them.

THE CORONARY CARE PLAN

Planning a care plan for patients on the coronary care unit needs to take into account the following (McGurn, 1981):

1. *Reduction of stress.* The reduction of noxious physical (e.g. temperature and pain) and sensory (e.g. noise, lighting and intrusion) stimuli is desirable. Specific sources should be identified in the assessment plan.

2. *Preservation of routines.* Care should be planned so that patients' routines are preserved as far as possible. In coronary care units, patients' eating, toileting and resting habits are often dramatically changed, sometimes resulting in disorientation and physical complications.

3. *Prevention of non-compliance.* Complex dietary and drug regimens will result in non-compliance, as will failure to explain the reasons for interventions. The nurse needs to ensure that the patient listens to, understands and retains information.

4. *Control of pain.* The nurse must ensure that the patient is free from pain. In coronary care, this often means the liberal use of analgesics and anxiolytic agents, such as diamorphine, diazepam and nitrates.

5. *Provision of adequate rest.* Needless disturbance of patients should be avoided, with provision of rest periods. Patients on high-dependency units are often seriously and needlessly deprived of sleep.

6. *Education of the patient.* The nurse should ensure that the patient understands what is happening and encourage him to take responsibility for his own health.

There are many types of format for recording data, defining problems and outlining goals and intervention strategies. Although different units or wards may have their own care plans, it is desirable to have some degree of standardisation to facilitate the transfer of patients between wards, units and hospitals, if required. The care plan is the major tool for communicating instructions and providing a permanent and legal record. Entries should be written concisely, legibly and systematically, avoiding jargon and abbreviations to minimise ambiguity about care. The care plan should be kept up to date and made flexible to meet patients' changing needs.

COMMUNICATION

For nursing intervention to be effective, communication between the nurse, the patient, the family and other personnel involved in care has to be effective. Communication can take many forms – structured or informal, verbal or non-verbal – and tends to be a continuous process in situations in which individuals are working within the same environment. Thus, much of nursing management will be directly or indirectly concerned with communication at some level. Contact at the bedside whilst performing physical and technical tasks forms an important part of such communication between nurses and patients, and the nurse is in a unique position in being at the bedside for most of the time. She will, therefore, be regarded as a prime source of communication (Cassem et al, 1970).

There is some evidence that the quality of communication that patients on coronary care receive can influence the speed of recovery and feeling of well-being (Garrity and Klein, 1975), and it is a shame that communication skills have not always been seen as a legitimate part of nursing work.

There are various reasons why nurse–patient communication is often inadequate in coronary care. These include the short duration of the patient's stay on the unit, the severity of his condition and, often, the nurse's preoccupation with handling technical rather than personal requirements. In her review of staff–patient communication in coronary care, Ashworth (1984) sees the aims of communication as being:

1. For the patient to perceive the nurse as:

   ● friendly
   ● helpful
   ● competent
   ● reliable

2. For the nurse to recognise patients':

   ● individuality
   ● perceived needs
   ● other needs

Coronary care patients are often brought suddenly into the unfamiliar environment of hospital. They change from a position of being in control of their lives to one of having to accept the submissive role of a patient. Effective communication can really only be achieved if the patient is allowed to retain his individuality. The nurse should work with the patient to affect positive adaptation and coping mechanisms, by education and counselling. Liaison with the patient and family is required to ensure that they are aware of the objective of the cardiac unit and understand the various procedures and treatments. A realistic outlook for the future, based on knowledge and understanding, may then be achieved. It is important for communication to be clear and comprehensible, using language familiar to the patient (at whatever level) and avoiding the use of jargon. Simple explanations need to be reiterated, since retention of verbal information in medical matters is seldom for long. An atmosphere of optimism should be encouraged by reassuring patients that survival and recovery are fully anticipated.

Cardiac nurses themselves need to be able to demonstrate credibility in their role as communicators. Communication is a two-way process, and there is a need to interact with the patient, adapting the approach to meet changing needs. 'Primary nursing' is the ideal method of maximising nurse–patient contact and increases the likelihood of getting to know the patient as an individual rather than a bed number. The nurse should be able to listen to the patient in a calm, unhurried, sympathetic manner and be genuinely interested in what the patient is saying.

Reassurance is a term frequently used in nursing, often without clarification or evaluation. Broad promises such as, 'Don't worry, everything will be OK' serve little purpose if the patient lacks a basic understanding of his condition, and may only lessen the nurse's credibility. The majority of patients can be placed at ease during their stay on coronary care providing the right approach is used, even if many are clinically anxious or depressed.

Some patients may not possess the necessary skills to be able to communicate successfully. They may be too ill or anxious to present themselves as they would wish, they may be physically or mentally handicapped or they may lack the knowledge and understanding to be able to make realistic decisions regarding their future. This may equally apply to the relatives, who can find the hospital environment imposing. Nurses have an important role to play as advocates of the patient and relatives, basing advice on experience, knowledge of the illness and the individual patient. As well as structured planned communication to convey specific points, there is also day-to-day conversation, interaction and non-verbal communication. Human contact is possibly more important in a technical environment, such as coronary care, than on the general medical ward. Patients are likely to appreciate knowing that a nurse is near at hand, especially if they are bedridden, when communication is perhaps the only way in which some patients can influence their environment and routine.

In the highly technical and invasive atmosphere of coronary care, there is sometimes a need to stand back and think carefully about what is the best treatment or strategy for the patient. Allowing a critically ill patient to die with peace and dignity is not a failure and may be a better course of action then prolonging life with multiple therapies, which mislead the relatives into thinking there is hope. Discussing such subjects openly in a constructive fashion with medical colleagues, in a detached and unemotional manner, involves a sensitive and professional approach, which is necessary but seldom easy.

Three main approaches have been suggested (Ashworth, 1984) that might improve nurse–patient communication on coronary care:

1. Planned education to develop communication knowledge and skills

2. Selective scientific reading, and the use of relevant research-based nursing practice information

3. Further research into staff–patient communication

Smooth and effective communication between nurses and other personnel is likely to result in better nurse–patient communication. There is, perhaps, a need to change the emphasis of priorities on intensive care units away from the technical aspects and towards the physical and emotional requirements of patients in our care.

ASSESSMENT OF PAIN

Pain is a complex and personal experience, and it is usually the nursing staff in hospital who are near at hand when the patient experiences pain. It is they who are frequently responsible for its evaluation and for providing relief. In the context of coronary care units, this should be on the nurses' own initiative, and it is, therefore, important that they have formed a proper assessment of the pain the patient is suffering. Inappropriate analgesia is dangerous: it may mask alternative diagnoses or produce cardiac and respiratory depression.

It is clear that the word 'pain' may apply to a variety of qualities, although it is still frequently considered in regard to a single attribute: the intensity of the experience. This, of course, ignores the qualitative dimensions of the pain experienced (Table 7.1), but it is nevertheless a useful indication. Moreover, it lends itself to numerical or graphic measurement for research purposes, by using a visual analogue scale (VAS) or a 'pain ruler' (Scott and Huskisson, 1976; Bourbonnais, 1981). Such methods are especially useful for the assessment of acute pain, such as that

Table 7.1 Words used to describe the quality of pain (Melzack, 1975)

Words describing the sensory qualities of the pain experienced in terms of:
- time (e.g. constant)
- space (e.g. radiating)
- pressure (e.g. compressing)
- temperature (e.g. hot)

Words describing the affective qualities of pain in terms of:
- tension (e.g. tiring)
- fear (e.g. terrifying)
- autonomic properties (e.g. nausea)

Words describing the subjective overall intensity, for example:
- excruciating

commonly accompanying acute myocardial infarction. They are sensitive and reliable indicators for pain evaluation, as well as being easy to use by both the person experiencing the pain and the observer (Huskisson, 1974; Revill et al, 1976).

The relief of pain is a major part of patient care and is essential for patient comfort and well-being. A careful and detailed assessment of the pain a patient is experiencing is essential if effective relief is to be provided in the minimum of time and will be more effective if the nurse establishes a rapport with the patient. The assessment should include the patient's own description of the pain and an observation of his reaction to it. It is not always possible to make this evaluation on admission to coronary care if the patient is critically ill, but later on it will be important to determine whether the pain the patient is still suffering is ischaemic or pericarditic pain or is just due to anxiety. Each of these will have different specific antidotes (such as aspirin or indomethacin for pericarditis, diazepam for anxiety), although the disinterested may simply choose to obliterate all possibilities with a large dose of diamorphine. The nurse and doctor must appreciate that the patient is the authority on his own pain. Above all, the patient must be believed; all pain is real, and calling pain imaginary does not make it go away.

In addition to the traditional provision of analgesia with drug therapy, there is a wide range of pain-relieving strategies that can be instituted by the nurse:

- Ensuring peace and comfort
- Careful positioning of the patient
- Reassurance
- Protection from stressful situations
- Limitation of unnecessary activity
- Promotion of sleep

If the patient fully understands the pain and its cause, it may then become less distressing. Coping strategies such as therapeutic touch, relaxation techniques and distraction are useful if they are performed by a skilled nurse. There are other useful methods for the relief of acute pain, which may be used alone or in conjunction with drugs. These include guided imagery, hypnosis and transcutaneous electric nerve stimulation (TENS) and have been discussed elsewhere (Peric-Knowlton, 1984; Wells, 1984).

The nurse needs to be aware of the limitations, as well as the benefits, of the non-pharmacological interventions available. Whereas a small study by Bourbonnais and MacKay (1981) showed that over half the nursing interventions used for the relief of chest pain were ineffective, an approach based upon a holistic approach to the patient resulted in a high degree of pain relief prior to the administration of medication and greater pain relief than medication alone (Diers et al, 1972).

COMFORT

The promotion of relaxation and comfort is an essential and fundamental component of nursing. Unfortunately, such skills tend to be overlooked on coronary care units. Careful positioning of the patient, reassurance and the presence of a caring nurse assume a high priority to ensure complete comfort (Wilson-Barnett, 1984). Careful bed-making, regulation of light, temperature and noise, and the provision of hot milky drinks in the evening may seem mundane and obvious but are often delegated to the most junior nurse as a low priority in the 'high-tech' environment of coronary care. The inability to get comfortable is a major reason for poor sleep (Jones et al, 1979). This is often due to poor hospital beds, their hard mattresses covered in plastic causing the patient to feel uncomfortable, hot and sweaty. It may be more beneficial for the patient if he sits in a supportive chain instead of lying in bed. However, it is no use providing such fundamental measures if the patient is in pain. Pain relief should assume the highest priority.

Patient discomfort may be compounded by invasive techniques, such as intravenous cannulation, and the frequent disturbances that occur when routine observations are made or recorded. Invasive monitoring devices and intravenous lines often result in the general enforced immobilisation of the patient, which carries with it the attendant risk of pressure sores. Thus, frequent changing of the patient's position in bed and the use of pressure-relieving devices are important in reducing discomfort. Consideration should be given to the siting of intravenous cannulae and the use of nasal cannulae rather than oxygen masks.

Rest has to be both physical and mental and can be achieved by a variety of factors including:

● Adequate pain relief
● Promotion of relaxation, comfort and sleep
● Ensuring that noise is kept at a low level
● Control of temperature, light and humidity
● Planned rest periods during the day

A warm, stimulating environment should be encouraged, where patients feel they can relax and chat with fellow patients, staff and relatives.

BED-REST AND ACTIVITY

Bed-rest is usual, but recent trends are towards early mobilisation, with slower schedules being reserved for those with complications. Hospitalisation and enforced bed-rest can produce their own problems, such as constipation, bone resorption, thromboembolism, pulmonary atelectasis, pressure sores and urinary retention. It is, therefore, important that patients mobilise as soon as possible, particularly the elderly who fare worse from complications due to enforced rest than they would otherwise do as a result of myocardial infarction alone. Active and passive leg movements should be encouraged, and early chest physiotherapy is advisable, especially in smokers. Rotation of the shoulders is also advisable to prevent 'frozen' shoulders and the shoulder–hand syndrome.

Although the coronary care unit should theoretically be the ideal environment for resting, in practice it rarely is because of the non-stop activity in and around the patients. Amongst its many other benefits, the purpose of rest following myocardial infarction is to decrease the myocardial demand for oxygen and limit myocardial work. Inactivity is a major problem, in that it serves as a source of frustration and boredom. It is, therefore, important to stress to the patient the need for temporary limitation but to reassure him that bed-rest is only temporary and is in his own best interest. Enforced bed-rest will only have adverse effects on someone who is normally active, by making him perceive himself as more seriously ill. Relaxation, deep breathing and active and passive leg exercises are useful in reducing boredom and mood changes, as well as the risk of physical complications of bed-rest. Such activities will boost patients' morale by making them feel that they are playing an active part in the recovery process.

It is preferable that the patient sits upright in bed rather than lying flat, because the latter requires more myocardial work to pump blood through the excess pool of tissue fluid in the lungs. Thus, patients with uncomplicated infarcts should sit out as early as possible. Some patients may feel reluctant or hesitant to resume activity, whereas others are over-zealous.

There is no reason why most patients cannot wash, eat and shave themselves. In fact, it is likely that there is danger of more stress resulting from not being allowed to do such activities than the actual performance of them. Patients may require some assistance from the nurse if they are severely restricted by equipment, such as short monitor cables, intravenous infusions, pacemaker units, etc., or if they are feeling weak or are generally too ill. The nurse should, in any case, offer to assist, as some patients may feel unable to ask. If the patient is bed-bound, the nurse needs to ensure that he has everything needed within easy reach.

EARLY AMBULATION

Only 30 years ago, patients with acute myocardial infarction were kept on strict bed-rest for 2 months, all activities being performed by attending nursing staff. Hospitalisation often lasted for 3–4 months, with limited mobilisation over the following year. The concern was that early mobilisation would lead to dysrhythmia, heart failure, rupture of the heart or formation of a left ventricular aneurysm. The period of strict rest was based upon pathological studies, which indicated that 6 weeks were required for a firm scar to form from the necrotic myocardium. However, it soon became apparent that this form of therapy led to an increased incidence of thromboembolic disorders, chest infections and musculoskeletal disorders. Alteration in vasomotor reflexes and hypovolaemia also occur with prolonged bed-rest, leading to tachycardia, hypotension and unsteadiness on standing. The highly controversial approach to early mobilisation in the early 1960s (Cain et al, 1961) was regarded as reckless and dangerous: uncomplicated infarct patients were allowed out of bed after only 15 days.

The emphasis today is on early mobilisation and discharge, especially for those who have an uncomplicated hospital course. This type of approach minimises physical and psychological disability, and reduces the risk of thromboembolism.

There is no doubt that peri-infarction mortality is higher in patients who have had complications (Norris et al, 1974), such as:

- Prolonged or recurrent chest pain
- Left ventricular failure
- Cardiogenic shock
- Significant dysrhythmia (e.g. ventricular tachycardia or fibrillation)
- Heart block
- Severe pericarditis
- Extensive infarcts
- Complicating disease (e.g. diabetes)

Early mobilisation should certainly be delayed in these patients, even when the underlying complication has been corrected. However, most of these potential high-risk cases may be identified in the first 24 hours following admission, and provisional selection for early discharge may be made within 48 hours.

Nursing should reflect the current pattern of care for coronary patients, which has been characterised by an increase in physical activity soon after infarction and has led to a decrease in imposed invalidism and an earlier discharge from hospital. Patients with an uncomplicated infarct are kept in bed for a maximum of 24–48 hours only. Indeed, in some units, patients are encouraged to sit out on the day of admission, providing they are free of pain and significant dysrhythmia. Gradual but early mobilisation should, certainly, encourage patients to walk around the ward by the end of a few days, and it is important that an individualised approach takes preference over a strict regimen.

When the patient resumes activity, it is helpful if the nurse knows the normal activity levels and habits of the patient. This should have been ascertained during the nursing assessment. A plan can then be developed by the nurse and patient to provide a framework as to what level of activity he can realistically be expected to achieve by a specific time. This will need to be a tentative plan, and it is important to stress that only guidelines and not strict regimens can be formulated, because each patient will be different in his abilities. An ideal method for quantifying the energy spent undertaking various activities is the metabolic equivalent (MET) system. One MET is equal to the resting oxygen uptake of approximately 3.5 ml/kg per minute. The average male can attain a level of 12 METs, and an uncomplicated post-infarct patient can probably achieve no more than 9 METs.

The stress that various activities have on the body can be assessed by observing heart rate and rhythm, respiratory rate and blood pressure. However, these should be monitored in an informal manner to avoid unduly worrying the patient. The development of symptoms such as chest pain, shortness of breath, palpitations or faintness are indications to cease activity. The patient should be made aware of this and encouraged to inform the nurse if such symptoms occur.

In uncomplicated cases, patients should be encouraged to climb one or two flights of stairs before they are discharged home. They will need to be advised about what they will be able to do at home, including information on eating, drinking and driving. A realistic appraisal of the prospect of a full recovery and early return to work is essential.

SLEEP

The function of sleep is unknown. It is thought to be a period of bodily and brain restitution (Adam and Oswald, 1984), although Meddis (1977) challenges the idea that sleep is necessary at all, believing that sleep is an instinct that merely serves as a means of segregating periods of inactivity and activity.

Sleep may be roughly divided into two broad stages:

- *Non-REM* (rapid eye movement) or orthodox sleep
- *REM* or paradoxical sleep

Non-REM sleep is characterised by lowering of the blood pressure, heart and respiratory rates, whilst REM sleep is characterised by the opposite and is strongly correlated with dreaming.

Many people experience onset or worsening of an illness during the night. Cardiovascular events often occur with a high frequency during sleep, especially REM sleep. Patients with nocturnal angina are more likely to suffer their attacks during periods of REM sleep (King et al, 1973), and there is also an increase in the frequency of premature ventricular contractions (Rosenblatt et al, 1973). The onset of symptoms of acute myocardial infarction is more frequent in bed, especially just after falling asleep and on waking (Thompson et al, 1991).

It is clear that coronary patients experience marked sleep disturbances in hospital, particularly in specialised units (Broughton and Baron, 1978). Additionally, much of this sleep is desynchronised and, therefore, less effective. The reasons for this poor sleep are many. Sleep may be affected by several factors, including age, noise, temperature, comfort, pain and anxiety (Webster and Thompson, 1986). Noise, mainly due to electromechanical equipment, staff movement and conversation, is a major problem in specialised units (Hilton, 1976). Bentley et al (1977) found that noise levels in three hospital areas, including an intensive care unit, were about 25–40 dB higher than internationally-recommended limits (30 dB at night, 40 dB during the evening and 45 dB during the daytime).

Patients will be able to sleep better if they are comfortable, free from pain and in a quiet and peaceful environment. The promotion of comfort and relaxation are important, as discussed in the previous section, with control of environmental factors (e.g. reduced noise, regulated room temperature and dimmed lights) needed. Pain relief is, of course, essential. Unnecessary nursing or medical observations or interventions disrupt the continuity and efficiency of patients' sleep, and essential procedures should be organised in a fashion that ensures that patients are only minimally disturbed. With current advanced technology, multichannel monitoring facilities make many routine observations easy to perform without waking the patient.

Nursing assessment should incorporate information about the patient's usual sleeping habits and patterns, such as quality and quantity of normal sleep, and the identification of any routines that the patient feels will enhance his ability to sleep. Hot milky drinks such as Ovaltine and Horlicks often form part of the nighttime ritual and have been shown significantly to improve sleep (Brezinova and Oswald,

1972). The use of a sleep questionnaire (such as the St Mary's Hospital Sleep Questionnaire, Ellis et al, 1981) is a useful adjunct in the assessment of sleeping habits.

DIET

Although diet is not usually considered in the early stages following myocardial infarction, there are many reasons why adjustments may need to be made. In the early hours following admission, nausea and vomiting are common, and there is a higher risk of cardiorespiratory arrest, which may lead to bronchial aspiration of gastric contents. A liquid diet is, therefore, probably best given initially until a normal diet can be instituted. Caffeine should be avoided because of its possible dysrhythmic effect, and salt should be avoided because of its deleterious effect on cardiac failure. In order to assist the healing process, adequate and appropriate nutrition is essential. The nurse should possess some of the knowledge and skills necessary to assess and advise on the nutritional requirements of the patient. Nurses, by the very nature of their close involvement with the patient and family, are ideally placed, yet all too often they seem to ignore their responsibility in this area, prematurely enlisting the help of a usually overworked dietitian. A careful assessment of the patient's usual eating habits and life-style is essential. Many patients will have preconceived ideas obtained from their relatives and the media about good dietary habits. Nurses play a major role in nutrition education and often have to perform the notoriously difficult task of persuading the patient to consider a change in dietary habits. The major difficulty is not in giving the advice to patients and their relatives, but in achieving the appropriate behavioural responses that should be in their own interests.

Many misconceptions regarding diet litter the popular press and even the fringe scientific literature. The problem is compounded by conflicting and unsubstantiated information and advice given by friends, relatives or health professionals, particularly with regard to coronary heart disease.

Other considerations in relation to diet include the following:

1. Patients on coronary care units feel nauseated or not hungry. Nourishing drinks and small snacks at times other than established meal times may be more appreciated.

2. Ethnic minorities will require special consideration, and relatives need to be consulted, as they can offer valuable advice and assistance by bringing in meals.

3. Although some patients may require parenteral or nasogastric feeding, these methods should not be undertaken lightly. Not only are they likely to be stressful to the patient, but they may also be associated with metabolic disturbance and infection.

4. Fluid restriction may be warranted if the patient is in heart failure. Such patients will require thoughtful mouth care, including mouth washes and sips of cold or iced water. Confiscating the water jug is not sufficient; the patient should be informed of what is being done and why. A notice concerning fluid restriction is needed above the bed to remind others that fluids are being monitored, and the patient will be able to prevent the tea-lady filling him up with fluid if he is aware of what the fluid restriction is trying to achieve.

Nurses should be aware that they are serving as role models in providing credibility to any health education. It is difficult to convince patients of such change if the nurse herself is overweight or smokes.

ELIMINATION

Prolonged bed-rest or general physical inactivity should be avoided, as this inhibits gastrointestinal motility and leads to constipation. The faeces may, additionally, become hardened because of increased water resorption or use of diuretics. The constipated patient will strain at stool, with excessive isometric work, which leads to vagal stimulation. This is likely to produce bradycardia or heart block and may severely compromise venous return, with dramatic falls in cardiac output. A 'bedpan' vasovagal collapse may result, but staff should be aware that patients with acute pulmonary emboli often call for a bedpan as a terminal event. Similar vasovagal effects may result with the use of a bedpan, upon which most patients seem to strain, whether constipated or not. They are most uncomfortable and stressful contraptions, which probably need banning. Using a bedside commode is easier and more comfortable and places the patient in a more familiar position for defaecation (Winslow et al, 1984). In fact, there appears to be little scientific evidence to support the use of a bedpan in preference to the commode. Laxatives may be warranted to prevent excessive straining at stool and may be helped by careful attention to the fluid and fibre content of the diet. The patient needs to be reassured that many patients have altered bowel habit following admission to hospital. This may simply be due to different dietary habits or enforced bed-rest, but certain drugs can alter normal elimination habits. For instance, opiates cause constipation and broad-spectrum antibiotics may cause diarrhoea. Additionally, many patients feel extremely embarrassed about using a commode or urinal in the vicinity of others. This in itself may give rise to constipation or retention. They are more likely to feel at ease in a private room or cubicle than in the middle of an open-plan area, even if they do have the benefit of partially-closed curtains through which different faces keep appearing. Perhaps more patients should be permitted to use a toilet at an earlier stage.

Careful recording of fluid balance is essential for patients on diuretic therapy. Daily weighing of the patient may be more accurate than a fluid balance chart for assessment in congestive cardiac failure. The patient should be warned of the resulting increase in quantity and frequency of urine. Consideration regarding the timing of diuretic administration should be given so that the patient is minimally disturbed during the night. Bumetanide (Burinex) is probably a shorter-acting loop diuretic than frusemide (Lasix) and will limit the duration of diuresis.

HYGIENE

Bathing and hygiene

Many patients admitted to coronary care have been unprepared for admission because of the sudden onset of symptoms and may feel acutely embarrassed and uncomfortable, particularly if they are sweating, have vomited or are partly naked. Patients are likely to be feeling too unwell in the immediate stages to look after themselves, and although the nurse will need to assist acutely, she should avoid encouraging the patient to become dependent on her help. The psychological aspects of bathing and hygiene are important. For example, patients feel better after a shower or bath and appreciate simple things such as being offered hand-washing facilities after using the commode, without having to ask.

Oral hygiene

Mouth toilet should be offered to all patients, especially those who wear dentures, are on fluid restriction or have been vomiting. Patients with dentures are often very embarrassed about cleaning them in the presence of others and should be afforded the necessary privacy and facilities.

Use of the bath and shower

It appears that coronary patients move more slowly and deliberately than normal when bathing in order to conserve energy (Winslow et al, 1985). Patients may prefer to shower if this has been their normal domestic routine, particularly during the later stages of their stay in hospital. However, oxygen consumption of coronary patients is higher in patients who shower than in those who use a bath (Johnston et al, 1981), and this should be taken into consideration. The isometric activity required by some patients to get out of a bath may result in a steep rise in arterial blood pressure, which increases myocardial work. Hence, before a patient is first bathed, the nurse needs to evaluate any potential difficulties. If the patient is weak, obese or generally likely to have difficulties, bathing is probably contra-indicated.

EMOTIONAL DISTURBANCES

Emotional disturbances after infarction may adversely influence subsequent mortality, speed of rehabilitation and ability to return to work. The manner in which a patient adapts emotionally to having sustained a myocardial infarction will be determined to a large extent by his premorbid personality (Totman, 1979; Byrne and Whyte, 1980). Emotional disturbances are extremely common in patients admitted to coronary care. Anxiety is, not surprisingly, very common, especially in women, and many patients are depressed, agitated or even openly hostile (Hackett et al, 1968; Cay et al, 1972). Many complain of difficulty in concentrating, and nearly half the patients will have difficulty with sleep. If anxiety is unrelieved, depression usually supervenes, and both may persist for long periods of time in many patients (Cay et al, 1973).

The nurse is often the first and ideal person to identify the emotional disturbances that may affect the patient in hospital. She needs to be able to recognise verbal and non-verbal cues to emotional distress and understand the basic mechanisms that the patient is using to cope. The profound emotional distress that often accompanies acute myocardial infarction can adversely affect the recovery process. For instance, severe anxiety during the initial phase of the illness results in an increased heart rate, blood pressure and myocardial oxygen demand. These cardiac effects, mediated through the sympathetic nervous system, may lead to life-threatening complications, including dysrhythmias, heart failure, pulmonary embolism and extension of the infarct. Moreover, the patient's emotional adjustment during the period on coronary care significantly influences rehabilitation and long-term survival.

Three of the most common acute emotional responses following acute myocardial infarction are fear, dependency and disorientation. These may later be replaced by anxiety and depression.

Fear

The patient's immediate reaction is usually fear, not only of death, but also of the threat the illness poses to his life-style (Thompson, 1995). This fear can be reduced by an explanation of the purpose of coronary care, the monitoring equipment and the high nurse:patient ratio. Patients need to be warned of and informed about routine observations, investigations and drug administration. Knowing the names of staff and the ease of summoning them increases their security. In general, the unit environment should become more reassuring than frightening to the patient and later his family, too.

Dependency

This can be reduced by encouraging the resumption of usual activities as soon as possible in an attempt to minimise the sense of damage and helplessness. Involving the patient in planning his own care helps to increase feelings of self-worth and independence. Involving the partner or other family members is a useful adjunct.

Disorientation

Disorientation, together with social isolation, can be reduced by the provision of a suitable environment, which includes calendars, clocks, radios, televisions, newspapers and windows with a view of the outside world. The additional comforts and provision of items such as personal photographs indicate extra thoughtfulness.

Anxiety

Anxiety is a normal but complex human phenomenon, which is difficult to define exactly. Mild anxiety is part of normal everyday life, but, in excess, it impairs physical and mental performance. Empirically, anxiety is used to describe an unpleasant emotional state, although it is also used to describe differences in anxiety-proneness as a personal characteristic.

Various studies have reported raised anxiety levels in coronary patients. Dellipiani et al (1976) compared patients admitted to a coronary care unit in Edinburgh and patients in the Teesside coronary survey, who were treated at home, on a coronary care unit or on general medical wards. The pattern of anxiety was similar in both groups, regardless of where they were treated, although throughout the study period the Teesside patients were more anxious. Their level of anxiety was high early in the illness, fell rapidly and rose again towards the end of their stay in hospital. Anxiety soon after admission to coronary care units is no higher than for patients admitted as emergencies to general medical wards (Vetter et al, 1977).

Anxiety is certainly the most common initial response to acute myocardial infarction. Its main source is the prospect of sudden death, and the signs of anxiety are more likely to be noticed during the initial phase of the illness, when recurrent symptoms such as chest pain or shortness of breath develop, or when special procedures such as the insertion of a temporary pacemaker or cardioversion are required. A less obvious symptom that evokes anxiety is the feeling of weakness and complete exhaustion. Patients who have normally been fit and strong, but are now feeling weak as a consequence of an infarct, may experience extreme anxiety and frustration. Anxiety about transfer to the ward and discharge home is likely to be particularly high if the patient is discharged abruptly with little or no warning.

Anxiety can be identified subjectively and objectively. Subjectively, patients will appear tense, apprehensive and restless. They may have a sustained tachycardia, sweat freely and constantly seek reassurance. Care must be taken not to mistake these symptoms for heart failure. Objectively, anxiety can be measured in a variety of ways, including physiological and biochemical indices, such as blood pressure, heart rate and plasma or urinary catecholamine levels. However, in cardiac patients, such methods are more likely to reflect the physical than the psychological state. Questionnaires such as the Hospital Anxiety and Depression (HAD) Scale (Zigmond and Snaith, 1983) or visual analogue scales may prove more practical and quicker to use.

Once anxiety has been assessed, intervention can be more specifically tailored to the patient's needs. The patient with a mild level of anxiety is usually alert and able to absorb information and solve problems, even though he may be restless and irritable. In contrast, the patient with a very high level of anxiety is often terrified and much too distressed to perceive and communicate normally.

A reduction of anxiety can usually be achieved in the majority of patients by considerate, attentive and competent nurses, who can be a major source of reassurance. Close and consistent nurse–patient contact increases the patient's feelings of security (Thompson, 1990). Relaxation techniques involving progressive muscle relaxation may be effective in minimising undue stress.

Depression

Depression is common in coronary patients and will often follow anxiety, especially if the latter is untreated. This is particularly so after a second myocardial infarction (Cay et al, 1972). It is a reactive rather than endogenous depression and seldom assumes psychotic status. It is an understandable response to myocardial infarction because of the implied loss of health, loss of earning capacity, impairment of physical activity and diminution of general status within family and society. It is important that depression is recognised and dealt with promptly, because it may interfere with the recovery process. Patients who are depressed make the poorest long-term recovery, as measured by their ability to return to work and resume sexual activity. They may experience sadness, disinterest, sleep disturbances and loss of appetite. In the acute phase, depression usually appears on the third to fifth day, when the patient is at an emotional low ebb. Denial is the most common coping mechanism and can often be recognised by statements the patient makes. There may be refusal to acknowledge that he has suffered a heart attack and is becoming depressed as a consequence. Denial is usually a temporary phenomenon and may serve to protect the patient from further psychological deterioration. Gradual acceptance of the illness and active participation in recovery usually follows. However, denial is dangerous to the patient when its presence allows him to engage in some form of behaviour that threatens his welfare, for example trying to take too much exercise too soon. The nurse needs to examine to what extent denial is interfering with the treatment and endangering the patient.

Depression is often accompanied by anxiety. Some patients may be irritable, oversensitive or prone to bouts of tearfulness. Others may experience feelings of hopelessness and helplessness, which results in them forming a generally pessimistic outlook. A full assessment of the patient's situation is required to ascertain whether the depression is part of the normal process of adapting to illness or whether it is related to other events. It may be helpful for the nurse to sit quietly with the patient and attempt to determine the major worries. Many of his fears may be quite realistic and are likely to prove difficult to resolve or alleviate. Some concerns may be unfounded, and once these are identified, the nurse can help correct any misconceptions that the patient may hold. Having someone to talk with, or to hold or cry with, may enable the patient to organise his thinking and help him positively to reassess his future. An optimistic but realistic outlook, which conveys hope and gives him energy and enthusiasm, is usually what is required. Probably the best antidote is early mobilisation, to counter the physical and psychological problems associated with immobility. The sooner the patient is back on his feet, the sooner will feelings of self-worth and self-esteem return. The nurse will need to avoid overprotection or the encouragement of dependency.

Anger and hostility

Once patients are aware of the fact that they have had a heart attack (and what this may imply), it is possible that their reaction may be one of anger, hostility or both. There is much emphasis and media coverage today on healthy living, and patients who consider that they have taken special care of their health may feel cheated that this has happened to them. Anger occurs in response to frustration, threat or injury. It may be expressed actively or passively or may be self-directed. Active expressions of anger include sarcasm, criticism, irritability and argument. Passively, it may be expressed through non-compliance, boredom, withdrawal or forgetfulness. Self-directed anger is manifested as depression, self-depreciation, accident proneness and somatic symptoms such as headaches and dizziness.

It is often difficult to remain objective, especially when the patient is critical of the care he is receiving or of the personnel who provide it. The attending medical staff and others may feel powerless or may experience anger themselves. They need to try to help the patient clarify his ideas and feelings, and explain constructive ways of dealing with such feelings. A consistent approach should be adopted towards the patient, and staff should not allow themselves to be played off against each other.

THE REACTION OF THE FAMILY

Hospital is a frightening place for the majority of the general public, especially cardiac intensive care and high-dependency units, their very titles suggestive of danger and bodily assault. The family will have more time to sit and think about the implications of these titles and may actually fear the coronary care unit more than the patient, who is usually too busy being ill. Relatives often feel that their loved one has been taken away and isolated from them. They frequently feel helpless, frightened and unnecessarily excluded from close involvement with their loved one. All members of the family (especially the partner) may fear that the patient may die, and there may be many recriminations and feeling of guilt if there have been recent family arguments or upsets. Friction or tension within the family unit prior to myocardial infarction is mentioned by about 20% of patients (Solomon et al, 1969), and this may be unresolved if the patient dies, causing untold guilt in the future.

Professional support from nurses and doctors is sadly lacking where the family is concerned (Skelton and Dominian, 1973), and that which they do get is often inadequate or inappropriate (Thompson and Cordle, 1988). Nursing intervention is aimed at assessing and supporting the family's coping mechanisms by providing information and reassurance and involving other appropriate professional help and opinion. Family members may view the patient's illness as a loss; they may feel they have lost the security of having certain needs, especially economic and emotional security, consistently and reliably met. They are, therefore, likely to need information, reassurance and support, but often feel reluctant to seek out staff and indicate their concerns. Many feel that by doing so they may be in the way, stopping important work, or that they may cause friction with the staff, resulting in a deterioration of their relative's care. It is, therefore, important for the coronary care staff to take the initiative in making and maintaining contact with the family, especially the partner, who is most likely to benefit from involvement in the care of the patient (Thompson, 1990). She can also provide a unique service by giving insight into the patient's preferences, dislikes and frame of mind and by generally supporting him in his recovery. Unnecessary distress may be prevented by including the partner in discharge planning and preparing the family for the patient's homecoming. Anticipation of any difficulties will facilitate a smooth and continuous transition from hospital to home.

The reaction of the partner to the illness is likely to be influenced by a number of factors, not least of which will be the general stage of the marriage (Skelton and Dominian, 1973). She will need to be warned that she is likely to experience emotional and physical responses to her husband's illness, such as fatigue, anxiety, depression, difficulty in sleeping, weight loss and sexual difficulties. These are expected stress reactions to the patient's return home. The partner will often feel that if she shows concern, she may be accused of being overprotective, and if she does not, she may be regarded as callous and unsympathetic.

Once the patient returns home, family members are often afraid to express their true feelings to the patient in case they induce another heart attack. Such cautious suppression of feelings inhibits frank and easy communication within the family and often results in a general atmosphere of tension. Both partners and their families should be invited to follow-up visits to continue education and to provide an opportunity to discuss their problems and receive advice about possible resolution. Groups for the partners of post-infarction patients may be beneficial in offering support, providing information and encouraging changes in life-style.

TRANSFER FROM THE CORONARY CARE UNIT

Although transfer to the ward may be interpreted by the patient as evidence of improvement, it may sometimes be viewed as an indication of lack of care or rejection. Anxiety and even fear about transfer are not uncommon, and these are likely to be compounded if the patient is transferred abruptly or during the night. Such negative reactions can be reduced by careful preparation and explanation at the time of transfer. Anxiety levels in patients who receive structured pretransfer teaching are significantly less than in those who do not (Toth, 1980). A pretransfer teaching programme should, therefore, be incorporated into the training of coronary care personnel and become a routine in the management of acute myocardial infarction. The incidence of cardiovascular complications is reduced in patients who are prepared for transfer from the unit, especially if cared for by the same nurses and doctors throughout their stay in hospital (Klein et al, 1968). There is also evidence that family support during the transfer phase can reduce associated cardiovascular morbidity and patient stress (Schwarz and Brenner, 1979). Predischarge management can be further improved if the patient's nurse follows the patient from the coronary care unit to the ward, to serve as a liaison between the patient and the ward staff.

It is important to warn the patient and family that, after transfer, there is usually a marked change in daily routine, with greatly reduced nursing and medical attention and possible changes in medication, diet and activity. Although it may be thought that the majority of coronary patients would be concerned about no longer being closely monitored, this does not seem to be the case (Thompson et al, 1986). Most assume that they must have virtually recovered, since they no longer have monitoring equipment, cannulae or high nurse:patient ratios. Perhaps worse still, ward staff may perceive the patient in the same light, and there is a real danger that the post-coronary patient will be left alone to 'self-care', in the belief that he requires minimal nursing contact. It is vital that, during handover from the unit to the ward, a full explanation of what has happened to the patient, and what is required in terms of care and treatment, is given. A fully documented up-to-date care plan, with a suggested plan of further management and expected outcome, is highly desirable. Ideally, such a handover should involve the patient, who can clarify any points and make a valid contribution.

Preparing patients for transfer from coronary care forms an important part of nursing management and requires more attention than it is frequently afforded. There is certainly a need for a systematic evaluation of this process.

References

Adam K and Oswald I (1984) Sleep helps healing. *British Medical Journal*, **289:** 1400–1401.
Ashworth P M (1984) Staff–patient communication in coronary care units. *Journal of Advanced Nursing,* **9:** 35–42.
Bentley S, Murphy F and Dudley H (1977) Perceived noise in surgical wards and an intensive care area: an objective analysis. *British Medical Journal,* **ii:** 1503–1506.
Bourbonnais F (1981) Pain assessment: development of a tool for the nurse and the patient. *Journal of Advanced Nursing,* **6:** 277–282.
Bourbonnais F and MacKay R C (1981) The influence of nursing interventions on chest pain. *Nursing Papers,* **13:** 38–48.
Brezinova V and Oswald I (1972) Sleep after bedtime beverage. *British Medical Journal,* **ii:** 431–433.
Broughton R and Baron R (1978) Sleep patterns in the ICU and on the ward after acute myocardial infarction. *Electroencephalography and Clinical Neurophysiology,* **45:** 348–360.
Byrne D G and Whyte H M (1980) Life events and myocardial infarction revisited. The role of measures of individual impact. *Psychosomatic Medicine,* **42:** 1–10.
Cain H D, Frasher W G and Stivelman R (1961) Graded activity program for safe return to self-care after myocardial infarction. *Journal of the American Medical Association,* **171:** 111.
Cassem N H, Hackett T P, Bascom C and Wishnie H (1970) Reactions of coronary patients to the CCU nurse. *American Journal of Nursing,* **70:** 319–325.
Cay E L (1982) Psychological aspects of cardiac rehabilitation. *Hospital Update,* **8:** 161–170.
Cay E L, Vetter N J, Philip A E and Dugard P (1972) Psychological reactions to a coronary care unit. *Journal of Psychosomatic Research,* **16:** 437–447.
Cay E L, Vetter N J, Philip A E and Dugard P (1973) Return to work after a heart attack. *Journal of Psychosomatic Research,* **17:** 231–243.
Dellipiani A W, Cay E L, Philip A E, Vetter N J, Colling W A, Donaldson R J and McCormack P (1976) Anxiety after a heart attack. *British Heart Journal,* **38:** 752–757.
Diers D, Schmidt R L, McBridge M A B and Davis B L (1972) The effect of nursing interaction on patients in pain. *Nursing Research,* **21:** 419–428.
Ellis B W, Johns M W, Lancaster R, Raptopoulos P, Angelopoulos N and Priest R G (1981) The St Mary's Hospital Sleep Questionnaire: a study of reliability. *Sleep,* **4:** 93–97.
Garrity T F and Klein R F (1975) Emotional responses and clinical severity as early determinants of six-month mortality after myocardial infarction. *Heart and Lung,* **4:** 730–737.
Hackett T P, Cassem N H and Wishnie H A (1968) The coronary care unit, a reappraisal of its psychologic hazards. *New England Journal of Medicine,* **279:** 1365–1370.
Hilton B A (1976) Quantity and quality of patients' sleep, and sleep disturbing factors in a respiratory intensive care unit. *Journal of Advanced Nursing,* **1:** 453–468.

Huskisson E C (1974) Measurement of pain. *Lancet*, **ii:** 1127–1131.

Johnston B, Watt E W and Fletcher G F (1981) Oxygen consumption and hemodynamic and electrocardiographic responses to bathing in recent post-myocardial infarction patients. *Heart and Lung*, **10:** 666–671.

Jones J, Hoggart B, Withey J, Donaghue K and Ellis B W (1979) What the patients say: a study of reactions to an intensive care unit. *Intensive Care Medicine*, **5:** 89–92.

King M J, Zir L M, Kaltman A J and Fox A C (1973) Variant angina associated with angiographically demonstrated coronary artery spasm in REM sleep. *American Journal of Medical Science*, **265:** 419–422.

Klein R F, Kliner V A, Zipes D P, Troyer W G and Wallace A G (1968) Transfer from a coronary care unit. *Archives of Internal Medicine*, **122:** 104–108.

McGurn W C (1981) The nursing process applied to people with cardiac problems. In *People with Cardiac Problems: Nursing Concepts*, McGurn W C (ed.), pp. 76–100. Philadelphia: J B Lippincott.

Meddis R (1977) *The Sleep Instinct*. London: Routledge and Kegan Paul.

Melzack R (1975) The McGill Pain Questionnaire: major properties and scoring methods. *Pain*, **1:** 277–299.

Norris R M, Caughey D E, Mercer C J and Scott P J (1974) Prognosis after myocardial infarction: six year follow up. *British Heart Journal*, **36:** 786–790.

Peric-Knowlton W (1984) The understanding and management of acute pain in adults: the nursing contribution. *International Journal of Nursing Studies*, **21:** 131–143.

Revill S I, Robinson J O, Rosen M and Hogg M I J (1976) The reliability of a linear analogue for evaluating pain. *Anaesthesia*, **31:** 1191–1198.

Rosenblatt G, Hartmann E and Zwilling G R (1973) Cardiac irritability during sleep and dreaming. *Journal of Psychosomatic Research*, **17:** 129–134.

Schwarz L P and Brenner Z R (1979) Critical care transfer: reducing patient stress through nursing interventions. *Heart and Lung*, **8:** 540–546.

Scott J and Huskisson E C (1976) Graphic representation of pain. *Pain*, **2:** 175–184.

Skelton M and Dominian J (1973) Psychological stress on wives of patients with myocardial infarction. *British Medical Journal*, **ii:** 101–103.

Solomon H A, Edwards A L and Killip T (1969) Prodromata in acute myocardial infarction. *Circulation*, **40:** 463–471.

Thompson D R (1990) *Counselling the Coronary Patient and Partner*. London: Scutari Press.

Thompson D R (1995) Fear of death. In *The Cardiac Patient: Nursing Interventions*, O'Connor S (ed), pp. 117–126. London: Mosby.

Thompson D R and Cordle C J (1988) Support of wives of myocardial infarction patients. *Journal of Advanced Nursing*, **13:** 223–228.

Thompson D R, Bailey S W and Webster R A (1986) Patients' views about cardiac monitoring. *Nursing Times*, Occasional Paper, **82(9):** 54–55.

Thompson D R, Sutton T W, Jowett N I and Pohl J E F (1991) Circadian variation in the frequency of onset of chest pain in acute myocardial infarction. *British Heart Journal*, **65:** 177–178.

Toth J C (1980) Effect of structured preparation for transfer on patient anxiety on leaving coronary care unit. *Nursing Research*, **29:** 28–34.

Totman R (1979) What makes 'life events' stressful? A retrospective study of patients who have suffered a first myocardial infarction. *Journal of Psychosomatic Research*, **23:** 193–200.

Vetter N J, Cay E L, Philip A E and Strange R C (1977) Anxiety on admission to a coronary care unit. *Journal of Psychosomatic Research*, **21:** 73–78.

Webster R A and Thompson D R (1986) Sleep in hospital. *Journal of Advanced Nursing*, **11:** 447–459.

Webster R A and Thompson D R (1992) *Caring for the Coronary Patient*. Oxford: Butterworth Heinemann.

Wells N (1984) Response to acute pain and the nursing implications. *Journal of Advanced Nursing* **9:** 51–58.

Wilson-Barnett J (1984) *Key Functions in Nursing* (Fourth Winifred Raphael Memorial Lecture). London: Royal College of Nursing.

Winslow E H, Lane L D and Gaffney F A (1984) Oxygen consumption and cardiovascular response in patients and normal adults during in-bed and out-of-bed toileting. *Journal of Cardiac Rehabilitation*, **4**: 348–354.

Winslow E H, Lane L D and Gaffney F A (1985) Oxygen uptake and cardiovascular responses in control adults and acute myocardial infarction patients during bathing. *Nursing Research*, **34**: 164–169.

Zigmond A S and Snaith R P (1983) The Hospital Anxiety Depression Scale. *Acta Psychiatrica Scandinavica*, **67**: 361–370.

8

Management of Other Causes of Chest Pain on the Coronary Care Unit

Acute chest pain is one of the most common reasons for patients being admitted to hospital; most are sent directly to the coronary care unit. The prevalence of central chest pain in the community in the 40–60-year-old age group is about 8%. Half of these patients have typical anginal pain, but only one quarter will have coronary heart disease. The negative coronary angiography rate in the UK is 10% (and in the USA, 30%). Thus, many people suffer chest pain initially believed to be due to coronary heart disease but later shown to have other causes.

Formulating the initial diagnosis is sometimes very difficult in view of the number of possible sources of pain, including the heart, the pericardium, the lungs and pleura, the oesophagus, the spine and the chest wall. Many patients who arrive on the coronary care unit prove subsequently not to have had a heart attack, and many do not even have a cardiac cause of pain (Table 8.1). Effective triage and strategies for improved referral to coronary care could significantly reduce the cost of acute care (Fineberg et al, 1984). Whilst many patients may not have suffered myocardial infarction, other serious conditions may require urgent diagnosis and treatment. The most important of these are:

- Unstable angina
- Pulmonary embolism

Table 8.1 Some causes of chest pain

Cardiovascular causes	Non-cardiac causes
Myocardial ischaemia	Herpes zoster
Coronary artery spasm	Oesophageal reflux
Myocardial infarction	Oesophageal spasm
Pericarditis	Hiatus hernia
Dissecting aortic aneurysm	Pneumonia
Pulmonary embolism	Pneumothorax
Mitral valve prolapse	Pleurisy
	Peptic ulceration
	Gall-bladder disease
	Musculoskeletal pain
	Da Costa's syndrome (cardioneurosis)

- Dissecting aortic aneurysm
- Pericarditis
- Oesophageal pain
- Abdominal pain

UNSTABLE ANGINA

About half of all the patients who sustain a myocardial infarction have warning symptoms, the most common of which is worsening angina. Up to 60% of patients recall antecedent anginal pains, although the significance was often unrealised. Indeed, many patients without previous cardiac disease are not admitted to hospital because the diagnosis of myocardial ischaemia is not considered.

Anginal pain at rest or during minimal exertion is known as unstable, crescendo or pre-infarction angina. Despite the last term, not all patients with this syndrome subsequently sustain a myocardial infarct, but its occurrence does highlight a group of patients at increased risk. In a recent series, 27% of patients developed myocardial infarction within 3 days of hospital admission, and a further 11% within 1 year (Karlson et al, 1993). In-hospital mortality is about 7%. An episode of unstable angina within 1 week of myocardial infarction conveys a 1-year mortality of over 20%. Recognition of this condition with appropriate therapy may prevent myocardial infarction and its sequelae.

Definition

There is no agreed definition of unstable angina. It may be used to describe symptoms in patients (usually males aged between 40 and 60 years) caused by myocardial ischaemia that are:

- Of recent onset (within 4 weeks)
- Occurring at rest or with minimal activity
- Different from previous anginal pain (in duration or by accompanying symptoms)
- Accompanied by ECG changes of ischaemia

Of course, all these findings may occur with myocardial infarction, and, indeed, subclinical myocardial infarction ('micro-infarction'), which may be detectable by measurement of the sensitive serum marker enzyme, troponin T (see Chapter 6), probably occurs in patients with unstable angina. Patients with unstable angina and raised levels of troponin T are more likely to develop problems (Hamm et al, 1993).

Pathophysiology

Typical exercise-induced angina results from an imbalance between myocardial oxygen supply and its demand, because of a fixed stenosis in one or more coronary arteries. Thallium scanning during pain may show temporary perfusion defects, suggesting that unstable angina is due to a reduction in coronary flow rather than increased myocardial demand. However, there appears to be no difference in the severity or distribution of coronary atheromata in patients with stable and unstable angina, so coronary artery spasm may be the prime initiating factor or perhaps a collateral circulation has not had time to form. Coronary arterial spasm, usually occurs in association with eccentric type I atheromatous lesions (see Chapter 3), but coronary angiography may be normal in many cases, (Waters et al, 1983), showing the large part that isolated coronary artery spasm plays in unstable angina. In most cases, however, the vessels show type II plaques undergoing fissuring, often with non-occlusive luminal thrombus. Distal micro-embolisation into small myocardial vessels is very common and may prove fatal (Davies et al, 1986). The extent of thrombus formation may be affected by the size of the plaque disruption and the blood flow in the affected artery. Coexisting coronary artery disease may reduce flow, as may increased blood viscosity due to activation of coagulation factors and platelets. Higher levels of fibrinogen have been identified in patients with unstable angina. Recent evidence suggests that unstable angina is a hypercoagulable state, marked by increased thrombin generation.

It is not known whether acute cardiac events occur spontaneously or whether they are precipitated by trigger events, but a definite circadian pattern to cardiac events is recognised, with particularly susceptible times in the early morning, on waking, and also around bedtime (Thompson et al, 1991). This matches the diurnal variation in blood viscosity and coagulability (Tofler et al, 1987).

Chest pain is the usual presenting symptom. It is typically anginal in nature but worse in respect of intensity, duration and accompanying symptoms (e.g. nausea and sweating). Attacks typically occur at rest and are probably caused by coronary artery spasm. Examination may reveal signs of ischaemia, such as dysrhythmias, a third or fourth heart sound, reversed splitting of the second heart sound and transient mitral systolic murmurs. Blood pressure and pulse are normal but may rise transiently at the onset of pain. If hypotension and pyrexia are present, myocardial infarction has probably already occurred.

Investigations

The electrocardiogram (ECG)

Between episodes of ischaemic pain, the 12-lead ECG may be normal, although non-specific changes are often present. During pain, the ECG may show ST elevation (Prinzmetal changes) or, more usually, planar or down-sloping ST depression. T wave flattening, peaking and inversion may also occur with pain. Serial ECGs may show both ST elevation and depression. The appearance of Q waves usually implies infarction, although even these can be a transient manifestation of ischaemia (Goldberger, 1979). The ischaemic changes in the ECG during pain do not always predict subsequent angiographic findings, but ST depression and anterior T wave inversion are associated with a poorer outcome.

Holter monitoring

Continuous ST monitoring via Holter monitors can be used to detect transient ST changes compatible with ischaemia. Even those patients on optimal treatment may continue to have asymptomatic episodes of ischaemia, which may adversely affect prognosis (Langer et al, 1989). Silent myocardial ischaemia is common in patients with ischaemic heart disease, often occurring at rest, and is probably caused by altered coronary arterial tone. It is thought to contribute towards what is termed the 'total ischaemic burden' on the heart (a combination of symptomatic and asymptomatic ischaemia), which may relate to prognosis (Cohn, 1987). Various theories have been advanced to explain why some ischaemic episodes are perceived whilst others are not. It may be that silent episodes involve smaller areas of myocardium, or perhaps the patient's pain threshold is higher. Alternatively, the pain mechanism may be defective, as occurs in diabetes. The Framingham study has suggested that as many as one third of myocardial infarcts are silent (Kannel and Abbott, 1984), and their 10-year mortality is higher than that of symptomatic myocardial infarction. This is possibly because the painless infarct patients are not diagnosed and do not receive appropriate post-infarction care and intervention.

Cardiac enzymes

Increases in the cardiac enzyme levels usually signify myocardial necrosis. Minor elevations of highly cardiospecific enzymes are probably compatible with the diagnosis of unstable angina, particularly if they are unaccompanied by ECG changes, but the diagnostic criteria of unstable angina and myocardial infarction have very indistinct boundaries.

Management

Unstable angina is a cardiological emergency, and admission to a specialist unit is required for therapy to avert myocardial infarction and any sequelae. In addition, other clinical manifestations of severe myocardial ischaemia (e.g. dysrhythmias or heart failure) need controlling, and important precipitants (e.g. anaemia, hypertension and valve disease) need excluding.

It may not be possible to exclude myocardial infarction on admission, but differentiation may be important because emergency bypass surgery can be carried out in centres where immediate coronary angiography and surgery are available (Rahimtoola, 1984).

Drug therapy

It is possible to stabilise the majority of patients with medical therapy using a combination of anti-anginal therapy (beta-blockers, nitrates and calcium antagonists) and antithrombotic therapy (aspirin and heparin).

Beta-adrenergic blocking agents

Beta-blockers are the mainstay of therapy for unstable angina and will control pain in about three-quarters of patients and probably decrease progression to myocardial infarction by about 10%. They act predominantly by reducing the heart rate and myocardial oxygen consumption. There is a small theoretical disadvantage of unopposed alpha-adrenergic vasoconstriction, precipitating coronary arterial spasm and leading to worsening myocardial ischaemia. However, since most patients will concurrently be treated with nitrates and calcium antagonists, this is rarely a clinical problem. The main practical consideration is, therefore, the risk of impaired left ventricular function, by direct action on the myocardium or secondary to an induced bradycardia. Beta-blocking agents should, therefore, be given in small and frequent doses to reduce the pulse rate to about 60 beats per minute, and it is probably better to select an agent with a short duration of action, as it is not possible to anticipate which patients will react adversely. The ultra-short acting beta-blocker esmolol is safe and effective if there is any doubt about cardiac decompensation. Cardioselective beta-blockers are preferred, since coronary sympathetic vasodilator tone is mediated by the beta-2 receptor; this is particularly important if coronary artery spasm is suspected.

Nitrates

Nitrates reduce cardiac work and oxygen consumption by reducing preload and some afterload. Subendocardial blood flow is also improved. Some of these effects may be offset by an increase in heart rate, so nitrates may need to be given with a beta-blocker or diltiazem. Although nitrates may be given orally, intravenous nitrates are easier to titrate against blood pressure and headaches. Buccal glyceryl trinitrate (GTN) (5 mg, 6 hourly) may achieve as good blood nitrate levels without the need for an intravenous infusion. The starting dose of intravenous nitrate should be low (around 2–5 µg/min), increasing to as much as 300 µg/min, depending on systemic blood pressure. The systolic blood pressure should not be allowed to fall below 100 mmHg or coronary perfusion pressures will fall, which may precipitate myocardial infarction. If hypotension develops at low doses of nitrate therapy, it may be advisable to insert a Swan–Ganz catheter, so that unsuspected hypovolaemia is not missed, and to ensure that the patient has an adequate left ventricular filling pressure.

Nitrates are of major value in patients with coronary vasospasm and should be administered to all those who show ST elevation on the ECG when in pain.

Calcium-channel blockers

Calcium antagonists probably do not offer any major therapeutic benefit over nitrates and, used as monotherapy, may be harmful (Lubsen and Tijssen, 1987). Verapamil and diltiazem are particularly useful if there is a fast pulse rate unresponsive to beta-blockade, and diltiazem may have a protective effect, as in non-transmural myocardial infarction (Gibson et al, 1986). Nicardipine has the least cardiodepressant activity, which may be an important consideration when co-prescribing with beta-blockers.

Anticoagulants

Since non-occlusive thrombi are present in many patients with unstable angina, there is a rational basis for acute administration of anticoagulants. Intravenous heparin needs to be started early in the course of unstable angina, and continuous infusion is better then intermittent boluses for inhibiting thrombin formation. A loading bolus of 5000 U should be followed by an infusion to maintain the activated partial thromboplastin time (APTT) at approximately twice the control value. Heparin often has a swift analgesic action and may be effective in preventing progression to myocardial infarction (Telford and Wilson, 1981). The optimum duration of therapy is unknown. If the heparin infusion is withdrawn suddenly, there may be a significant risk of return of symptoms, unless aspirin is given (Theroux et al, 1992). Whilst the combination of heparin with aspirin may increase the risk of bleeding, it reduces the risk of myocardial infarction and sudden death in comparison to those treated by aspirin alone or placebo (Wallentin, 1989).

Heparin is a non-specific thrombin inhibitor; the new specific antithrombotic agents, such as hirudin, may prove to be advantageous..

Aspirin

Unstable angina is associated with enhanced platelet reactivity and increased production of the powerful vasoconstrictor thromboxane A2, which may aggravate the degree of coronary obstruction. Administration of aspirin will reduce the risk of myocardial infarction by more than 50%, as well as cardiac mortality (Anti-platelet Trialists' Collaboration, 1994). Low-dose treatment (75 mg per day) is probably sufficient, provided a loading dose of at least 300 mg has been given.

Thrombolytic agents

Although the role of fresh thrombus is well established in unstable angina, thrombolytic agents have not yet been shown to be of value in the treatment of unstable angina (Bar et al, 1992).

Intra-aortic balloon counterpulsation

Some centres still advocate the use of counterpulse balloon pumping if other medical therapies have failed. However, there is an appreciable insertion mortality and morbidity, particularly with regard to vascular injury and lower limb ischaemia. Most patients with unstable angina can be controlled for short periods, but they cannot usually be weaned off the balloon pump without a sudden deterioration, often associated with cardiogenic shock. As a consequence, once the balloon has been inserted, there is little choice but to proceed to cardiac catheterisation and surgery (either coronary artery bypass grafting or angioplasty).

Surgery

The majority of patients settle with conservative management in the first 24 hours. Many of these will suffer pain later, and about one third will need coronary artery surgery within 2 years. Early angiography should, therefore, be carried out in most cases, particularly younger patients and those whose symptoms fail to settle promptly. Those found to have left main stem disease, triple coronary artery disease or ventricular aneurysms are usually considered for early bypass surgery (ACC/AHA, 1991).

Those patients who do not settle with conservative therapy should be assessed for emergency coronary artery bypass surgery or coronary angioplasty. Angioplasty has a success rate of restoring patency of the affected artery in up to 93% of cases, with a low mortality (less than 2%). The success rate is higher for patients on heparin (Bittl and Ryan, 1992).

PULMONARY EMBOLISM

Pulmonary emboli are common, and up to one third are fatal, contributing to approximately 15–20% of all hospital deaths. In the UK, there are an estimated 20 000 deaths per year from pulmonary embolism, as well as a further 40 000 non-fatal cases. Most patients have the usual clinical risk factors, including immobility, recent surgery or recent myocardial infarction. The most common source of emboli are the deep veins of the legs, although clinical evidence will be present in less than half the patients presenting with pulmonary embolism. Emboli may originate from the right ventricle in some patients, following myocardial infarction.

Signs and symptoms

Pulmonary emboli cause a varying degree of symptoms and signs, depending upon their size; many may not be detected clinically. Acute *minor* pulmonary emboli present with pleuritic chest pain and some breathlessness, but little haemodynamic disturbance. Acute *major* pulmonary emboli significantly obstruct the major pulmonary vessels and produce sudden, and often dramatic, effects. Massive emboli will result in circulatory arrest, syncope, cyanosis and cardiac arrest (often marked by electromechanical dissociation on the ECG). Smaller emboli may cause dyspnoea, with dull central chest pain (undistinguishable from angina), tachycardia, gallop rhythm and a raised jugular venous pressure.

Investigations

The diagnosis of pulmonary embolism is not easy. Most diagnostic tests are non-specific and are prone to misinterpretation, and many patients correctly diagnosed have negative investigations.

Electrocardiography

The ECG is vital to exclude myocardial infarction, but there are no changes diagnostic of pulmonary embolism. The ECG is usually normal in acute minor pulmonary embolism. Non-specific findings include sinus tachycardia, widespread T wave inversion (especially in leads V1–V4), right axis deviation, right bundle branch block and the classical (but rare) S1, Q3, T3 pattern of acute cor pulmonale. Atrial fibrillation is precipitated in about 5% of cases.

Chest radiography

The chest X-ray is often normal but may reveal an alternative diagnosis, such as pneumothorax or pneumonia. If the X-ray is abnormal, loss of lung volume (e.g. elevated hemidiaphragm) is the most common sign. There may be pulmonary opacities (not necessarily wedge shaped) or linear atelectasis with a small pleural effusion. Larger emboli will produce an area of oligaemia with a 'plump' hilum.

Arterial blood gases

Since pulmonary emboli can give rise to both vascular and airway changes, blood gas changes are variable and are often within normal limits. Patients with heart failure or chronic lung disease may also have pre-existing abnormalities. The classical abnormalities are hypoxaemia and hypocapnia.

Radioisotope lung scanning

A combined ventilation/perfusion (V/Q) scan (Figure 8.1) is the best generally-available technique for the diagnosis of pulmonary embolism. The patient is

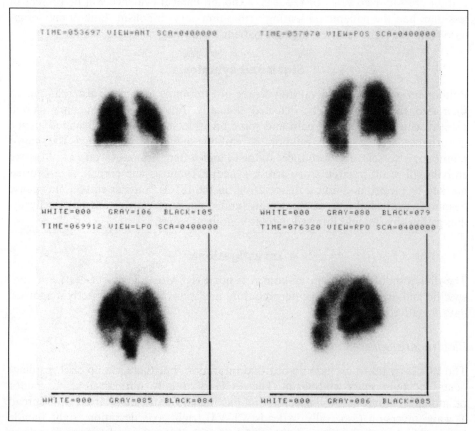

Fig. 8.1 A perfusion lung scan. Note the multiple defects, which may be due to pulmonary embolism; a ventilation scan is required for confirmation

injected with technetium-labelled macro-aggregates of albumin, which lodge in the pulmonary capillaries. The distribution of the trapped macro-aggregates is determined with a gamma camera, to produce multiple views of pulmonary perfusion. Significant perfusion defects are seen as 'cold' spots. Whilst a normal perfusion scan excludes pulmonary embolism, false positive scans are common. Perfusion defects may be produced by numerous conditions affecting pulmonary blood flow, including chronic obstructive airway disease, pneumonia and pleural effusions. In these cases, a ventilation scan is needed to clarify the diagnosis.

During a ventilation scan, the patient inhales radioactive xenon (133-Xe or 127-Xe) or uses a technetium aerosol. The gamma camera records the distribution of alveolar gas in a multiple view series, which is compared directly with the perfusion scan. Ventilation should be preserved in the areas of abnormal perfusion in cases of pulmonary embolism, i.e. there will be a ventilation/perfusion mismatch. If the area of hypoperfusion is due to primary lung disease, ventilation to the same area will be impaired, resulting in a matched defect. Radionuclide scans are usually reported as representing a low, moderate or high likelihood of pulmonary embolism. When suggestive of pulmonary embolism, it is likely that the scan underestimates the size of the embolus.

Pulmonary arteriography

Pulmonary angiography is the definitive way of making the diagnosis, although it is seldom required. It is indicated in severely-ill patients where the diagnosis is not clear, particularly if pulmonary embolectomy or thrombolysis is being considered. It is also useful where clinical suspicion is high but the lung scan is equivocal.

Management

The treatment of pulmonary embolism is determined by the symptoms and degree of haemodynamic upset (Gray and Firoozan, 1992). Most emboli will lyse spontaneously with time, and management should be directed towards sustaining life and preventing recurrence. Pain and anxiety should be treated by diamorphine, and 100% oxygen should be given. Vasodilators are contraindicated, and a high central venous pressure should be maintained.

There are three treatment options:

● Anticoagulation
● Thrombolysis
● Surgery

Anticoagulation

Heparin accelerates the action of antithrombin III and prevents further fibrin deposition, allowing spontaneous endogenous thrombolysis. Heparin should be given in sufficient dose to keep the APTT at two to three times control values. A loading dose of 5000–10 000 U should be followed by a continuous intravenous infusion of 1000–2000 U/hr. This should be given until the patient stabilises, and perhaps for as long as a week, after which warfarin may be substituted.

Thrombolysis

Massive pulmonary emboli are associated with a high mortality, and every attempt should be made to relieve the obstruction. Thrombolysis is very effective and may be better administered via a pulmonary arterial catheter. Streptokinase 250 000–500 000 U given over half an hour, followed by 100 000 U/hr for up to 72 hours is the usually-recommended dosage. It is not known whether 1.5 million units, as normally prescribed in acute myocardial infarction, is equally effective. Other thrombolytic agents may also be used, and the usual precautions and contraindications apply, as for coronary thrombolysis.

Surgery

Embolectomy is very effective in selected cases but requires cardiopulmonary bypass and is associated with a high mortality (over 50%). Prior pulmonary angiography is mandatory. Those normally considered are patients who continue to deteriorate despite thrombolytic therapy, those in whom thrombolysis is contraindicated and those with respiratory failure and shock.

Prognosis

Most deaths from pulmonary emboli occur in the first hour, and the overall mortality is about 10%. Spontaneous thrombolysis starts within hours, and small emboli will not be detectable after 5 days. About 50% of lung scans will be normal by 2 weeks.

DISSECTING AORTIC ANEURYSM

An aneurysm is a sac produced by dilatation of the wall of an artery, which is filled with blood to form a pulsatile mass. It can present with leakage or rupture (producing shock) or may be found on routine examination.

An acute dissecting aneurysm is the most frequent and most lethal disorder of the thoracic aorta. There is an incidence of 5–10 per million, and it is thus twice as common as rupture of an abdominal aortic aneurysm. It is more common in men, and there is usually a previous history of hypertension.

Dissection is initiated by a small tear in the aortic intima, which is a degenerative event. Most dissections (66%) arise in the ascending aorta, and the blood passes into the medial layer of the aortic wall. The blood may then flow proximally into the pericardium (with fatal tamponade) or distally to involve the aortic arch, descending and abdominal aorta and its branches.

Clinical features

The presentation is usually dramatic and dominated by pain. There is sudden excruciating ('tearing') pain felt anywhere from the epigastrium to the neck. It radiates to the back and, sometimes, all four limbs. The patient is cold, clammy and paradoxically hypertensive, with systolic blood pressures often in excess of 200 mmHg. Peripheral pulses may be absent, reduced or asymmetrical. Subsequent signs and symptoms depend upon which branches of the aorta are involved in the dissection process. For example, there may be a hemiplegia due to involvement of a carotid artery, or inferior myocardial infarction when the right coronary artery is involved (occlusion of the left coronary artery is usually fatal). Blood in the pericardial sac may give rise to a pericardial friction rub, and the murmur of aortic incompetence may develop secondary to dilatation of the aortic ring. Such presentations often serve to confuse the diagnosis, as may the ECG, which can show ST elevation, dysrhythmias, left ventricular hypertrophy or conduction defects. Thrombolytic therapy may be given in error (Blankenship and Almquist, 1989). The chest X-ray is diagnostic in two-thirds of cases, showing a widened superior mediastinum and sometimes a left-sided pleural effusion caused by extravasated blood. Care must be taken in interpreting the emergency anteroposterior (portable) chest film; apparent mediastinal widening may be seen in a normal patient. Echocardiography, particularly transoesophageal echocardiography, is useful in confirming the diagnosis, and whilst a CAT scan helps to localise the dissection, angiography is the usual definitive investigation.

Management

The two leading problems are pain and shock. Large doses of diamorphine, probably best given by intravenous infusion, are often required to control the severe pain. Shock is usually secondary to the severe pain, since there will be only slight blood loss unless there is aortic rupture.

After pain relief, the next vital step is to reduce the blood pressure. Sodium nitroprusside is useful in view of its short half-life and should be titrated to keep the systolic blood pressure below 100 mmHg. Beta-blockade is particularly useful, since it will lead to the reduction of both systolic blood pressure and pulse pressure. The reduced force of cardiac contraction may further limit intimal tearing. Labetalol is suitable for infusion, and the alpha-blocking activity of the drug helps to maintain peripheral vasodilatation.

With successful hypotensive treatment, up to half the patients can survive, particularly those with small, distal dissections. If complications emerge, or the blood pressure cannot be controlled, surgical intervention is required, and this is always needed if the ascending aorta is involved.

The most successful surgical techniques are fenestration and circumferential intimal anchorage. Fenestration involves opening the aorta and cutting a window in the intimal dissection flap, enabling blood to re-enter the aortic lumen. The other procedure involves opening the aorta, dividing the dissection flap and suturing it around the outer wall of the aorta.

Prognosis

Untreated, the mortality is 30% in the first day, increasing to 70% in 7 days and 90% by 3 months. With medical and surgical intervention, this has been reduced to 15%, many patients surviving for more than 3 years.

PERICARDITIS

Acute pericardial disease has many causes, the most common being acute viral pericarditis and post-infarction pericarditis. The diagnosis should be suspected if the pain is worse on lying flat and may be confirmed by an audible pericardial friction rub. The rub is high pitched, superficial and scratchy and is similar to the sound made by stroking the hair above the ear. It has a to-and-fro sound passing between diastole and systole as the ventricles fill. It may be missed since it is often soft, transient, localised and intermittent. Shoulder-tip pain is common if the inferior surface of the heart is involved.

Post-infarction pericarditis

About 20% of transmural myocardial infarcts are complicated by pericarditis within the first week. Small effusions may be detectable on echocardiography. Pericarditis may also recur within 3 months, in association with plural effusions and systemic symptoms, including malaise and fever (Dressler's syndrome). Dysrhythmias are less common. The mechanism is thought to be autoimmune, triggered by a response to the products of myocardial damage. Antiheart antibodies can be found. A similar condition may complicate cardiac surgery (post-cardiotomy syndrome) and may relate to blood in the pericardial cavity. The response to steroids is often dramatic, although non-steroidal anti-inflammatory drugs should be tried first. Relapses may occur up to 2 years after myocardial infarction.

Viral pericarditis

Acute viral pericarditis affects young adults, and the usual viruses are Coxsackie B, echovirus, influenza and infectious mononucleosis. Following a typical flu-like illness, there is fever and chest pain, which is sharp, retrosternal and radiates to the left shoulder. The pain may be mild or excruciating. Atrial dysrhythmias are common, possibly caused by inflammation of the superficially-located sinus node. The ECG may show sinus tachycardia and widespread ST elevation, which is concave upwards in the leads facing the affected cardiac surface (Figure 8.2).

Treatment

Treatment depends on the severity of the symptoms. In most cases simple analgesia or non-steroidal inflammatory agents are enough, with bed-rest. More severe cases require steroids, which will quickly control pain, fever and any resistant atrial dysrhythmias. If there is an associated myocarditis, bed-rest is important. Anticoagulation therapy should be reduced or stopped to avoid haemorrhagic pericarditis with effusion. Any blood in the pericardial cavity may lead to Dressler's syndrome. It is obviously important that patients who present with viral pericarditis are not inadvertently thrombolysed, since fatal tamponade can result.

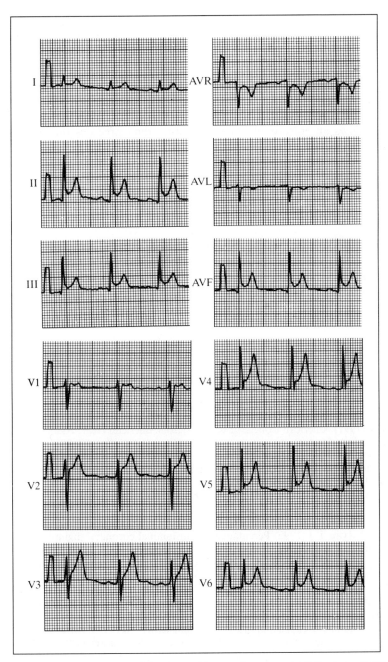

Fig. 8.2   ECG: acute viral pericarditis. Note widespread concave 'saddle-shaped' ST segment elevation

OESOPHAGEAL PAIN

Reflux oesophagitis is probably the most common cause of chest pain and can be demonstrated in about 40% of the general adult population. It, therefore, frequently coexists with ischaemic chest pain, and the diagnosis of reflux oesophagitis should not exclude coexistent myocardial ischaemia.

Oesophageal rupture is an uncommon disorder, which may easily be confused with myocardial infarction. The pain is severe, central and often radiates to the back. It follows an episode of vomiting, rather than precedes the vomiting, as in myocardial infarction.

ABDOMINAL PAIN

Peptic ulcer disease or *gall-bladder disease* may present with lower chest/upper abdominal pain, which may be referred to the shoulders. Chronic cholecystitis may have many symptomatic similarities to angina. A perforated peptic ulcer may mimic myocardial infarction or even cause it.

Occult *gastrointestinal bleeding* may present with pain and shock and can be easily confused with acute myocardial infarction.

Acute pancreatitis may present with shock, hypoxia and severe upper abdominal/lower chest pain. The pain may be eased by sitting forward, rather as in pericarditis.

References

ACC/AHA (1991) American College of Cardiologists/American Heart Association guidelines and indications for coronary artery bypass grafting. *Circulation,* **83:** 285–382.

Anti-platelet Trialists' Collaboration (1994) Overview I: Prevention of death, myocardial infarction and stroke by prolonged anti-platelet therapy in various categories of patients. *British Medical Journal,* **308:** 81–106.

Bar F W, Verhugt F W, Col J et al (1992) Thrombolysis in patients with unstable angina improves the angiographic but not the clinical outcome. Results of UNASEM – a multicentre randomised placebo controlled trial with anistreplase. *Circulation,* **86:** 131–137.

Bittl J A and Ryan T J (1992) Percutaneous transluminal coronary angioplasty for unstable angina. In *Unstable Angina,* Rutherford J D (ed.), pp. 191–209. Boston: Marcel Dekker.

Blankenship J C and Almquist A K (1989) Cardiovascular complications of thrombolytic therapy in patients with a mistaken diagnosis of acute myocardial infarction. *Journal of the American College of Cardiology,* **14:** 1579–1582.

Cohn P F (1987) Total ischaemic burden: pathophysiology and prognosis. *American Journal of Cardiology,* **59:** 3C–6C.

Davies M J, Thomas A C, Knapman P A and Hangartner J R (1986) Intramyocardial platelet aggregation in patients with unstable angina suffering sudden ischaemic death. *Circulation,* **73:** 418–427.

Fineberg H V, Scadden D and Goldman L (1984) Care of patients with a low probability of acute myocardial infarction. *New England Journal of Medicine,* **310:** 1301–1307.

Gibson R S, Boden W E, Theroux P, Strauss H D and Pratt C M (1986) Diltiazem and reinfarction in patients with non-Q-wave myocardial infarction. *New England Journal of Medicine,* **315:** 423–429.

Goldberger A L (1979) *Myocardial Infarction: Electrocardiographic Differential Diagnosis.* St Louis: C V Mosby.

Gray H H and Firoozan S (1992) Management of pulmonary embolism. *Thorax,* **47:** 825–832.

Hamm C W, Ravkilde J, Gerhardt W et al (1993) The prognostic value of serum troponin T in unstable angina. *New England Journal of Medicine,* **327:** 146–150.

Kannel W B and Abbott R D (1984) Incidence and prognosis of unrecognised myocardial infarction: an update on the Framingham study. *New England Journal of Medicine,* **311:** 1144–1147.

Karlson B W, Herlitz J and Pettersson P (1993) One year prognosis in patients hospitalised with a history of unstable angina pectoris. *Clinical Cardiology,* **16:** 397–402.

Langer A, Freeman M R and Armstrong P W (1989) ST segment shift in unstable angina: pathophysiology and association with coronary anatomy and hospital outcome. *Journal of the American College of Cardiology,* **13:** 1495–1502.

Lubsen J and Tijssen J P (1987) Efficacy of nifedipine and metoprolol in the early treatment of unstable angina in the coronary care unit: findings of the Holland Inter-university Nifedipine/metoprolol Trial (HINT). *American Journal of Cardiology,* **60:** 18a–25a.

Rahimtoola S H (1984) Coronary bypass surgery for unstable angina. *Circulation,* **69:** 842–848.

Telford A M and Wilson C (1981) A trial of heparin versus atenolol in the prevention of myocardial infarction in the intermediate coronary syndrome. *Lancet,* **i:** 1225–1228.

Theroux P, Waters D, Lam J, Juneau M and McCans J (1992). Re-activation of unstable angina after the discontinuation of heparin. *New England Journal of Medicine,* **327:** 141–145.

Thompson D R, Sutton T W, Jowett N I and Pohl J E F (1991) Circadian variation in the frequency of onset of chest pain in acute myocardial infarction. *British Heart Journal,* **65:** 177–178.

Tofler G H, Brezinski D A, Schafer A J, Czeisler C A, Rutherford J D and Willich S N (1987) Concurrent morning increase in platelet aggregability and the risk of myocardial infarction and sudden death. *New England Journal of Medicine,* **316:** 1514–1518.

Wallentin L, for the Risk Study Group in South East Sweden (1989) Aspirin 75 mg after an episode of unstable coronary artery disease – risk for myocardial infarction death in a randomised placebo-controlled study. *Circulation,* **80** (supplement 11): 419.

Waters D D, Miller D D, Szlachcic J, Bouchard A, Methe M, Kreeft J and Theroux P (1983) Factors influencing the long-term prognosis of treated patients with variant angina. *Circulation,* **68:** 258–265.

9

Complications of Acute Myocardial Infarction and their Management

There are numerous complications that may arise as a consequence of acute myocardial infarction (Chatterjee, 1993). The risk of complications is mostly dependent upon:

- The size of the acute myocardial infarction
- The cumulative loss of functional myocardium if there has been previous ischaemic damage
- The extent and severity of coronary arterial disease

Abnormal electrical activity in ischaemic or necrotic cardiac tissue can precipitate disturbances in cardiac rate, rhythm and conduction (the 'dysrhythmias'), whilst the loss of left ventricular myocardium leads to pump failure ('heart failure').

Dysrhythmias are the most common complication of myocardial infarction, occurring in about 90% of patients. These will need treating if there is a deterioration in circulatory function (hypotension, heart failure or syncope) or if the rate is increasing myocardial work such that ischaemia is worsened. Most dysrhythmias can be prevented or abolished by relief of pain and anxiety, correction of hypoxaemia and treatment of heart failure.

Cardiac arrest complicates about 3% of cases that reach hospital and may be recurrent. Circulatory standstill is usually associated with ventricular fibrillation, asystole or electromechanical dissociation (EMD), although many other dysrhythmias (e.g. ventricular tachycardia or complete heart block) can have serious haemodynamic consequences during the acute phase of myocardial infarction.

Heart failure complicates about one quarter to one half of myocardial infarcts and arises from the loss of contractility in the damaged myocardium. As a result, the ejection fraction falls and there is a concomitant rise in the left ventricular end diastolic pressure (LVEDP). A fall in the intra-aortic pressure reduces coronary artery perfusion, and this, with arterial hypoxaemia and acidosis, leads to a further reduction in myocardial performance. The development of heart failure is primarily determined by the extent of myocardial necrosis, although hypoperfusion of the adjacent surviving myocardium may compromise its contractility – so-called 'stunned' myocardium (Braunwald, 1991).

THE DYSRHYTHMIAS

Acute myocardial infarction is commonly associated with fatal dysrhythmias, and the detection and treatment of these was the primary reason for the creation of coronary care units. It is probable that both the size and the location of the infarction play an important part in their aetiology. Dysrhythmias need swift and effective therapy if there is circulatory impairment or compromised ischaemic myocardium, or if they predispose to more severe (malignant) dysrhythmias, such as ventricular tachycardia or ventricular fibrillation. Dysrhythmias may arise because of abnormal impulse formation, abnormal conduction or ectopic activity. A classification is shown in Table 9.1.

Following acute myocardial infarction, patients almost invariably show overactivity of the autonomic nervous system. Parasympathetic (vagal) overactivity is particularly common with inferior and posterior myocardial infarction, manifesting as a sinus bradycardia, AV blockade or hypotension. Sympathetic overactivity (tachycardia and transient hypertension) may be present in nearly half of all patients (particularly those with anterior infarction) and lowers the threshold for ventricular fibrillation.

Consequences of cardiac dysrhythmias

Clinical consequences of dysrhythmias arise because of impairment of circulation or myocardial oxygenation. Such consequences are extremely variable but are

Table 9.1   A classification of cardiac dysrhythmias

Abnormal impulse formation and ectopic beats	Conduction disturbances
At the Sinus node Sinus arrhythmia Sinus bradycardia Sinus tachycardia Sinus arrest	*In the Sinus node* SA block *In the AV node* First-, second- and third-degree AV block
In the atria Atrial ectopic beats Atrial tachycardia Atrial flutter Atrial fibrillation Wandering atrial pacemaker	*In the bundle of His* Left bundle branch block Right bundle branch block Left anterior and posterior hemiblocks *Others* Intra-atrial block
In the AV node Nodal ectopic beats Junctional rhythm Junctional tachycardia	Ventricular pre-excitation Atrioventricular dissociation
In the ventricles Ventricular ectopic beats Idioventricular rhythm Ventricular tachycardia Ventricular fibrillation	

always more pronounced in patients with cardiac disease. Whilst the healthy heart can withstand many abnormal rhythms, the diseased heart cannot, and sustained tachycardias may lead to circulatory collapse or ischaemic pain. Any circulatory embarrassment is serious following acute myocardial infarction, since it may compromise perfusion in areas of marginally ischaemic myocardium. If these then become infarcted, the cycle may be repeated.

Tachycardias are particularly serious, since increases in heart rate lead to a reduction in diastolic timing. Ventricular filling is, therefore, reduced, with a fall in cardiac output. Coronary arterial blood flow also takes place during diastole, and a shortened perfusion time reduces oxygen supply to the myocardium at a time when demand is high, which may precipitate ischaemic pain or even myocardial infarction.

Management of acute dysrhythmias

The treatment of acute rhythm disturbances on coronary care units usually aims to restore normal sinus rhythm and prevent recurrence of the dysrhythmia. Establishment of sinus rhythm is sometimes not possible (e.g. in atrial fibrillation), and treatment is then designed to slow the ventricular rate and improve cardiac output. Treatment is either electrical or pharmacological. If drugs are used, they are usually given intravenously, since absorption by other routes may be slowed because of a low cardiac output, which impairs tissue perfusion, particularly in muscle and the gut. Wherever possible, attention should be directed towards the precipitating cause. Pain, fear, hypoxia, acidosis and electrolyte imbalance should be considered. Restoration of normal rhythm will be difficult if these factors remain uncorrected.

THE BRADYCARDIAS

Slow heart rates (bradycardias) usually occur as a result of sino-atrial dysfunction, when generation of the impulse at the sinus node is inhibited, or when conduction through the heart is slowed or blocked (heart block). Bradycardia predisposes to cardiac standstill.

Sinus bradycardia

Sinus bradycardia is arbitrarily defined as a sinus rhythm slower than 60 beats per minute. Bradycardia occurs in about 30% of patients following acute myocardial infarction and normally indicates parasympathetic overactivity, with release of acetylcholine from autonomic fibres in the atria and AV node. Because afferent vagal fibres are more common on the inferior surface of the heart, inferior myocardial infarction is often accompanied by vagal overactivity and consequent bradycardia. Whilst slowing of the heart is useful in protecting the injured heart, by limiting myocardial work, it may result in hypotension secondary to a reduced cardiac output. Coronary perfusion may also be reduced. Escape rhythms are more likely to occur, which can predispose to ventricular tachycardia and fibrillation. Sinus bradycardia is usually asymptomatic, but sudden onset of any bradycardia may result in hypotension with dizziness or syncope.

No treatment is required unless there are signs of low cardiac output, when a single dose of atropine (0.3–0.6 mg) is usually sufficient to raise the pulse and restore the blood pressure to normal. Further doses may be given at 2–3 minute intervals, up to a total dose of 2.4 mg. Isoprenaline may be used to maintain heart rate but should be administered with care in acute myocardial infarction; increased myocardial work may extend the infarct or even precipitate ventricular dysrhythmias.

Cardiac pacing may be considered to raise the sinus rate if there is evidence of ectopic (escape) ventricular activity, such as ventricular ectopics or ventricular tachycardia. This will often control the ectopic rhythm without resort to antidysrhythmic agents. If sinus bradycardia complicates anterior myocardial infarction, insertion of a temporary pacing wire may be needed, since sudden complete block may follow (Jowett et al, 1989).

Sino-atrial (SA) block

If the sinus node fails to initiate one or more stimuli, or if there is block of transmission of the impulse into the atria, SA block is said to occur (Figure 9.1). The atria and ventricles will not be depolarised, and long pauses in the pulse may result.

Block at the sinus node is classified in the same way as block at the AV node (see p. 213), although first-degree SA block cannot be recognised electrically.

Second-degree SA block may occur in one of two forms:

● The PP interval becomes progressively shorter until a long pause occurs between two beats (sino-atrial Wenckebach). This is very similar in appearance to sinus arrest
● Long pauses occur regularly following multiple normal PP cycles. Whilst this most frequently happens every 3–4 beats and has little effect on the pulse rate, the pulse rate will be halved if it occurs with alternate beats

Third-degree SA block (commonly known as 'sinus arrest') is characterised by cardiac standstill for varying periods of time. Escape beats from the atria, AV node or ventricles then take over pacemaker function (escape rhythm).

Since, in most patients, the right coronary artery supplies the sinus node, SA block is particularly common following acute inferior myocardial infarction. Drugs may sometimes be implicated.

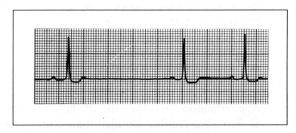

Fig. 9.1 ECG: SA block

No treatment is required if the pauses are short and asymptomatic, but dropped beats are often felt by the patient, and syncope may accompany prolonged pauses. If drugs are responsible, the dose should be reduced or completely stopped. Atropine, isoprenaline and pacing may occasionally be required, as for sinus bradycardia.

Junctional bradycardia (Figure 9.2)

The AV junction is the second major site of impulse formation. If the sinus node fails to initiate an impulse, and no other focus arises in the atria, the AV junction takes over the pacemaker function. This most commonly arises following acute myocardial infarction, particularly if the patient is acidotic or hypoxic. AV junctional rhythms are relatively slow (40–60 beats per minute) but may speed up by enhanced automaticity to produce relative junctional tachycardias (60–100 beats per minute), or junctional tachycardias (> 100 beats per minute).

If junctional rhythm is present, the atria and ventricles may be stimulated at the same time by the nodal pacemaker. The stimulus passes normally into the ventricles, producing a normal QRS complex, but there is also retrograde activation of the atria by the same impulse, such that a P wave may appear slightly before, after or buried in the QRS complex, depending upon the velocity of forward (antegrade) and backward (retrograde) conduction. The retrograde spread of the atrial impulse may also be recognised by the shape of the P wave, which is abnormal and usually inverted.

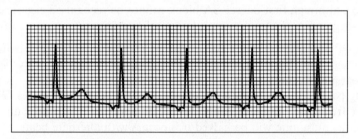

Fig. 9.2   ECG: junctional bradycardia, lead aVF. The junctional focus has also activated the atria, as shown by the fact that each ventricular complex is preceded by an inverted P wave

Because the atria and ventricles beat simultaneously, atrial contraction takes place against closed mitral and tricuspid valves. Blood is then pumped backwards into the superior vena cava, resulting in giant venous 'v' waves in the venous pulse. This dysrhythmia is usually short lived, and no treatment is required apart from stopping any medication that may be depressing the Sinus node. Atropine or isoprenaline may restore sinus rhythm, if necessary.

HEART BLOCK

Heart block exists when conduction from the atria to the ventricles is either slowed down or completely blocked. The conduction disturbance may arise within or just below the AV node (high block) or below the divisions of the bundle of His and involving the bundle branches (low block). Inter-His and multisite blocks may occur. Heart block usually results in bradycardia, with or without hypotension, and a reduced cardiac output. Alternatively, there may be ventricular standstill and sudden death.

Heart block complicates approximately 10% of cases of acute myocardial infarction. Inferior infarction is usually associated with high block, and anterior infarction is associated with low block.

Atrioventricular (AV) block

Atrioventricular heart block may be transient, intermittent or permanent, and the dysfunction has been classified as first-, second- or third-degree AV block.

First-degree heart block (Figure 9.3)

During first-degree heart block, the impulse passing from the atria to the ventricles is delayed at the AV node (or rarely in the atria or bundle of His), resulting in prolongation of the PR interval. The PR interval varies with age but does not usually exceed 0.2 second. First-degree heart block is asymptomatic, since it produces no change in heart rate, and the abnormality may only be appreciated electrocardiographically. It complicates up to 14% of acute myocardial infarcts and is more common with inferior myocardial infarction. Any cause of increased parasympathetic (vagal) tone, e.g. carotid sinus massage, can delay AV conduction and prolong the PR interval. Drugs, such as digoxin, diltiazem and beta-blockers, that affect the AV node may also produce first-degree heart block.

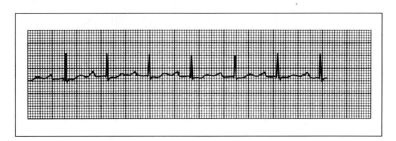

Fig. 9.3   ECG: first-degree AV block

Second-degree heart block

This is a partial AV block, which results in some atrial impulses failing to reach the ventricles. It is usually asymptomatic, unless it is associated with a slow ventricular rate.

There are two clinically-recognised types of second-degree heart block, although histological and electrophysiological distinctions are not quite so clear cut.

Mobitz Type I (Wenckebach) AV block (Figure 9.4)

This is the more common (90% of cases) form of second-degree heart block. Each successive stimulus from the atria finds it more difficult to pass through the AV junction, reflected as a progressive prolongation of the PR interval on the ECG. Eventually, the stimulus is unable to pass through to the ventricles, and the atrial P wave is not followed by a QRS complex. When the next atrial impulse arrives at the AV junction, it is able to pass through normally, since conductivity is restored, and the cycle then repeats. The frequency of dropped beats varies, and they may be numerous or very few.

This dysrhythmia often complicates inferior myocardial infarction and may precede complete heart block.

Other causes include electrolyte imbalance or drugs that suppress AV conduction, such as digoxin and diltiazem.

Mobitz Type II AV block (Figure 9.5)

Here, the AV junction does not respond to every atrial stimulus because of infranodal blockade. The PR interval is constant and the pulse regular, although the QRS complex is often widened because simultaneous blockade of the bundle branches often coexists. This is why this form of block is more serious, being associated with slow ventricular rates, Stokes–Adams attacks and sudden death. The observed rhythm may be called 2:1 or 4:1 heart block, to denote the ratio of atrial to ventricular beats.

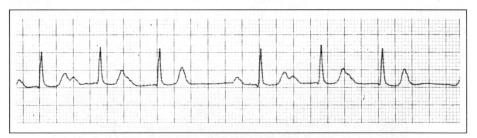

Fig. 9.4   ECG: second-degree AV block (Mobitz type I)

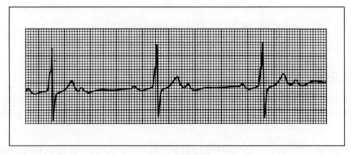

Fig. 9.5   ECG: second-degree AV block (Mobitz type II), with 2:1 AV conduction

This type of heart block is always associated with advanced myocardial disease and often progresses to complete heart block or asystole. Pacemaker insertion is usually necessary.

Third-degree (complete) heart block (Figure 9.6)

In complete heart block, atrial impulses are totally blocked, either at or below the AV junction. An escape rhythm takes over from within the distal AV node, the His–Purkinje system or the ventricles. P waves occur regularly but have no relationship to the slower ventricular QRS complexes. Complete heart block can also occur with atrial fibrillation, in which case there are no P waves, and it can then only be recognised by appreciation of the ectopic ventricular pacemaker, which will be slow and with abnormal QRS morphology.

The heart rate and QRS morphology vary in complete heart block, depending upon the origin of the secondary pacemaker. If the block is within the AV node, the QRS complex is usually normal, unless there is coexistent bundle branch block. However, if the block is infranodal, the ectopic pacemaker usually arises in either the left or right bundle, producing widened QRS complexes at a slower rate. In general, the lower down the conducting system that the secondary pacemaker arises, the slower the rate, the wider the complex and the higher the associated mortality. Lower pacemakers are often irregular, with a propensity to interposed ventricular ectopic beats and ventricular standstill.

Following acute inferior infarction, the pacemaker is usually high nodal and develops slowly following first- and second-degree heart block. The rate is usually regular and haemodynamically stable, at 40–60 beats per minute. However, complete heart block following acute anterior myocardial infarction is more serious and is associated with a high (75%) mortality. Blockade in these cases usually results from infarction of the bundle branches, and escape rhythms originate low down in the ventricles. As such, they are slow (less than 45 beats/minute) and irregular, and their onset often occurs without warning.

Complete heart block may be asymptomatic if there is a fast regular ventricular escape rhythm, and not all cases of AV block require pacing (Jowett et al, 1989). Drugs affecting AV conduction, such as digoxin, diltiazem and beta-adrenergic blocking agents, should be stopped.

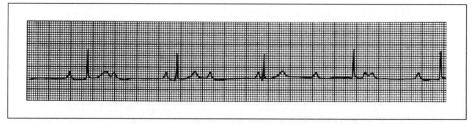

Fig. 9.6   ECG: third-degree AV block

In patients without myocardial infarction, fibrosis of the AV junction is the most common cause of complete heart block. It is probably a degenerative process and predominantly affects men.

First- and second-degree (Wenckebach) block usually require observation only. Cardiodepressant drugs should be stopped. Mobitz type II heart block carries a poor prognosis and needs pacing. Symptomatic heart block requires temporary pacing, although an atropine bolus or isoprenaline infusion may help as a temporary measure to raise the ventricular rate. Pacemakers and indications for permanent cardiac pacing are discussed in detail in Chapter 11.

Atrioventricular dissociation (Figure 9.7)

Atrioventricular dissociation (AVD) is a non-specific term used when the atria and ventricles are activated by independent pacemakers, the ventricular rate being the same or slightly faster than the atrial rate. The rhythm is mostly regular and manifests as normal P waves that bear no relation to the QRS complexes. As the atrial rate is slower than the ventricular rate, the P-P interval is longer than the R-R interval, and the P waves gradually overtake, or 'march through', the QRS complexes; the PR interval diminishes, until the P wave becomes superimposed upon the QRS complex and eventually appears on the other side. When the P wave is far enough beyond the QRS complex, the sinus beat will 'capture' the next QRS complex, resulting in an early PQRST complex. Hence, AVD should always be expected when the PR interval progressively shortens. Occasionally, synchronous discharge of the atria and ventricles will result in the two impulses meeting and interfering with each other's progress, resulting in a wide, abnormal QRS complex or 'fusion beat'. Demonstrating AVD is very important in the diagnosis of ventricular tachycardia (see p. 230).

AVD is usually benign but is often confused with complete heart block, as both show independent atrial and ventricular activity. However, in AVD, the ventricular rate is faster than the atrial rate, and there is no block at the AV junction, unless both the ventricular and atrial impulse stimulate the AV node at the same time, when it will become refractory.

AVD is usually precipitated by drugs or myocardial infarction. No treatment is required, unless drugs are the underlying cause, when these should be withdrawn.

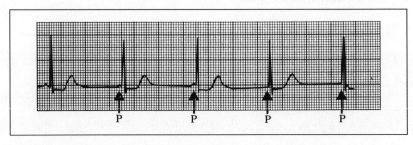

Fig. 9.7   ECG: atrioventricular dissociation, with respective atrial and ventricular rates of 49 and 51 per minute. The last two P waves are covered by superimposed QRS waves

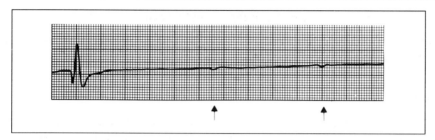

Fig. 9.8 ECG: ventricular asystole. The arrows indicate residual atrial complexes

Ventricular standstill and asystole (Figure 9.8)

If impulses fail to reach the ventricles, or impulse formation ceases, ventricular standstill results. If the problem is primarily in the conduction system, atrial P waves may continue to occur, but there will be no ventricular activity unless a ventricular pacemaker takes over. If this does not happen, the ventricles are left without electrical stimulation, and ventricular standstill occurs. There is no cardiac output, and cardiac arrest results. More often, no electrical activity (either atrial or ventricular) is seen, and the term asystole is used.

This form of cardiac arrest has a poor prognosis and has many causes, such as metabolic acidosis, electrolyte imbalance, hypoxia and drugs, apart from acute myocardial infarction. About 25% of in-hospital and 10% of out-of-hospital cardiac arrests are due to asystole. It complicates up to 14% of cases of acute myocardial infarction admitted to coronary care, and the mortality exceeds 90%. Management is for cardiac arrest, as described in Chapter 10.

Following cardiac arrest, an apparent rhythm called 'dying heart rhythm' is sometimes seen terminally. True stimulation of the heart does not occur, and irregular, bizarre complexes continue for several minutes, even though the patient is dead. For this reason, it may be better to turn the monitor off if relatives are present.

THE TACHYCARDIAS

An increase in pulse rate (tachycardia) is the normal response of the heart to increased physical work, so that cardiac output may be increased. However, abnormal tachycardias are often associated with a diminished cardiac output. At different heart rates, systolic timing remains remarkably constant, so that increases in heart rate occur at the expense of diastolic timing. Since ventricular filling takes place in diastole, ventricular filling time falls as the heart rate increases, and hence cardiac output is diminished. Furthermore, since coronary blood flow takes place during diastole, coronary insufficiency may result, causing ischaemic chest pain. Symptoms provoked by tachycardia may thus include angina, dyspnoea, palpitation or syncope.

Mechanisms of tachycardias

Most tachycardias are produced by one of two pathophysiological mechanisms: re-entry or enhanced automaticity.

Re-entry

Re-entry may occur within the atria or the ventricles or may involve the AV junction. A circuit exists by the presence of two or more conduction pathways with different electrical characteristics. This is best understood by explaining the mechanism in relation to junctional tachycardias.

Junctional tachycardias are caused by the circulation of an impulse between the atria and the ventricles ('circus movement' or 're-entry'). This occurs if there are two separate connections between the atria and the ventricles, one allowing forward (antegrade) conduction and the other allowing return (retrograde) conduction. In the minority of cases, this is due to an anatomically-separate conduction pathway, such as occurs in the Wolff–Parkinson–White or Lown–Ganong–Levine syndrome (AV re-entry tachycardias). However, most are caused by the establishment of a circuit within, or around, the AV node itself (AV nodal re-entry tachycardias). These are probably caused by part of the node becoming refractory, allowing a bypass circuit to be established around itself (Figure 9.9).

The rapid passage of the circulating impulse between the atria and ventricles results in what is sometimes called a 'reciprocating tachycardia'.

Enhanced automaticity

Automaticity describes the inherent ability of specialised cardiac tissue to initiate electrical impulses. The cells responsible are known as pacemaker or automatic cells. In the sinus node, these will discharge spontaneously at about 80 times per minute, but elsewhere automatic cells have a slower discharge rate. For example, in the AV node, this may be at about 60 times per minute, and within the ventricles, 30 times per minute. This back-up system of 'escape rhythms' exists to prevent rhythm failure should the sinus node fail to discharge. In this instance, an alternative pacemaker usually takes over, and although the rate will initially be slow, there is a tendency for the rate of this abnormal pacemaker to speed up because of 'enhanced automaticity'. When an ectopic site takes over pacemaker function, it is denoted by the prefix 'idio', for example idionodal tachycardia and idioventricular tachycardia.

Attempting to terminate these dysrhythmias using drugs that suppress re-entry circuits (e.g. verapamil) will be ineffective, although the ventricular response may be slowed.

Narrow-complex tachycardias

The main abnormal narrow-complex tachycardias are junctional tachycardias, atrial flutter and atrial fibrillation. Each may present acutely as a sustained or paroxysmal tachycardia. Treatment is usually directed towards the restoration of

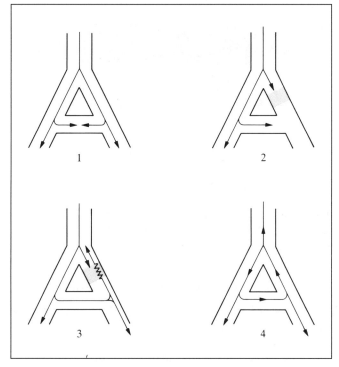

Fig. 9.9 Circus movement during re-entry tachycardia
(1) Normal electrical conduction through a common proximal piece of tissue, which splits into two pathways.
(2) A unidirectional block develops in one limb of tissue (possibly because of a slowing in the refractory period) and this fails to conduct the impulse. The other pathway conducts normally.
(3) The normal conduction wave is carried round to the proximal side of the block, which, if it has recovered functionally, will transmit the impulse in a retrograde direction.
(4) If the normal limb of tissue has recovered, it can be stimulated by the returning impulse and a circus movement about the area of conducting tissue is set up, which is self-propagating. This gives rise to a re-entrant dysrhythmia.

sinus rhythm, although in chronic or unstable rhythms, treatment aims to control the ventricular rate. Other atrial causes of fast or irregular pulses include sinus tachycardia and multiple ectopic beats.

Junctional tachycardias

Sometimes it is not possible to determine the exact atrial rhythm during tachycardias unless specialised leads are used. Whilst narrow-complex tachycardias are commonly labelled 'supraventricular tachycardias' (SVTs) (Figure 9.10), they incorporate both ventricular and atrial myocardium within the circuit (with the exception of a true atrial tachycardia), and the term 'junctional tachycardia' is a better term. The dysrhythmia is characterised by the sudden onset of a tachycardia greater than 150 beats per minute. In some patients, there may be no symptoms, but in the context of acute myocardial infarction, there is often ischaemic pain, dyspnoea or syncope.

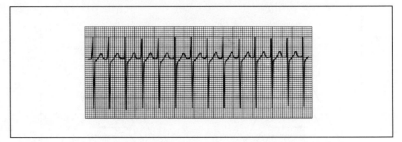

Fig. 9.10 ECG: junctional tachycardia

There are three forms of junctional tachycardia:

● AV nodal re-entry tachycardia (AVNRT)
● AV re-entry (reciprocating) tachycardia (AVRT)
● True paroxysmal atrial tachycardia (PAT)

AV nodal re-entry tachycardia (AVNRT)

Most junctional tachycardias are due to AV nodal re-entry. AVNRTs originate from a focus within, or immediately adjacent to, the AV node. The re-entry circuit usually comprises a slow forward limb and a fast retrograde limb, resulting in almost simultaneous atrial and ventricular activation. The ECG shows rapid normal QRS complexes at a rate of 160–220 beats per minute, with the P wave buried in the QRS complex. The onset (if recorded) is usually associated with a premature atrial beat, which conducts to the ventricles with a prolonged PR interval.

AV re-entry tachycardia (AVRT)

AVRTs are associated with the presence of an accessory AV connection or pathway, such as the bundle of Kent in the Wolff–Parkinson–White syndrome. This diagnosis is often made from the sinus rhythm ECG (short PR interval and delta wave). During the tachycardia, antegrade conduction occurs through the AV node, and the retrograde pathway is through the extranodal accessory pathway. Atrial and ventricular activation are thus separated in time, which results in the P wave occurring between the QRS complexes. The rate is typically 150–250 beats per minute, with a 1:1 AV conduction relationship. The P waves may be difficult to see, but brief interruptions of the tachycardia (for example by carotid sinus massage) may be very helpful.

Paroxysmal atrial tachycardia (Figure 9.11)

The term paroxysmal atrial tachycardia (PAT) was often incorrectly applied to AVNRTs in the past. True paroxysmal atrial tachycardia is much less common and is caused by the rapid discharge of an atrial pacemaker arising from one or more foci in the atria (usually the interatrial septum). An intra-atrial re-entry

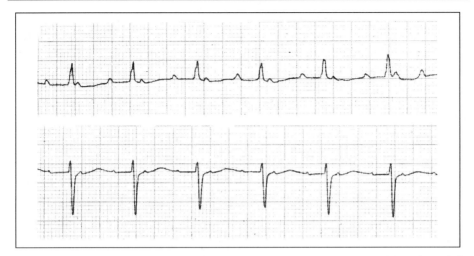

Fig. 9.11 ECG: atrial tachycardia with 2:1 AV block (leads AVF and V1). Atrial rate is 175/min

circuit is usually present, although a few cases of atrial tachycardia may be caused by enhanced automaticity of an atrial focus that speeds up. Second- or third-degree atrioventricular block is often present, so the ventricular response is usually not rapid and causes little systemic upset. Whilst 'PAT with block' is described classically in relation to digitalis toxicity, this is only the case in about 10% of episodes.

The treatment of junctional tachycardias

The urgency of treatment depends upon symptoms. Cardiac output falls as the heart rate rises, due to loss of atrial transport. Ischaemic pain may be produced, and in the peri-infarction period, ventricular work must be limited to prevent infarct extension.

Carotid sinus massage may terminate re-entry tachycardias or increase AV block to allow differentiation from atrial flutter (see Figure 9.12). The carotid sinus is located anterior to the sternomastoid muscle, at the upper level of, or just above, the thyroid cartilage. The carotid artery is massaged against the transverse process of the 6th vertebra for 10–20 seconds by direct (and sometimes uncomfor-

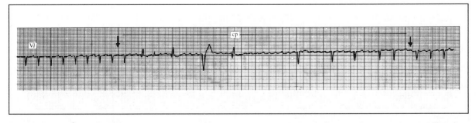

Fig. 9.12 ECG: SVT slowed by pressure on the carotid sinus (cp = carotid pressure). This has increased block at the AV node, showing that the underlying rhythm is atrial flutter

table) pressure. Other methods of vagal stimulation are the Valsalva manoeuvre, splashing cold water on the face or stimulation of the soft palate (the gag reflex).

Electrical cardioversion is the treatment of choice if there is rapid haemodynamic deterioration, regardless of prior digitalisation.

Drug treatment is usually very effective, and long-term treatment should be considered for repeated and poorly-tolerated attacks. The drug of choice for acute narrow-complex tachycardias is adenosine, particularly if there is left ventricular dysfunction or hypotension (Garratt et al, 1992). Adenosine is sometimes used in broad-complex tachycardias if they are thought to be due to an aberrantly-conducted supraventricular tachycardia. It may induce atrial fibrillation or even asystole, which is usually short lived. Flushing or transient chest pain may occur. When given to patients in sinus rhythm, adenosine may reveal otherwise latent pre-excitation (e.g. Wolff–Parkinson–White syndrome).

A bolus injection of verapamil (5–10 mg) may be preferable in patients with asthma (adenosine can cause bronchospasm) and usually restores sinus rhythm within 2 minutes in over 90% of cases. It should never be given for broad-complex tachycardias.

Beta-blockers are often successful but should be avoided if there is cardiac failure or in patients who have been pretreated by verapamil. Refractory tachycardias usually respond to amiodarone. Overdrive or underdrive cardiac pacing may be effective in selected cases.

Atrial flutter (Figure 9.13)

During atrial flutter, the atria contract at a rate of 220–350 (usually about 300) beats per minute, in response to a macro re-entry circuit within the atrium. The ECG shows flutter (F) waves, which have a saw-tooth appearance in the inferior leads. Leads V1 and V2 often appear to show large, discrete biphasic P waves. Flutter waves may be obscured by the QRST complex if the rate is very fast, and because atrial activity is concealed, sinus tachycardia of 150 beats per minute may be diagnosed. In such cases, flutter waves may be revealed by carotid sinus massage, which will transiently increase AV blockade and slow the ventricular response. If this is not effective, alternate F waves should be sought, which are often found hidden in the preceding T wave. This may be confirmed by measuring the interval between the P wave and the following T wave peak. It should be precisely the same as the interval between the T wave peak and the following P wave.

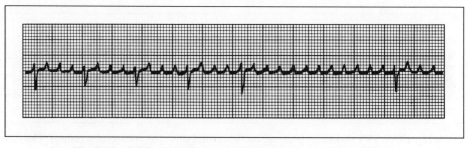

Fig. 9.13   ECG: atrial flutter, with varying degrees of AV block

Although the AV node can respond to atrial rates of about 300 beats per minute, there is usually some degree of AV blockade. In the healthy AV node unaffected by drugs, this results in a ventricular rate of about 150 beats per minute (i.e. there is 2:1 block). Higher degrees of AV blockade usually occur in the presence of drugs or when there is damage to the conducting system, although 3:1 conduction is unusual. Whilst the pulse is usually regular, AV conduction ratios may vary, giving rise to varying RR intervals on the ECG and an irregular pulse. Exercise decreases AV blockade and may lead to a doubling of the pulse rate. As a result, the apparently normal patient with a pulse rate of 75 beats per minute may feel faint on exercise when switching from 4:1 block to 2:1 conduction. During 2:1 conduction, ventricular conduction may become aberrant, and the widened QRS complexes may give the appearance of ventricular tachycardia.

Atrial flutter is unstable and should always be converted to sinus rhythm, unless it has been present for years. Carotid sinus massage will not usually restore sinus rhythm but may reveal the true nature of the atrial dysrhythmia by increasing AV block, allowing flutter waves to be seen more easily. Verapamil can also be used to increase AV block temporarily, and it produces sinus rhythm in 20% of cases. Otherwise, the treatment of atrial flutter is the same as for atrial fibrillation. DC cardioversion is especially useful.

Atrial fibrillation (Figure 9.14)

Paroxysmal or sustained atrial fibrillation is one of the most common cardiac dysrhythmias. It is more frequent with increasing age, affecting about 2% of people over 60 years of age. It complicates between 10 and 15% of myocardial infarcts and is associated with a poor prognosis (reflecting cardiac failure from extensive myocardial damage).

During atrial fibrillation, normal atrial contraction is replaced by a disorganised and continuous series of irregular fibrillation waves (350–600 per minute), caused by multiple and changing micro re-entry circuits. Myocardial contraction is ineffective for atrial emptying, and the atria remain functionally in diastole. Because the ventricles are incompletely filled by atrial systole prior to ventricular contraction, the presence of atrial fibrillation reduces cardiac output by about 10–20%.

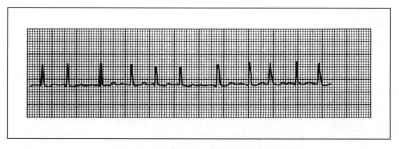

Fig. 9.14 ECG: atrial fibrillation

Although atrial fibrillation makes the heart less efficient, the most important consequence is that of thromboembolism, especially stroke. The incidence of peripheral embolisation is particularly high in patients with paroxysmal atrial fibrillation, atrial infarction or rheumatic heart disease.

The ECG in atrial fibrillation shows the replacement of P waves by small irregular undulations of the baseline (f waves), which represent the only evidence of atrial activity. These are not always visible in all leads. At fast heart rates, the ventricular response becomes more regular, and f waves are usually not visible. Differentiation from a nodal tachycardia may then be difficult, and often it is only a slight irregularity in the ventricular rate that allows the correct diagnosis to be made. Sometimes, the f waves are very coarse and may be mistaken for normal P waves or flutter waves. If the atrial f waves have a rate of more than 350 per minute, atrial fibrillation is more likely, particularly if the ventricular response is totally irregular. The ventricular response in the untreated patient is usually at a rate of about 100–180 beats per minute, and the QRS is normal, except when the rate is so fast that aberrant conduction occurs.

Atrial fibrillation complicating myocardial infarction is often transient, and it may be enough to control the ventricular rate with a small dose of beta-blocker, if required. Digoxin should probably be avoided, because its positive inotropic activity may worsen acute ischaemia.

In patients with atrial fibrillation of more than a few days' duration, the risks of embolisation following cardioversion (either electrically or pharmacologically) is 3–5%. Prior anticoagulation is, therefore, advisable.

If atrial fibrillation is producing haemodynamic deterioration, intravenous amiodarone or DC cardioversion should be considered. The energy required to cardiovert atrial fibrillation is very variable (100–360 J), and treatment with drugs may be needed before, during or after cardioversion; maintenance of sinus rhythm could be by amiodarone or sotolol (plus disopyramide or flecainide, if needed). Patients taking disopyramide or flecainide should be initially monitored to look for pro-arrythmic effects of the drug in the peri-infarction period.

Sinus tachycardia

Sinus tachycardia is arbitrarily defined as a sinus rhythm greater than 100 beats per minute and commonly ranges between 100 and 150 beats per minute. The P waves are normal and have a 1:1 relationship with the QRS complexes. The PR and QT intervals decrease as the heart rate increases, such that, during tachycardia, the P wave tends to merge with the preceding T wave. It may then be difficult to ascertain whether the rhythm is arising from the sinus node or elsewhere, but there may be clues. During sinus tachycardia, the heart rate is usually less than 140 beats per minute at rest and varies with respiration (sinus arrhythmia). The tachycardia does not start or finish abruptly. 'Sinus' rates of 150 beats per minute are, on closer inspection, usually due to atrial flutter with 2:1 block.

A sinus tachycardia is found in one third of patients with acute myocardial infarction and represents an attempt to maintain cardiac output in the face of reduced stroke volume. The tachycardia may be worsened by fear, anxiety or pain.

A sinus tachycardia may be a sign of impending left ventricular failure. Incipient heart failure is more likely in the presence of tachypnoea, a wide pulse pressure and a loud first heart sound.

Adequate analgesia will often settle a sinus tachycardia following myocardial infarction and also helps with associated anxiety. The use of intravenous beta-blockade has been shown to improve prognosis in patients with acute myocardial infarction (ISIS-1, 1988); limiting heart rate and myocardial work may reduce infarct size, as well as myocardial oxygen consumption. The mortality of patients with sinus tachycardia is higher than for those with sinus bradycardia, and death is usually due to left ventricular failure (Bigger et al, 1977). Beta-blocking agents should, therefore, be given in small and frequent doses to reduce the pulse rate to about 60 beats per minute, and it is probably better to select an agent with a short duration of action (e.g. metoprolol), since it is not possible to anticipate which patients will react adversely. The ultra-short acting beta-blocker esmolol is safe and effective if there is any doubt about cardiac decompensation.

Atrial ectopic beats (Figure 9.15)

Atrial extrasystoles are very common in both health and disease and occur when an atrial focus discharges before the sinus pacemaker. Atrial ectopic beats (premature atrial contractions) are seen on the ECG as premature (often abnormally shaped) P waves, usually followed by normal QRS complexes. The further the ectopic focus is from the sinus node, the greater the abnormality in shape of the P wave and the shorter the PR interval. An incomplete compensatory pause follows the ectopic beat, because the premature impulse depolarises the SA node, which must recover before it is able to initiate another sinus beat. The PP interval between three consecutive P waves (i.e. two complete PQRST complexes) is only, therefore, slightly longer than the interval between two normal PQRST complexes. Complete compensatory pauses are a feature of ventricular ectopic beats.

Conduction of atrial impulses to the ventricles depends upon the recovery status of the AV node. If the atrial ectopic beat arises near the AV node (seen as an abnormal P wave and short PR interval), the AV node may be refractory. The

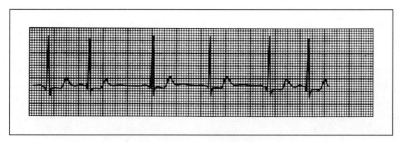

Fig. 9.15 ECG: atrial ectopic beats. Note that the ectopic P waves are slightly different from those of SA origin

impulse is, therefore, blocked, and no QRS follows. If the AV node is partially refractory, a prolonged PR interval is seen, because conduction of the ectopic beat is delayed. Other parts of the conducting system below the AV node may also be refractory, even when the AV node is able to convey the supraventricular impulse, and an aberrantly-conducted impulse is then seen on the ECG (see definition below).

Atrial ectopics are very commonly seen following acute myocardial infarction, often indicating sympathetic overactivity, hypoxia or anxiety. They are usually asymptomatic and cause no haemodynamic upset. With relief of pain, sedation and beta-blockade, they usually disappear, but where they reflect progressive atrial dilatation, treatment of heart failure is necessary. Atrial ectopics often precede reciprocating tachycardias by initiation of a re-entry circuit and may need treatment to prevent this.

> **Aberrant conduction** is the term applied when a widened and abnormal QRS complex is seen following a supraventricular impulse. It is the result of the unequal recovery periods of the right and left bundle branches. If a supraventricular stimulus is conducted to the bundles before both have recovered, bundle branch block will occur. This is usually of the right bundle branch block pattern, since the right bundle has a longer refractory period than the left bundle. Differentiating ventricular ectopic beats from aberrantly-conducted supraventricular beats may be difficult. With aberrantly-conducted beats, P waves may be seen, and the QRS is usually of the right bundle branch block pattern. In the chest lead V1, the R′ wave is larger than the secondary R wave (i.e. the right 'rabbit's ear' is longer). In contrast, ventricular ectopics usually show monophasic or biphasic QRS patterns in chest lead V1, and the left 'rabbit's ear' is larger. P waves are not seen, and the ectopic beat is followed by a full, rather than an incomplete, compensatory pause.

Idionodal tachycardia (Figure 9.16)

The normal discharge rate from the AV node is about 50–60 beats per minute. If there is suppression of sinus or atrial pacemaker function, the AV node may take over as the pacemaker. Because of enhanced automaticity, the rate may increase gradually to 70–100 beats per minute. The sinus node often continues to discharge at a slower rate, and there is a propensity to atrioventricular dissociation.

Idionodal rhythm arises as a consequence of sinus node depression following myocardial infarction, or secondary to drugs.

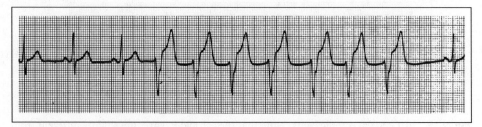

Fig. 9.16   ECG: accelerated idioventricular rhythm

VENTRICULAR DYSRHYTHMIAS

Ventricular dysrhythmias include ventricular ectopics (VEs), ventricular tachycardia (VT), ventricular flutter and ventricular fibrillation (VF). A number of factors predispose patients to the development of ventricular dysrhythmias following acute myocardial infarction, including myocardial ischaemia, electrolyte imbalance, acid/base abnormalities, hypoxia and drug therapy. The detection and prompt treatment of serious ventricular dysrhythmias was the primary reason for the creation of coronary care units.

Factors predisposing to ventricular dysrhythmias

Myocardial ischaemia

Myocardial ischaemia may result from occlusive or non-occlusive changes in the coronary vasculature that impair the blood supply to the myocardium. Ischaemia predisposes to cardiac dysrhythmias, regardless of whether or not myocardial necrosis takes place. Normal electrical conduction pathways may alter with ischaemia, providing a focus for dysrhythmias. Myocardial irritability following acute myocardial infarction is, of course, the major cause of ventricular dysrhythmia. Necrotic myocardial tissue provides a focus for this ectopic activity, and myocardial hypoxia associated with exaggerated catecholamine release compounds the situation.

Electrolyte and acid/base imbalance

A low serum potassium concentration is probably the most common electrolyte disturbance seen on the coronary care unit, and is usually associated with prior diuretic therapy, although the infarction itself may produce a transient fall in the serum potassium. This hypokalaemia probably reflects a catecholamine-induced shift of potassium into cells and may thus be a marker for the severity of the infarct. Hypokalaemia can lead to complex ventricular ectopic beats, ventricular tachycardia and, eventually, ventricular fibrillation. The risk of ventricular fibrillation is approximately 10-fold in patients with a serum potassium of less than 3 mmol/l following acute myocardial infarction, compared to those whose potassium level is greater than 4 mmol/l (Campbell et al, 1987). Potassium replacement depends upon the initial serum level and the urgency of the situation. The maximum safe intravenous infusion rate of potassium chloride is about 30 mmol/h. Potassium canrenoate can be given faster than other potassium salts (400 mg i.v. over 5 minutes) in urgent situations.

Hyperkalaemia may be found in those on ACE-inhibitors, in renal failure or because of acidaemia following cardiac arrest. The QRS widens, indicating an intraventricular conduction block. If untreated, the QRS duration continues to increase, and ventricular fibrillation ensues.

Intravenous calcium gluconate (10 ml of a 10% solution given over 3 minutes) will protect the heart from asystolic arrest, and glucose and insulin may then be used to control the serum potassium level.

The effect of drugs

Many drugs, both cardiovascular and non-cardiovascular, may predispose the patient to cardiac dysrhythmias. Furthermore, many drugs prescribed as antidysrhythmic agents may sometimes produce serious dysrhythmias (pro-dysrhythmic effect). Episodes of torsade de pointes may be precipitated by drugs that affect the QT interval, such as the Class 1 antidysrhythmic agents (disopyramide, quinidine and flecainide) and phenothiazines, as well as low levels of calcium, potassium and magnesium. It is likely that severe left ventricular dysfunction predisposes to this dysrhythmia, which is often self-terminating but may progress to ventricular fibrillation.

Ventricular ectopics (Figure 9.17)

Ventricular extrasystoles (premature ventricular complexes, PVCs) occur when an ectopic ventricular focus discharges prematurely anywhere within the His–Purkinje system or the ventricles. They can occur at any time in diastole. The QRS complex is premature, widened (>0.12 second), slurred and usually notched. There is no preceding P wave, and the following T wave usually points in the opposite direction.

Although infrequent ventricular ectopics do not adversely affect cardiac output, attention has previously been focused on them as 'warning dysrhythmias' (Lown et al, 1967). Ventricular ectopic beats that are frequent, multifocal, occurring in salvoes or showing the R-on-T phenomenon (ventricular ectopics occurring on the apex of the preceding T wave) are termed 'complex'. Such complex ventricular ectopics are often considered to be precursors of ventricular fibrillation. However, these warning dysrhythmias only occur in about half of patients who develop ventricular fibrillation (Noneman and Rodgers, 1978). In addition, successful abolition of these ventricular ectopics with lignocaine does not affect mortality, compared to those who are not treated (May et al, 1983). It is usual practice, now, to await the development of ventricular fibrillation and reverse this rapidly by cardioversion, although it is important to correct hypokalaemia and hypoxia. All patients with low serum potassium levels should also receive magnesium supplements.

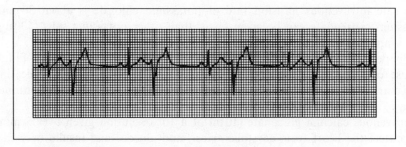

Fig. 9.17   ECG: ventricular ectopic beats (ventricular bigeminy)

Treatment of ventricular ectopic beats

Whilst no antidysrhythmic drug has yet been shown to decrease mortality when used to suppress ventricular ectopics (apart from beta-blockade), drug therapy should be considered for ventricular ectopics producing haemodynamic disturbances, repetitive short episodes of ventricular tachycardia and perhaps R-on-T ectopics (Surawicz, 1986). Clinical findings such as a persistent third heart sound, early heart failure and prolonged ST elevation may well be better predictors of malignant dysrhythmias. Lignocaine is probably the most frequently and most controversially-used prophylactic agent. Administration of lignocaine before hospital admission is probably not justified (Kertes and Hunt, 1984), and the intramuscular route of administration is, anyway, contraindicated because of thrombolytic therapy later on. Care is needed in the elderly and those with hypotension or conduction defects. Lignocaine may be of value following cardiac arrest due to ventricular fibrillation, to prevent recurrence, although the trend these days is to give smaller doses for shorter times (up to 12 hours). The incidence of side-effects if then very much reduced, without an apparent increase in further episodes of ventricular fibrillation.

Many other drugs (e.g. flecainide, encainide, mexiletine and moricizine) have been tried as prophylaxis against ventricular dysrhythmias, but short-term mortality does not seem to differ with or without treatment (Reiffel et al, 1994). Amiodraone may be the exception to this (CASCADE, 1993). The use of beta-blockade in the acute phase of myocardial infarction seems to reduce the incidence of serious dysrhythmias (attributable, in part, to their inherent antidysrhythmic properties), as well as limiting infarct size (Hjalmarson and Olsson, 1991). Sotalol may be of particular advantage where recurrent ventricular tachycardia or fibrillation has complicated myocardial infarction (Reiffel et al, 1994). Antidysrhythmic therapy is usually continued for about 3 months.

Serious ventricular dysrhythmias can occur after patients leave hospital, and these patients are difficult to identify. Early exercise stress tests, 24-hour monitoring or signal-averaged ECGs may be helpful in identifying patients at risk (see Chapter 13). Patients with ventricular aneurysms may benefit from surgery, as may those with chronic recurrent ventricular tachycardia. Scarred or ischaemic areas of the myocardium may act as a focus for dysrhythmias, and coronary artery bypass grafting, with or without removal of an irritable focus, may be of benefit (Anderson and Mason, 1983). Epicardial and endocardial mapping are often required to locate these areas, which can also be tackled non-invasively using low-energy radio-frequency ablation. Resistant, life-threatening dysrhythmias may be an indication for overdrive pacing or implantation of cardioverter defibrillators (see Chapter 14).

Parasystole (Figure 9.18)

Parasystole is a relatively uncommon dysrhythmia but is often seen following myocardial infarction, particularly in patients taking digoxin.

It is a dual rhythm, in which two pacemakers concurrently and independently govern the rhythm of the heart. During parasystole, an ectopic ventricular focus discharges regularly and competes with another focus, which may be in either the atria or the ventricles. The competition is usually with normal sinus rhythm, the

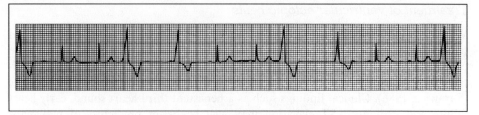

Fig. 9.18   ECG: parasystole

ventricular rhythm mostly being at a slightly faster rate. The interval between successive ventricular ectopic beats is the same or a multiple of that interval, and since this parasystolic focus is independent of the regular heart rhythm, there is no fixed relationship between the two rhythms, and the coupling interval (i.e. the interval between the ectopic beat and the sinus beat) varies.

It might be expected that the dominant pacemaker would take over cardiac rhythm and suppress the ectopic focus. However, during parasystole, the ectopic focus is protected by 'entrance block', a unidirectional block in the vicinity of the ectopic focus. Outward conduction from the ectopic focus is normal and forms the secondary pacemaker. Two pacemakers, therefore, exist, each discharging at its own independent rate and depolarising the myocardium if it is in a responsive state. If the two pacemakers discharge simultaneously, each activates the adjacent myocardium, and a 'fusion beat' will arise as the two discharge wavefronts collide. A QRS complex intermediate in appearance between a normal sinus beat and a ventricular ectopic results.

No treatment is required, and parasystole normally resolves spontaneously.

Ventricular tachycardia

Ventricular tachycardia (VT) is a life-threatening re-entry dysrhythmia, which may be defined as a succession of three or more beats arising from one or more foci in the ventricles at a rate of over 100 beats per minute. The QRS complexes are wide (>0.12 second) and regular, at a rate of 100–220 beats per minute. During ventricular tachycardia, the atria continue to beat and dissociated P waves may be seen (AV dissociation). The atrial rate is usually slower than the ventricular rate, as it originates at the sinus node. However, there may be coexistent atrial tachycardia, junctional rhythm or atrial fibrillation. Occasionally, ventricular beats may pass back through the AV node to stimulate the atria, and P waves then appear after the QRS complex. Fusion and capture beats may be present, which helps in distinguishing ventricular tachycardia from other broad-complex tachycardias.

- *Fusion beats* occur when a normal supraventricular stimulus meets a ventricular stimulus being conducted retrogradely. The resulting QRS complex looks partly like a normal QRS complex and partly like a ventricular ectopic beat
- *Capture beats* occur when an atrial stimulus arrives at a non-refractory AV node and is conducted normally to the ventricles. This results in a normal P wave followed by a normal (narrow) QRS complex

There are four types of ventricular tachycardia:

- Monomorphic ventricular tachycardia
- Polymorphic ventricular tachycardia
- Accelerated idioventricular tachycardia
- Ventricular flutter

Monomorphic ventricular tachycardia (Figure 9.19)

This is the most common form of ventricular tachycardia. The ventricular complexes are of uniform appearance (monomorphic), and each episode of ventricular tachycardia continues for a variable time, usually terminating in a long pause before sinus rhythm returns. Each paroxysm of tachycardia starts with a ventricular ectopic beat, which occurs at the same fixed interval from the previous QRS complex.

Polymorphic ventricular tachycardia (Figure 9.20)

Torsade de pointes ('turning of the points') is a dangerous polymorphic dysrhythmia characterised by paroxysms of ventricular tachycardia following a QRST complex with a prolonged QT interval. The QRS complexes undulate around the isoelectric line, with a marked change of amplitude occurring every 5–30 beats. The episodes may be precipitated by drugs that prolong the QT interval, such as Class 1 antidysrhythmic agents (quinidine, procainamide and disopyramide), phenothiazines or electrolyte imbalance (hypokalaemia, hypomagnesaemia or hypocalcaemia). A congenital prolongation of the QT interval (e.g. the Romano Ward syndrome) may occasionally be the cause. Torsade de pointes usually terminates spontaneously but may precede ventricular fibrillation.

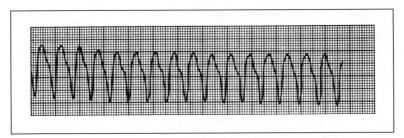

Fig. 9.19   ECG: monomorphic ventricular tachycardia

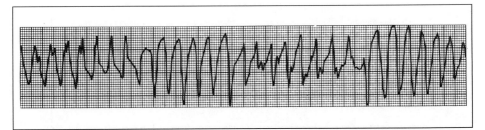

Fig. 9.20   ECG: torsade de pointes

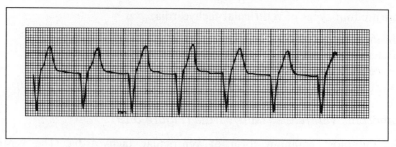

Fig. 9.21   ECG: idioventricular tachycardia

Accelerated idioventricular tachycardia (Figure 9.21)

When escape rhythms arise in the ventricles or His–Purkinje system, they are called idioventricular rhythms; they are usually slow, at about 60 beats per minute. Idioventricular rhythms often speed up, although the rate does not exceed 120 beats per minute. After about 30 beats, sinus rhythm usually takes over, although idioventricular tachycardia may be replaced by a sustained ventricular tachycardia or ventricular fibrillation.

Ventricular flutter (Figure 9.22)

This is characterised by a rapid ventricular rate of 180–250 beats per minute, in which it is not possible to differentiate the QRS complexes from the ST segments or T waves. The pattern of oscillating waves of large amplitude has been likened to rows of hair pins. It often precedes ventricular fibrillation.

The diagnosis of broad-complex tachycardias

Differentiating ventricular tachycardia from other broad-complex tachycardias is important, both in the management of the acute dysrhythmia and for long-term therapy to prevent recurrence.

Regular broad-complex tachycardias may be due to:

- Ventricular tachycardia
- Supraventricular tachycardia (SVT) with pre-existent bundle branch block
- SVT with rate-related bundle branch block

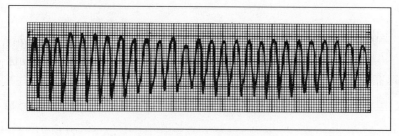

Fig. 9.22   ECG: ventricular flutter

Irregular broad-complex tachycardias may be due to:

● Atrial fibrillation with pre-existing bundle branch block
● Atrial fibrillation with rate-related bundle branch block
● Torsade de pointes

Ventricular tachycardia is often misdiagnosed as having a supraventricular origin (Dancy et al, 1985), which is of major concern, since treatment and prognosis are markedly different. Generally speaking, if the patient is known to have cardiac disease, the broad-complex tachycardia is due to ventricular tachycardia. If the patient is thought to have a normal heart, the tachycardia is likely to be supraventricular in origin.

Differentiation relies heavily on the demonstration of independent atrial and ventricular activity (AV dissociation). A full 12-lead ECG should always be recorded, providing the patient is well enough during the tachycardia. If the QRS in sinus rhythm is of normal duration, a QRS duration greater than 0.14 second indicates a ventricular origin of the tachycardia. Ventricular concordance (uniformly positive or negative QRS complexes) in the chest leads is virtually diagnostic of ventricular tachycardia. The RR interval is regular unless there are capture beats and, in contrast to supraventricular tachycardias (which are affected by respiration), does not vary by more than 0.04 second.

It is important to realise that the clinical condition of the patient is not helpful. Some patients tolerate ventricular tachycardia extremely well, whilst others may be severely haemodynamically compromised by a rapid supraventricular tachycardia. **If in doubt, broad-complex tachycardias should be treated as ventricular tachycardia.**

Guidelines for diagnosis are shown in Table 9.2.

Treatment of ventricular tachycardia

Treatment of ventricular tachycardia depends on the haemodynamic status of the

Table 9.2 Features of ventricular tachycardia

Clinically
● The venous pulse rate is slower than the arterial pulse rate
● There are irregular cannon waves seen in the venous pulse
● There is varying intensity of the first heart sound

In the 12-lead ECG
● There is left axis deviation (QRS < −30°)
● The QRS duration is >0.14 second (140 ms)
● There are multiple QRS morphologies
● There is concordance of the QRS vector in the chest leads (i.e. they are all in the same direction)
● In chest lead V1, the R wave is taller than the R[1] wave (the left 'rabbit's ear' is longer)
● Dissociated P waves may be seen (AV dissociation)
● Blocked, fusion and capture beats may be present
● There is a Q wave in V6 or a notch on the downstroke of the S wave in V1/V2

---

patient. Short salvoes do not usually require treatment. Hypokalaemia (and probably hypomagnesaemia) should be corrected.

Most sustained ventricular dysrhythmias are accompanied by moderate to severe haemodynamic decompensation and require rapid termination. The treatment of choice in such circumstances is cardioversion. An initial shock of no less than 100 J should be used; lesser charges may induce ventricular fibrillation. Where a defibrillator is not immediately available, a precordial blow is sometimes effective (Caldwell et al, 1985), as may coughing.

Stable ventricular tachydysrhythmias in the presence of good cardiac output and stable blood pressure can be treated either electrically or pharmacologically. An approach to the management of regular, acute, broad-complex tachycardias is shown in Figure 9.23.

Many antidysrhythmic drugs have been used for acute treatment and controlling of recurrent ventricular tachycardia, but lignocaine remains the first choice in most coronary care units. Although it is not the most effective of drugs, it is usually safe and has a short half-life (6 minutes). A 50–100 mg bolus is followed by a continuous infusion of 1–4 mg/min. Side-effects are rare and include dizziness, tremor and agitation. Amiodarone is highly effective and is a suitable second choice. Its long-term use must be carefully considered in view of the side-effect

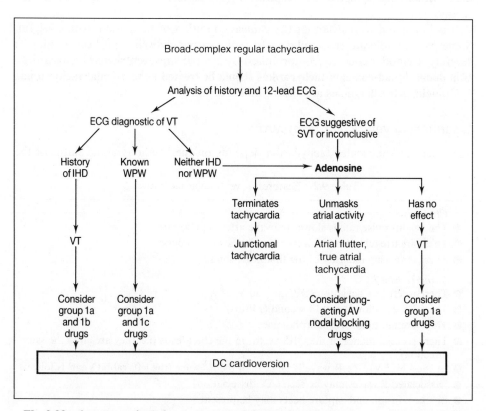

Fig. 9.23   An approach to the management of acute broad-complex regular tachycardia
WPW = Wolff–Parkinson–White syndrome

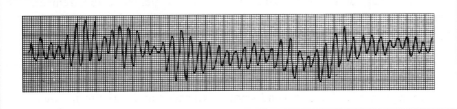

Fig. 9.24 ECG: ventricular fibrillation

profile (Shukla et al, 1994). Third choice drugs include flecainide, disopyramide and mexiletine. Bretylium is a final choice but may take 20–30 minutes for effect.

Special attention should be directed to concurrent drug therapy, particularly if the QT interval is prolonged. Torsade de pointes is often caused by antidysrhythmic therapy. Magnesium and potassium should be given, and consideration of isoprenaline infusion or atrial pacing, if needed.

Ventricular fibrillation (Figure 9.24)

Electrically and mechanically, the heart is completely disorganised when in ventricular fibrillation (VF), and cardiac arrest results. The ECG shows fine or coarse waves of irregular size, shape and rhythm. Fine VF may mimic asystole and produce an apparently flat line on the ECG.

About 90% of deaths following acute myocardial infarction are due to ventricular fibrillation, nearly half occurring in the first hour following onset of symptoms and most immediately (acute occlusional VF).

Primary VF describes fibrillation that occurs within the first 12 hours of acute myocardial infarction. It is usually associated with a good prognosis, as the heart is often still functioning well. Prophylaxis with lignocaine, beta-blockers and magnesium may reduce the incidence of primary ventricular fibrillation.

Reperfusional VF may occur following thrombolysis, but this probably reflects a good prognosis; the infarct-related artery has been opened.

Secondary or late VF describes fibrillation in hearts whose function has been severely compromised by the infarct (i.e. there is often heart failure or hypotension). The prognosis is poor.

The management of cardiac arrest from ventricular fibrillation is fully discussed in Chapter 10.

HEART FAILURE

Although very common complications of acute myocardial infarction, acute left ventricular failure and congestive heart failure are often the presenting problems of patients admitted directly to the coronary care unit. It is, therefore, important to have an understanding of both acute and acute-on-chronic heart failure.

Heart failure is a clinical syndrome that results from an inability of the heart to provide an adequate cardiac output for the body's metabolic requirements. The symptoms are not usually due to low cardiac output, but rather to the compensatory mechanisms that the body employs to maintain an adequate output. These compensatory responses include fluid retention and increased sympathetic activity, which may result in pulmonary and peripheral oedema. In the later stages, the heart adapts to increased intraventricular tension by dilatation and hypertrophy. These changes predispose to subendocardial ischaemia and may precipitate angina.

The prognosis of heart failure is poor, and the Framingham Heart Study showed that there was no evidence of improvement over the 40 years from 1948 to 1988. From the first onset of congestive heart failure symptoms, the median survival was 1.7 years in men and 3.2 years in women (Ho et al, 1993); the prognosis is, therefore, worse than for most cancers.

Fortunately, considerable progress has been made in the last few years in the understanding of the pathology of heart failure, as well as in the development of strategies that improve not only symptoms, but also prognosis. The aims of modern management of heart failure are based upon an accurate diagnosis, using simple non-invasive investigations, and institution of therapy to improve symptomatology, functional capacity, quality of life and prognosis.

Aetiology

Heart failure is usually caused by loss of myocardial tissue (as a result of myocardial infarction) or decreased myocardial contractility (as in ischaemia, hypertrophy or cardiomyopathy). A reduced cardiac output may result from dysrhythmias or from drugs that either depress myocardial contractility or produce salt and water retention (e.g. non-steroidal anti-inflammatory agents). Valvular disease and hypertension may also produce heart failure.

Whilst these causes of heart failure are usually associated with poor ventricular contraction, normal systolic function may be seen in some patients with heart failure. Diastolic dysfunction is often the earliest haemodynamic abnormality in patients with heart failure and can be the sole cause. Diastole is the energy-requiring relaxation phase of the cardiac cycle, and cardiac output is directly related to the end diastolic volume. Abnormal diastolic function may, therefore, have profound effects on cardiac output. It should be suspected in patients with normal-sized hearts and pulmonary congestion and is mainly prevalent in patients with long-standing hypertension or aortic valve disease. Diastolic dysfunction may be assessed non-invasively by echocardiography or nuclear scanning. Choosing appropriate therapy for heart failure will depend on whether the primary problem is systolic or diastolic dysfunction. Calcium-channel blockers are showing promise in treatment of the latter.

The response to heart failure

When the heart fails, several compensatory mechanisms are activated to maintain cardiac output and tissue perfusion. The fall in blood pressure caused by a diminished cardiac output stimulates the baroreceptors, which produces increased catecholamine secretion (leading to tachycardia and increased myocardial contractility).

However, the cardiac catecholamine supplies soon become exhausted, so selective arterial vasoconstriction redistributes the cardiac output. Flow to the gut and liver is reduced, so that supply to the heart and skeletal muscle can be increased. Dilatation of the heart causes a reflex increase in cardiac output, as increased myofibril stretching increases the force of myocardial contraction (Starling's Law). With chronic heart failure, the left ventricle hypertrophies to maintain pump action. This latter compensation is counterproductive, since the increased left ventricular mass has impaired contractility and, additionally, has a higher metabolic requirement. Stroke volume falls as a result. A further adaptation is seen in the arterioles, particularly those supplying the skeletal muscle and kidneys. The vessel walls become oedematous and less responsive to circulating vasodilators, such as adenosine. As a consequence, systemic vascular resistance is high, and the reduced renal blood flow stimulates the renin–angiotensin system, leading to production of high levels of angiotensin II, which causes further widespread vasoconstriction, with sodium and water retention secondary to secretion of aldosterone. Whilst this maintains cardiac preload, oedema usually results.

Symptoms of heart failure

The signs and symptoms of heart failure are caused by reduced cardiac output (forward heart failure) and an increased venous pressure in the lungs and peripheries, because of inadequate ventricular emptying (backward failure).

An increased awareness of respiration is the usual presentation of left ventricular failure; dyspnoea is caused by increased pulmonary vascular engorgement, with decreased compliance of the lungs. Paroxysmal nocturnal dyspnoea results when nocturnal absorption of oedema fluid increases the intravascular volume, waking the patient with gasping respiration, cough and wheeze. Fatigue and lethargy are marked, caused by low blood flow to exercising muscles.

Heart failure has been graded according to exercise limitation by the New York Heart Association Criteria Committee (1964). Symptoms such as fatigue, palpitations, dyspnoea and angina are used to record the degree of symptomatic heart failure:

- Class I – Heart disease with no limitation on ordinary physical activity
- Class II – Slight limitation. Ordinary physical activity (e.g. walking) produces symptoms
- Class III – Marked limitation. Unable to walk on the level without disability. Less than ordinary activity produces symptoms
- Class IV – Dyspnoea at rest. Inability to carry out any physical activity

Acute left ventricle failure (pulmonary oedema)

Acute left ventricular failure often presents very suddenly and is usually associated with pulmonary oedema, as a result of transudation of fluid into the pulmonary alveoli. This occurs when the pulmonary capillary pressure rises, secondary to raised left atrial pressure, and exceeds the pulmonary oncotic pressure (25–30 mmHg). There is decreased air flow to and from the alveoli, because oedema of the pulmonary membranes causes airway narrowing. The lung compliance ('stiffness') increases, making breathing more difficult, and alveolar flooding reduces gaseous exchange within the alveoli. This leads to dyspnoea, with arterial hypoxaemia. Increased mucus production may precipitate cough and wheeze (cardiac asthma), and the sputum may be tinged with blood from small haemorrhages in the congested bronchial mucosa.

Right ventricular failure

Right ventricular failure usually occurs secondary to left heart failure but can occur alone following right ventricular infarction, pulmonary embolism, pulmonary valve disease or chronic lung disease (cor pulmonale).

Symptoms are due to pulmonary hypertension, which is associated with high systemic venous pressure. Oedema, with elevation of the JVP, is usual. The liver becomes engorged and enlarged and may be tender. Functional tricuspid incompetence occurs, and the dilated right ventricle often produces a right parasternal heave. Pleural effusions and ascites are common.

Treating heart failure

The aims of treatment are to relieve symptoms by:

- Increasing salt and water excretion
- Reducing intracardiac pressures and volume overload
- Increasing myocardial contractility

The underlying cause should, wherever possible, always be treated.

Following acute myocardial infarction, attention should be paid to correcting hypoxaemia, since it will further worsen impaired left ventricular function by increasing areas of critical myocardial ischaemia. Ventilatory function will already be compromised by the combined action of reduced pulmonary compliance, pulmonary vascular congestion and respiratory depression from injected opiates. Although assisting impaired left ventricular contraction with positive inotropes would seem logical first-line therapy, these may increase the size of the myocardial infarct. Overstimulation increases myocardial work in the areas of borderline perfusion. Treatment is, therefore, aimed at reducing intravascular volume with diuretics and using drugs to produce peripheral vasodilatation, to thus reduce afterload.

Bed-rest promotes a diuresis and reduces myocardial work. However, passive legs exercises are recommended, to prevent deep vein thrombosis.

Salt and water restriction may also be necessary, as well as avoiding any drug that may potentiate this (e.g. indomethacin).

Diuretics

Diuretics provide the mainstay of treatment for left ventricular failure. They inhibit sodium resorption by the kidney and reduce intravascular volume and hence cardiac preload. There is loss of sodium from arteriolar walls, allowing vasodilatation and a reduction in afterload. Potassium intake needs to be increased to prevent hypokalaemia, which may precipitate dysrhythmias.

Loop diuretics, such as bumetanide and frusemide, are the usual diuretics used for heart failure. Given intravenously, they reduce pulmonary venous pressure within 15 minutes. This is before the onset of diuresis and is probably due to a direct vasodilatory effect on the capillary beds. The reduction in pulmonary capillary pressure eases dyspnoea, and the reduction in left ventricular wall tension reduces left ventricular work and oxygen demand. It is important that filling pressures are not reduced too much by dehydrating the patient; a filling pressure of 12–18 mmHg is probably required to optimise left ventricular function.

In severe heart failure, the gut wall becomes oedematous, limiting absorption of orally-administered drugs; this may be compounded by slowed gut transit time, secondary to opiate therapy. A switch to intravenous diuretics is often rewarded with a diuresis. Overdiuresis should be avoided, since a depleted plasma volume will reactivate the renin–angiotensin system, again producing fluid retention and vasoconstriction.

Oral dopamine agonists (such as ibopamine) are being explored as an alternative to diuretics in heart failure, since they do not activate the renin–angiotensin system, but much work still needs to be done (Parker et al, 1993).

Vasodilators

There are many vasodilatory agents that may be used in the management of heart failure (Franciosa et al, 1984). Their haemodynamic effects depend on their ability to affect arterioles or venules (Table 9.3). The most important vasodilator group is the angiotensin converting enzyme (ACE) inhibitors.

ACE-inhibitors

The benefits of ACE-inhibitors for patients with congestive heart failure has been unequivocally demonstrated (Packer, 1992). They lower venous and arterial blood pressure and increase cardiac output and renal blood flow. Aldosterone levels fall, reducing fluid retention and allowing a reduction in the dose of diuretics. ACE-inhibitors have been shown to improve symptomatic well-being in patients with all grades of heart failure who remain symptomatic despite diuretic therapy, as well as improving their prognosis.

Their use may be limited by side-effects, including cough, renal impairment and symptomatic hypotension, but ACE-inhibitors should now be prescribed for all patients with heart failure who do not have contraindications.

The role of ACE-inhibitors following acute myocardial infarction. The early routine use of ACE-inhibitors in unselected patients following acute myocardial infarction has been addressed by three major studies (ISIS-4, 1995; GISSI-3, 1994). Broadly speaking, the studies show a small benefit with ACE-inhibitor administration in the first 24 hours, but this is probably brought about by greater benefits in high-risk patients and no effect in the rest of the study population.

Table 9.3 Commonly used vasodilators

Drug	Mechanism	Dosage	Onset of action	Precautions
Nitroprusside	Direct action	IV only 0.5–1 µg/kg/min Titrate for effect	Immediate	Sudden hypotension – requires close monitoring Cyanide and thiocyanate toxicity
Nitrates	Direct action	IV, SL, B, O, TD Wide range of doses	Minutes	Headache, flushing, hypotension
Hydralazine	Direct action	IV, 10–20 mg IM, 10–20 mg O, 25–100 mg tid	Minutes	Tachycardia may produce angina Lupus-like syndrome Blood dyscrasias
Prazosin	Alpha-adrenergic blocker	O, 0.5–5.0 mg tid	0.5–2 hr	First-dose hypotension Tachyphlyaxis in heart failure
Captopril	ACE-inhibitor	O, 6.25–50.00 mg tid	0.5–1.5 hr	First-dose hypotension Altered taste Rashes Proteinuria
Enalapril	ACE-inhibitor	2.5–40.0 mg daily	1–2 hr	Hypotension if patient is sodium depleted
Nifedipine	Calcium-channel blocker	O, 5–160 mg tid SL, 5 mg	15–30 min 2–5 min	Hypotension and tachycardia Headache Ankle oedema Negative inotropic effect in high doses
Nicardipine	Calcium-channel blocker	O, 20–30 mg tid	30–60 min	As nifedipine, but little inotropic effect

IV = intravenous; IM = intramuscular; B = buccal; O = oral; SL = sublingual; TD = transdermal.

In patients with asymptomatic left ventricular dysfunction following acute myocardial infarction, ACE-inhibitors probably prevent progression to overt heart failure but may not improve survival (SOLVD Investigators, 1992; Sweberg et al, 1992).

For patients with overt heart failure or significant left ventricular damage (an ejection fraction under 40% of normal) following recent myocardial infarction, the results of the SAVE (Pfeffer et al, 1992) and AIRE (AIRE Investigators, 1993) studies are clear: ACE-inhibition should be commenced within 1 week of myocardial infarction to reduce mortality and serious subsequent cardiovascular events (St John Sutton, 1994).

Other vasodilators

Hydralazine raises cardiac output by arteriolar vasodilatation but may produce reflex tachycardia. This would be unhelpful in increasing myocardial work and oxygen consumption.

Nitrates predominantly affect venous capacitance vessels. Intravenous nitrates are particularly helpful in acute left ventricular failure to reduce cardiac preload.

Sodium nitroprusside is often used for the treatment of acute left ventricular failure and mitral incompetence following acute myocardial infarction. It is particularly useful in hypertensive heart failure. Administration requires close supervision.

Calcium-channel blocking agents may be useful in heart failure, particularly if it is complicated by hypertension. Usually, there is a favourable acute response, but long-term results with drugs such as verapamil and nifedipine have been disappointing, possibly because of negative inotropic activity. In contrast, the second-generation calcium antagonists, such as nicardipine and amlodipine, have little cardiodepressant activity and may prove to be beneficial in the long term.

Positive inotropic agents

Logically, the use of positively-acting inotropic agents should be of value in the treatment of heart failure to promote cardiac output. However, most drugs tried so far have been associated with decreased survival in the long term (Wilmshurst, 1993). Inotropic support may be of value in the short term in patients following acute myocardial infarction or cardiac surgery or for those awaiting operation (including transplantation).

Digoxin

The role of digoxin in heart failure, particularly following acute myocardial infarction, remains controversial (*Lancet*, 1989). In those with chronic heart failure, digoxin will reduce the diuretic requirements and improve symptoms and exercise time, regardless of whether or not the patient is in atrial fibrillation. It is not as potent as the ACE-inhibitors in this respect and should, therefore, be an optional add-in therapy, after diuretics and ACE-inhibitors, for patients in sinus rhythm.

Beta-adrenergic agonists

Whilst short-term haemodynamic improvements may be seen in patients with heart failure, long-term use of beta-adrenergic agonists is limited by peripheral vasoconstriction (Table 9.4). Dopamine and dobutamine are relatively cardioselective beta-1 stimulants and are especially useful in patients with heart failure and cardiogenic shock following myocardial infarction. Significant vasoconstriction is, fortunately, only present with higher doses of dopamine, allowing the benefits of positive inotropism to improve renal perfusion and cardiovascular haemodynamics. Dobutamine is similar and does not seem to affect the pulse rate so much.

Phosphodiesterase-inhibitors

Enoximone and milrinone are phosphodiesterase-inhibitors marketed for short-term intravenous use in patients with heart failure on intensive care units. They strengthen cardiac contraction and dilate peripheral vessels, reducing ventricular preload and afterload with little effect on blood pressure. Whilst they may be useful in the short term, there is no evidence that they improve survival. On the contrary, the PROMISE (Prospective Randomised Milrinone Survival) study, which used oral milrinone, was terminated prematurely because of a 27% excess death rate in the treated group (Packer et al, 1991).

Anticoagulants

Anticoagulants should be considered for patients with enlarged hearts, dysrhythmias or generally poor left ventricular function. This last group are prone to deep vein thrombosis and pulmonary embolism, with formation of left ventricular thrombus.

Table 9.4 Comparison of different inotropic agents

Receptor effects	Adrenaline	Dopamine	Dobutamine	Isoprenaline
Alpha				
Arteriolar vasoconstriction	+ + + +	+ + low dose + + + high dose	+	0
Dopaminergic				
Vasodilation in gut and kidney	0	+ +	0	0
Beta-1				
Increased myocardial contractility	+ + + +	+ + + +	+ + + +	+ + + +
Increased heart rate	+ + +	+ + +	+ +	+ + + +
Increased AV conduction	+ +	+ +	+ +	+ +
Beta-2				
Arteriolar vasodilation	0	+ +	+ +	+ + + +

Antidysrhythmic agents

Most patients with heart failure have complex ventricular dysrhythmias, which are not always symptomatic. Sudden death is responsible for half the deaths in patients with heart failure, presumably secondary to a malignant dysrhythmia. However, the role of antidysrhythmic agents is not clear; most agents are negatively inotropic. Amiodarone may be the exception and might improve prognosis (Dargie and Cleland, 1988). The use of beta-blockers to improve survival and symptoms is of current interest, but these are very difficult to introduce and use clinically (Bashir et al, 1993).

Ultrafiltration

Mechanical methods to remove fluid in heart failure have been used in refractory heart failure (Simpson et al, 1986). Ultrafiltration allows controlled removal of body water without the adverse haemodynamic effects of haemodialysis, since only venous access is needed.

POST-INFARCT ISCHAEMIA

If the infarct-related artery is not opened quickly or completely enough, there is a risk of reocclusion and reinfarction. In the ISIS-2 trial (1988), there were about 3% of patients with reinfarction. Post-infarction angina may affect up to one third of patients, and the risk of reinfarction is considerable, particularly in those who presented with non-Q wave infarction (Bosch et al, 1987). Symptomatic coronary reocclusion usually occurs within 24 hours, although asymptomatic reocclusion may occur later (Ohman et al, 1990). Cases of reinfarction are more likely to develop cardiogenic shock and have a poor prognosis; they have a 2.5 times greater risk of death or further myocardial infarction within 1 year.

A definite diagnosis needs to be made; chest pain may be due to other causes, such as pericarditis, pulmonary embolism or dyspepsia. Transient ECG changes and response to GTN are the main confirmatory features. In the first instance, sublingual, buccal or intravenous GTN should be given and the patient given intravenous beta-blockers if not already beta-blocked. The resting ECG should be inspected for signs of reinfarction. If the electrocardiogram has changes compatible with reinfarction, patients should receive further thrombolysis, but those treated with APSAC or streptokinase should not be rechallenged with the same drug after 3 days, because of the development of antistreptokinase antibodies, which render the streptokinase inert, as well as being more likely to induce anaphylaxis (Buchalter et al, 1992). TPA should be used in these circumstances, and the patient should be considered for early angiography and reperfusional intervention (percutaneous transluminal coronary angioplasty or coronary artery bypass grafting).

CARDIOGENIC SHOCK

Shock is a complex syndrome associated with inadequate perfusion of vital organs, most significantly the brain, the kidneys and the heart. Cardiogenic shock complicates about 7.5% of cases of acute myocardial infarction and carries a very high mortality (Goldberg et al, 1991).

Cardiogenic shock is essentially a disease of inadequate pump function and is nearly always associated with massive cardiac damage involving more than 40% of the left ventricular myocardium, but it can occur with pulmonary emboli, cardiac tamponade or following cardiac surgery.

There are four subgroups of post-coronary patients with cardiogenic shock:

1. *Recent massive myocardial infarction.* The affected vessel is usually the left main stem coronary artery, which results in 40–50% of the left ventricular myocardium being damaged.

2. *Acute-on-chronic infarction.* This occurs when there is a smaller myocardial infarction, which takes the cumulative damage to more than 40% of the ventricular myocardium. These patients are more likely to have pre-existing hypertension and multicoronary artery disease.

3. *Myocardial infarction with mechanical complications.* Here the myocardial infarction is complicated by a mechanical defect, such as a ruptured mitral valve, ruptured septum or acute left ventricular aneurysm. These lesions compromise the pumping action of the heart and lead to cardiogenic shock.

4. *Myocardial infarction with recurrent dysrhythmias.* Dysrhythmias (especially ventricular tachycardia) reduce cardiac output and increase myocardial work and oxygen consumption, so may extend the size of the originally infarcted area. Extension of the infarction is commonly seen in patients dying from cardiogenic shock.

Mortality from cardiogenic shock is in excess of 90%, in spite of recent advances in therapy. Some patients are admitted in shock, and 50% develop the syndrome in the first 24 hours. A small proportion (15%) may develop shock more than 7 days later.

The syndrome presents with:

- Systemic hypotension (systolic BP less than 90 mmHg)
- Oliguria (less than 20 ml urine per hour)
- Arterial vasoconstriction, leading to hypoperfusion of the vital organs and peripheries

The patient will be cold, sweaty and cyanosed, with rapid shallow respiration, hypotension and tachycardia. Mental changes reflecting poor cerebral perfusion are usually present, including irritability, restlessness and, later, coma.

The abrupt loss of myocardial contractility usually results in a significant rise in intracardiac pressures and a critical fall in arterial blood pressure and cardiac output. However, left ventricular filling pressures and the cardiac index can vary widely, and it is not wise to assume that cardiac output is low or the filling pressures high. Full clinical assessment with invasive monitoring is mandatory (Table 9.5).

Table 9.5   Assessment of cardiogenic shock

Determinant	Method
Preload	Swan–Ganz catheter
Afterload	Arterial catheter
Heart rate	ECG monitoring
Contractility	Echocardiography
Infarct size	ECG, cardiac enzymes and ventriculography

Management

Since the mortality of established cardiogenic shock is so high, the best approach is prevention. This relies on early intervention to bring about reperfusion of the ischaemic or infarcting myocardium (infarct limitation), in order to arrest the inevitable progress to myocardial necrosis, leading to loss of left ventricular myocardium. Unfortunately, the greatest difficulty in preventing cardiogenic shock arises because patients are seldom seen early enough.

Cardiogenic shock is a cardiological emergency and requires aggressive management (Table 9.6).

Cardiac dysrhythmias may precipitate shock in patients with borderline left ventricular function and should be controlled as soon as possible. Immediate echocardiography is vital to assess the major haemodynamic problems and may later be supplemented by insertion of a Swan–Ganz catheter. These steps may sometimes demonstrate unsuspected hypovolaemia, which is often found in patients with right ventricular infarction and patients taking diuretics or antihypertensive agents.

An arterial line is desirable for measurement of blood pressure and frequent blood gas estimation. A urinary catheter should be inserted to record hourly urine output.

Cardiovascular haemodynamics should be stabilised using a combination of intravenous fluids, vasodilators and sympathomimetic agents.

Emergency percutaneous transluminal coronary angioplasty (PTCA) may have a role in re-establishing coronary perfusion, if it can be carried out soon enough.

Patients with mechanical complications (e.g. ventricular septal defect, mitral valve disease or left ventricular aneurysm), may be temporarily stabilised by insertion of an intra-aortic balloon pump until surgery can be carried out.

Table 9.6   Management of cardiogenic shock

- Rapid admission to a coronary care unit
- Control dysrhythmias
- Immediate echocardiography
- Invasive haemodynamic assessment
- Haemodynamic stabilisation (fluids/inotropic support/vasodilators)
- Thrombolysis
- Cardiac catheterisation, to define coronary anatomy and mechanical defects
- Cardiac surgery or coronary angioplasty

Intra-aortic balloon pumping

Intra-aortic balloon pumping is used in the management of:

- Cardiogenic shock
- Haemodynamically unstable patients requiring support during preoperative investigation (mitral regurgitation or ventricular septal defects)
- Cases of crescendo angina unresponsive to maximal medical therapy (prior to angiography and/or surgery)
- Post-cardiac surgery for patients who cannot be weaned off cardiopulmonary bypass (because of 'stunned' myocardium)

A narrow balloon catheter is inserted via the femoral artery and advanced retrogradely to lie in the descending (thoracic) aorta, just below the aortic arch (Figure 9.25). When blood is ejected from the left ventricle, it passes unobstructed around the deflated balloon. At the onset of diastole, an ECG-activated trigger causes the balloon to inflate (with helium) so that it occludes the aorta. Approximately 50 ml of blood are pushed up towards the closed aortic valve. Since coronary blood flow occurs predominantly in diastole, the presence of the balloon aids myocardial perfusion and, additionally, improves cerebral blood supply. It also reduces cardiac afterload, so that, when the balloon deflates again, the intra-aortic pressure is low, and blood is ejected with minimal extra cardiac work and oxygen consumption. Pulmonary congestion is relieved, and global myocardial perfusion, often including collateral circulation to the infarcted area, is improved. Cardiac output may increase by up to 50%, allowing improved blood flow to the vital organs. The mean arterial blood pressure increases as myocardial function improves by up to 15 mmHg, and shock quickly stabilises.

Unfortunately, although pumping may improve the initial mortality for patients in cardiogenic shock, 'balloon dependence' is common, so that when this support is

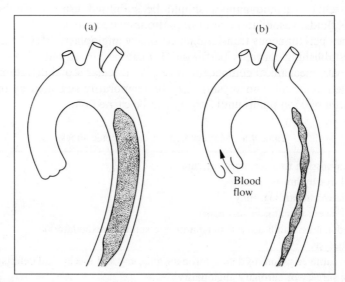

Fig. 9.25   Intra-aortic balloon counterpulsation in (a) diastole and (b) systole

withdrawn, shock returns. Since weaning patients off the pump is usually not possible, insertion should only be considered where surgical intervention is possible. Those who survive are those in whom surgery can be undertaken to repair mechanical defects (e.g. repair of the mitral valve or excision of an acute aneurysm). Such surgery is usually combined with simultaneous coronary artery bypass grafting.

CARDIAC RUPTURE

After dysrhythmias and cardiogenic shock, the most common cause of death following acute myocardial infarction is cardiac rupture, which complicates up to one quarter of cases. It usually occurs in the healing stages following infarction (3–5 days), although maximum risk seems to have moved towards the first 24 hours since the introduction of thrombolytic therapy (ISIS-2, 1988). It is associated with hypertension, diffuse coronary heart disease, anticoagulant therapy and extensive infarction, and is four times more common in women, especially the elderly, with a first infarct. The risk of cardiac rupture may be decreased by early treatment with beta-blockers (ISIS-1, 1988).

Rupture of the free wall of the left ventricle

The most common site for rupture is through the free left ventricular wall. It classically occurs in the first week following infarction, manifesting as chest pain, hypotension, dyspnoea and distended neck veins. Death is rapid and caused by an acute haemopericardium, leading to cardiac tamponade. This complication is responsible for about 15% of deaths following acute myocardial infarction. Recurrent chest pain without ECG changes may warn of imminent rupture, and cardiac collapse in the presence of normal complexes on the electrocardiogram (electromechanical dissociation) is typical.

Some patients may seem to have developed a left ventricular aneurysm, but the dilatation is in fact a pseudo-aneurysm of a partially contained rupture. The walls are formed by organised clot and fibrous tissue, which may be demonstrated by echocardiography or ventriculography. Differentiation from a true ventricular aneurysm is important, since complete rupture may occur at any time. Occasionally, these patients may present subacutely with a slowly-accumulating haemopericardium, giving rise to cardiac tamponade.

Cardiac tamponade presents with shock, an elevated JVP, muffled cardiac sounds, a small pulse pressure and pulsus paradoxus. Pulsus paradoxus is an exaggerated response to the normal reduction of cardiac output on inspiration (Table 9.7). Echocardiography helps to make the diagnosis. Pericardial aspiration should be carried out as soon as possible.

Rupture of the interventricular septum

The interventricular septum is supplied by both the left and the right coronary arteries or, occasionally, by the left coronary artery alone. Patients in this latter

Table 9.7   Measurement of pulsus paradoxus

1. Apply blood pressure cuff and measure the blood pressure
2. Reinflate the cuff to above the systolic point
3. Gradually deflate until the first Korotkoff sound can only be heard during expiration
4. Continue to deflate until the first Korotkoff sound is heard throughout the respiratory cycle
5. The difference between the two pressures is the degree of paradox and should not normally exceed 10 mmHg

group are at risk of septal infarction and subsequent rupture following thrombosis of the left coronary artery. Overall, rupture of the septum affects 2% of cases of acute myocardial infarction, and it is frequently a late complication, occurring in the healing phase. An intracardiac shunt is formed, blood being forced from the powerful left ventricle into the lower pressure right ventricle, resulting in a marked fall in cardiac output, with pulmonary circuit overload and severe pulmonary oedema. A loud pansystolic murmur is audible at the left sternal edge, with a systolic thrill. Chest pain is usual at the time of rupture, which typically occurs within 5 days of onset of the acute myocardial infarction.

Rupture of the papillary muscles

The papillary muscles may become ischaemic and infarcted, like any other part of the ventricular myocardium, and rupture in the healing stages. The posteromedial papillary muscle can rupture as a consequence of inferior myocardial infarction or, more rarely, the anterolateral papillary muscle may rupture following anteroseptal infarction. Acute mitral regurgitation results, with a fall in cardiac output and acute pulmonary oedema. An apical pansystolic murmur develops, which radiates to the axilla or sometimes the left sternal edge (the regurgitant jet is often eccentric). The degree of mitral dysfunction depends upon whether the rupture is partial or complete. The prognosis is better than for septal rupture and depends upon the degree of left ventricular dysfunction.

Management of cardiac rupture

The management of mechanical defects following acute myocardial infarction is surgical (see Chapter 14); without operation most patients with cardiac rupture will die.

RIGHT VENTRICULAR INFARCTION

Although coronary heart disease and subsequent infarction usually result in left ventricular dysfunction, the right ventricle may also be involved, either alone or with the left ventricle. Estimates from post mortem studies suggest an incidence of between 8 and 14% (Wartman and Hellerstein, 1948), but involvement via extension from acute inferior myocardial infarction is very common (Zehender et al,

1993). Early recognition of right ventricular infarction is required, since sudden and profound haemodynamic effects may develop, which can be treated or even averted by intravenous fluids. Despite high right-sided intracardiac pressures, these patients usually need expansion of the intravascular volume to maintain left-sided pressures and cardiac output. Inappropriate treatment with pressor agents (e.g. dopamine) or diuretics may be fatal.

Patients often demonstrate right ventricular failure disproportionate to left ventricular failure, and the clinical appearance may suggest cardiac tamponade. The right atrial pressure is elevated to about 20 mmHg, and systemic hypotension is common. The neck veins are distended and fail to empty on inspiration (Kussmaul's sign). A systolic murmur that increases with inspiration, caused by functional tricuspid regurgitation secondary to right ventricular dilatation, may be heard at the left sternal edge. Electrocardiography is frequently unhelpful unless right-sided chest leads are used, when ST elevation in leads V6R and V7R is of most value (Andersen et al, 1989). Echocardiography will exclude cardiac tamponade as a cause (which may not be suspected radiologically) and often shows a dilated right ventricle. Significant right ventricular infarction may be detected and followed by radionuclide ventriculography. Measurement of intracardiac pressures with a Swan–Ganz catheter will support the diagnosis and is of major value during therapy to optimise cardiac output.

Right ventricular involvement should be determined in all patients admitted with inferior myocardial infarction, since correct management decisions need to be made early to reduce the increased in-hospital morbidity and mortality that are associated with right ventricular infarction (Wellens, 1993).

LEFT VENTRICULAR ANEURYSM

Left ventricular remodelling following acute myocardial infarction comprises infarct expansion and global ventricular dilatation. With extensive transmural infarction, weakness of the wall can lead to formation of a left ventricular aneurysm. The incidence of left ventricular aneurysm following acute myocardial infarction is between 10 and 15%. They more commonly develop in the presence of diffuse coronary heart disease, in hypertensive patients or where there has been extensive myocardial damage. The site is usually anterolateral (60%), whilst 20% occur in the inferior wall. The apex and septum are sometimes also affected. During ventricular systole, the aneurysm bulges outwards and thus reduces the ejection fraction, by passively absorbing the force of myocardial contraction. The aneurysm itself may act as a focus for abnormal electrical activity (often ventricular tachycardia) and also as a site for thrombus formation. Systemic embolisation complicates about 50% of cases. Death in patients with cardiac aneurysms is associated with either a dysrhythmia or systemic embolisation, and it is rare for cardiac rupture to take place through a true left ventricular aneurysm.

Patients are often identified because of refractory left ventricular failure or because of persistent ST elevation on the ECG. Diagnosis may be confirmed by a standard chest X-ray, echocardiography or a MUGA scan. The definitive investigation is left ventriculography, which is normally performed with coronary angiography. Surgical excision (where possible) is often combined with revascularisation procedures, and postoperative mortality is about 7%. The 5-year survival is nearly 70% (Keenan et al, 1985).

LEFT VENTRICULAR MURAL THROMBI AND STROKE

Left ventricular mural thrombus may develop over areas of acutely-inflamed endocardium following acute myocardial infarction and is also found in association with most cases of left ventricular aneurysm. Clot may become dislodged (especially if there are paroxysmal dysrhythmias) and lead to peripheral arterial embolisation, predominantly stroke (50%). Left atrial thrombus often forms when the left atrium is dilated, as in mitral valve disease and left ventricular failure, especially in the presence of atrial fibrillation.

Stroke from cerebral embolism affects 1–3% of patients with myocardial infarction. This usually occurs within the first 10 days, but patients remain at risk for the first 12 weeks, particularly those with large anterior infarcts involving the apex, cardiac failure and dysrhythmias. Left ventricular mural thrombus may be visualised by echocardiography in many cases, and its occurrence may be minimised by routine anticoagulation with subcutaneous heparin (SCATI, 1989; Turpie et al, 1989). Patients at high risk should be fully anticoagulated with warfarin.

Silent myocardial infarcts with subsequent embolisation may present as a cerebrovascular accident, which is why an ECG should be carried out in all cases of stroke.

Cerebral haemorrhage is a recognised complication of thrombolytic therapy, and for some patients this may outweigh the potential benefits (Simoons et al, 1993).

DEEP VEIN THROMBOSIS AND PULMONARY EMBOLISM

The cause of deep vein thrombosis (DVT) is still not fully understood. Three classical risk factors (slowing of blood flow in the extremities, damage to the vessel walls and increased blood coagulability) are important, and there are thus many reasons why DVT is more likely following myocardial infarction, including immobility, increasing age, obesity and heart failure (THRIFT, 1992). DVT is thought to complicate as many as one third of cases of myocardial infarction. Many cases are asymptomatic, and the first sign may be a fatal pulmonary embolus (a finding in 10% of hospital autopsies). Thus, prophylaxis is of major importance.

Prophylaxis

Subcutaneous low-dose heparin (5000 U 8–12 hourly) should be used routinely in all admissions to coronary care and full anticoagulation considered for those with prolonged immobilisation and heart failure. Graded pressure (TED) stockings may also be useful. Early mobilisation is desirable for all patients (especially the elderly), provided there are no contraindications (Hirsh, 1981).

Diagnosis of established DVTs

Clinical signs are not always reliable but may include swelling, tenderness and redness of the affected limb. These signs are not specific. Venography is the best method of demonstrating thrombosis in the deep veins, and, with modern image enhancement, excellent quality films may be obtained right up to the inferior vena cava. The investigation is invasive and has the risk of producing thrombophlebitis in some patients. Other methods, including impedance phlebography and 125-I fibrinogen scanning, have limited application. MRI may be of value, but experience and availability are at present limited. Duplex ultrasound scanning is more promising, being cheap and easy to perform. It is an excellent investigation to detect thrombosis in the proximal veins, and since this is where 99% of pulmonary emboli arise from, it may become a very useful tool in the future (Mitchell et al, 1991).

Management

A bolus of heparin 5000 U followed by an infusion of about 40 000 U per day is required, adjusted to keep the activated partial thromboplastin time (APTT) approximately twice that of the control. Heparin should be continued for 5 days, and oral anticoagulants may be given at the same time, which take about 2–3 days for effect.

PERICARDITIS AND DRESSLER'S SYNDROME

Post-infarction pericarditis affects about 20% of patients in the first week following acute transmural myocardial infarction and is associated with larger infarcts, left ventricular failure and dysrhythmias. A small pericardial effusion may be seen on echocardiography. The ESR and white cell count may be elevated. Sometimes, pericarditis (and pleurisy) recurs 2 weeks to 3 months after myocardial infarction (Dressler's syndrome). There may be associated systemic symptoms, such as fever and malaise, and large pleural effusions may develop. The mechanism is thought to be autoimmune, triggered by blood in the pericardial cavity, or from antibodies to necrotic myocardium.

Treatment is with non-steroidal anti-inflammatory agents, such as aspirin or indomethacin, and bed-rest. The condition is self-limiting but may recur. It is best to discontinue anticoagulants, because of the risk of a haemorrhagic pericardial effusion. More resistant cases may need corticosteroid therapy. This will reduce pain and effusions more quickly.

SHOULDER–HAND SYNDROME

With early mobilisation of the post-coronary patient, this has become a rare complication. It presents with stiffness and pain in the shoulder (usually the left side) 2–8 weeks after acute myocardial infarction, sometimes accompanied by pain and swelling of the hand. Physiotherapy and analgesia are all that is required.

References

AIRE (Acute Infarction Ramipril Efficacy) Investigators (1993) Effect of Ramipril on mortality and morbidity of survivors of acute myocardial infarction with clinical evidence of heart failure. *Lancet*, **342:** 821–828.

Andersen H R, Falk E and Nielsen D (1989) Right ventricular infarction: diagnostic accuracy of electrocardiographic right chest leads V3R to V7R investigated prospectively in 43 consecutive fatal cases from a coronary care unit. *British Heart Journal*, **61:** 514–520.

Anderson K P and Mason J W (1983) Surgical management of ventricular tachydysrhythmias. *Clinical Cardiology*, **6:** 415–425.

Bashir Y, McKenna W J and Camm A J (1993) Beta-blockers and the failing heart: is it time for a U-turn? *British Heart Journal*, **70:** 8–12.

Bigger J T, Dresdale F J, Heissenbuttel R H, Weld F M and Wit A (1977) Ventricular arrhythmias in ischaemic heart disease: mechanism, prevalence, significance and management. *Progress in Cardiovascular Diseases*, **19:** 255–300.

Bosch X, Theroux P, Waters D D, Pelletier G B and Roy D (1987) Early post-infarction ischaemia: clinical, angiographic and prognostic significance. *Circulation*, **75:** 988–995.

Braunwald E (1991) Stunning of the myocardium: an update. *Cardiovascular Drugs and Therapy*, **5:** 849–851.

Buchalter M B, Suntharalingam G, Jennings I, Hart C, Luddington R J, Chakraverty R, Jacobson S K, Weissberg P L and Baglin T P (1992) Streptokinase resistance: when might streptokinase administration be ineffective? *British Heart Journal*, **68:** 449–453.

Caldwell G, Millar G, Quinn E, Vincent R and Chamberlain D A (1985) Simple mechanical methods for cardioversion: defence of the precordial thump and cough version. *British Medical Journal*, **291:** 627–630.

Campbell R W F, Higham D, Adams P and Murray A (1987) Potassium – its relevance for arrhythmias complicating acute myocardial infarction. *Journal of Cardiovascular Physiology*, **10:** S25–S27.

CASCADE Investigators (1993) Randomised anti-arrhythmic drug therapy in survivors of cardiac arrest – the CASCADE study. *American Journal of Cardiology*, **72:** 280–287.

Chatterjee K (1993) Complications of acute myocardial infarction. *Current Problems in Cardiology*, **18:** 1–79.

Dancy M, Camm A J and Ward D (1985) Misdiagnosis of chronic recurrent ventricular tachycardia. *Lancet*, **ii:** 320–323.

Dargie H J and Cleland J G (1988) Arrhythmias in heart failure: the role of amiodarone. *Clinical Cardiology*, **11**(supplement): 1126–1130.

Franciosa J A, Dunkman W B and Leddy C L (1984) Haemodynamic effects of vasodilators and long term response in heart failure. *Journal of the American College of Cardiology*, **3:** 1521–1530.

Garratt C J, Malcolm A D and Camm A J (1992) Adenosine and cardiac arrhythmias. *British Medical Journal*, **305:** 3–4.

GISSI-3 (1994) Effects of Lisinopril and transdermal glyceryl trinitrate singly and together on 6-week mortality and ventricular function after acute myocardial infarction. *Lancet*, **343:** 1115–1122.

Goldberg R J, Gore J M, Alpert J S, Osganian V, De Groot J, Bade J, Chen Z, Frid D and Dalen J E (1991) Cardiogenic shock after acute myocardial infarction – incidence and mortality from a community-wide perspective 1975–1988. *New England Journal of Medicine*, **325:** 1117–1122.

Hirsh J (1981) Prevention of deep vein thrombosis. *British Journal of Hospital Medicine*, **26:** 143–147.

Hjalmarson A and Olsson G (1991) Myocardial infarction. Effects of beta-blockade. *Circulation*, **84**(supplement 6): VI 101–107.

Ho K K, Anderson K M, Kannel W B, Grossman W and Levy D (1993) Survival after the onset of congestive heart failure in Framingham Heart Study subjects. *Circulation*, **88:** 107–115.

ISIS-1 Collaborative Group (1988) Mechanisms for the early mortality reduction produced by beta-blockade started early in acute myocardial infarction. *Lancet*, **i:** 921–923.

ISIS-2 Collaborative Group (1988) Randomised trial of intravenous streptokinase, oral aspirin, both or neither amongst 17,187 cases of suspected acute myocardial infarction. *Lancet*, **ii:** 349–360.

ISIS-4 Collaborative Group (1995) A randomised factorial trial assessing early oral Captopril, oral mononitrate, and intravenous magnesium sulphate in 58,050 patients with suspected acute myocardial infarction. *Lancet*, **345:** 669–685.

Jowett N I, Thompson D R and Pohl J E F (1989) Temporary transvenous endocardial pacing: six years experience in one coronary care unit. *Postgraduate Medical Journal*, **65:** 211–215.

Keenan D J M, Monro J L, Ross J K, Manners M, Conway N and Johnson A M (1985) Left ventricular aneurysm. *British Heart Journal*, **54:** 269–272.

Kertes P and Hunt D (1984) Prophylaxis of primary ventricular fibrillation in acute myocardial infarction. The case against lignocaine. *British Heart Journal*, **52:** 241–247.

Lancet Editorial (1989) Digoxin: new answers, new questions. *Lancet*, **ii:** 79–80.

Lown B, Fakhro A M, Hood W B and Thom G W (1967) The coronary care unit: new perspectives and developments. *Journal of the American Medical Association*, **199:** 188–198.

May G S, Furburg C D, Eberlein K A and Geraci B J (1983) Secondary prevention after acute myocardial infarction: a review of short-term acute phase trials. *Progress in Cardiovascular Diseases*, **25:** 335–359.

Mitchell D C, Grasty M S, Stebbings W S, Nockler I B, Lewars M D, Levison R A and Wood R F (1991) Comparison of duplex ultrasonography and venography in the diagnosis of deep vein thrombosis. *British Journal of Surgery*, **78:** 611–613.

New York Heart Association Criteria Committee (1964) *Diseases of the Heart and Blood Vessels; Nomenclature and Criteria for Diagnosis*, 6th edn. Boston: Little, Brown.

Noneman J W and Rodgers J F (1978) Lidocaine prophylaxis in acute myocardial infarction. *Medicine*, **57:** 501–515.

Ohman E M, Califf R M, Topol E J, Candela R, Abbottsmith C and Ellis P (1990) Consequences of re-occlusion after successful reperfusion therapy in acute myocardial infarction. *Circulation*, **82:** 781–791.

Packer M (1992) Patho-physiology of chronic heart failure and treatment of heart failure. *Lancet*, **340:** 88–95.

Packer M, Carver J R, Rodheffer R J, Ivanhoe R J, DiBianco R, Zeldis S M, Hendrix G H, Bommer W J, Elkayam U and Kukin M L (1991) Effect of oral milrinone in severe chronic heart failure. *New England Journal of Medicine*, **325:** 1468–1475.

Parker J O and the Ibopamine Study Group (1993) The effects of oral ibopamine in patients with mild heart failure: a double blind placebo controlled comparison with furosemide. *International Journal of Cardiology*, **40:** 221–227.

Pfeffer M A, Braunwald E, Moyle L A, Basta L, Brown E J, Cuddy T E, Davis R B, Geltman E M, Goldman S and Flakker G C (1992) Effect of captopril on mortality and morbidity in patients with left ventricular dysfunction after myocardial infarction: results of the survival and ventricular enlargement trial (SAVE). *New England Journal of Medicine*, **327:** 669–677.

Reiffel J A, Estes N A, Waldo A L, Prystowsky E N and DiBianco R (1994) A consensus report on antiarrhythmic drug use. *Clinical Cardiology*, **17:** 103–116.

SCATI Study Group (1989) Randomised controlled trial of subcutaneous calcium heparin in acute myocardial infarction. *Lancet*, **ii:** 182–186.

Shukla R, Jowett N I, Thompson D R and Pohl J E F (1994) Adverse effects with amiodarone therapy. *Postgraduate Medical Journal*, **70:** 492–498.

Simoons M L, Maggioni A P, Knatterud G, Leimberger J D, de Jaegere P, van Domburg R, Boersma E, Franzosi M G, Califfe R and Schroder R (1993) Individual risk assessment for intracranial haemorrhage during thrombolytic therapy. *Lancet*, **342:** 1523–1528.

Simpson I A, Rae A P, Simpson K, Gribben J, Boulton Jones J M, Allison M E and Hutton I (1986) Ultrafiltration in the management of refractory congestive heart failure. *British Heart Journal*, **55:** 344–347.

SOLVD Investigators (1992) Effects of enalapril on mortality and the development of heart failure in asymptomatic patients with reduced left ventricular ejection fractions. *New England Journal of Medicine*, **327:** 685–691.

Surawicz B (1986) R-on-T phenomenon: dangerous and harmless. *Journal of Applied Cardiology*, **1:** 39–61.

St John Sutton M (1994) Should ACE inhibitors be used routinely after infarction? Perspectives from the SAVE trial. *British Heart Journal*, **71:** 115–118.

Sweberg K, Held P, Kjekshus J, Rasmussen K, Ryden L and Wedel H (1992) Effects of the early administration of enalapril on mortality in patients with acute myocardial infarction – results of the Co-operative New Scandinavian Enalapril Survival Study II (Consensus II). *New England Journal of Medicine*, **327:** 678–684.

THRIFT (1992) The Thrombo-embolic Risk Factors Consensus Group. *British Medical Journal*, **305:** 567–574.

Turpie A G G, Robinson J G, Doyle D J, Muiji A S, Mishkel G J et al (1989) Comparison of high-dose with low-dose subcutaneous heparin in the prevention of left ventricular mural thrombosis in patients with acute anterior myocardial infarction. *New England Journal of Medicine*, **320:** 352–357.

Wartman W B and Hellerstein H K (1948) The incidence of heart disease in 2000 consecutive autopsies. *Annals of Internal Medicine*, **28:** 41–65.

Wellens H J J (1993) Right ventricular infarction. *New England Journal of Medicine*, **328:** 1036–1038.

Wilmshurst P (1993) Why inotropes continue to disappoint in heart failure. *British Heart Journal*, **70:** 4.

Zehender M, Kasper W, Kauder E, Schonthaler M, Geibel A, Olschewski M and Just H (1993) Right ventricular infarction as an independent predictor of prognosis after acute inferior myocardial infarction. *New England Journal of Medicine*, **328:** 981–988.

10
Cardiopulmonary
Resuscitation

Cardiorespiratory arrest occurs when there is sudden cessation of spontaneous respiration and circulation. The most common reason is a cardiac dysrhythmia secondary to coronary heart disease. Other causes include pulmonary emboli, massive haemorrhage and trauma. Coronary care units were developed primarily to treat ventricular fibrillation and other serious dysrhythmias in the first few hours following myocardial infarction. Unfortunately, many episodes occur before admission to hospital, and 40% of deaths relating to coronary heart disease (63% in young and middle-aged patients) occur within the first hour following the onset of symptoms, of which 90% are due to ventricular fibrillation. In addition, a large proportion of cardiac arrests occur on the hospital wards, where it is the nursing staff who have the responsibility for carrying out basic life support before the arrival of the 'arrest team'. Undoubtedly, open-plan wards permit the rapid recognition of circulatory arrest and, from the point of view of resuscitation, it is a shame that so many four-bed or single-bed wards now exist. Simulated cardiac arrests may help in identifying any deficiencies or difficulties in resuscitation within such areas (Sullivan and Guyatt, 1986).

Since resuscitation by nurses is usual on high-dependency units, and early steps are commonplace on general medical wards (especially at night), it is essential that the nursing staff can cope with this task competently. Although chances of resuscitation should be optimal within hospital, there are often deficiencies in the knowledge of basic resuscitation skills (Hershey and Fisher, 1982). Studies, both in the UK and in the USA, have highlighted this inadequacy, not only in nursing staff, but also in the junior medical staff (Gass and Curry, 1983; Casey, 1984; Skinner, 1985; Kaye and Mancini, 1986; Wynne et al, 1987; David and Prior-Willeard, 1993). One of the principal functions of the coronary care unit and its specialist staff must be to train personnel in the basic resuscitation procedures (Jowett and Thompson, 1988a). All hospital staff, whatever their work, need to learn the rudiments of cardiopulmonary resuscitation; it is one of the main life-saving procedures that can be carried out by everybody (Resuscitation Council, 1984). In addition, junior medical staff and those in specialist areas (e.g. CCU, ITU or accident and emergency) need to be checked on their proficiency at these basic skills, the use of simple equipment (oxygen, suction and airways) and defibrillation procedures (Royal College of Physicians, 1987). As staff become more senior and more experienced at attending arrests, increased confidence is not necessarily matched by an increase in skills (Marteau et al 1990; Berden et al, 1993), so that periods of retraining and retesting are required.

THE ETHICS OF RESUSCITATION

Most of the moral difficulties of resuscitation surround whether or not is should be undertaken in cases where there is serious underlying disease or debility. Resuscitation is best not attempted if a patient is found dead or if he is known to have a distressing or inevitably fatal illness. The age of the patient is immaterial. Failed attempts do little to enhance the dignity of death and may subject the patient and his relatives to added pain and misery (Baskett, 1986). It should be remembered that a large proportion of patients with cardiac arrest die despite intervention, and dramatic efforts may be inappropriate. A large British study (the BRESUS study) showed that for every eight attempted resuscitations, there were only three immediate survivors. One of these would die within 24 hours and another over the course of the following year (Tunstall-Pedoe et al, 1992). In-hospital survival was best in arrests in CCU, ITU or the accident and emergency department. 'Do not resuscitate' orders should be clearly understood by the patient's carers and recorded formally in both the medical and nursing notes. This is currently not a procedure that is well adhered to (Aarons and Beeching, 1991). The rationale for the order, and any patient consultation, should also be noted. Such orders should be reviewed frequently and changed if there is any relevant change in the patient's condition or circumstances. Hospitals should have written policies of when to start resuscitation (Doyal and Wilsher, 1993; Florin, 1993; Williams, 1993), which need understanding by all concerned. A recent study showed that one quarter of nurses did not know or did not understand such orders written in the patients' notes (Jones et al, 1993).

THE PRINCIPLES OF CARDIOPULMONARY RESUSCITATION

The basic principles of cardiopulmonary resuscitation (CPR) have only arisen from research work over the last 30–35 years. The sequence of airway management, artificial respiration and external chest compression is now well established. Early manual methods of ventilation (e.g. Holger–Neilson) have been surpassed by expired air resuscitation methods ('mouth-to-mouth'), which have been shown to improve arterial oxygenation (Safar et al, 1958; Elam and Greene, 1961), but support of the arrested circulation has changed little since early descriptions by Kouwenhoven et al (1960) and Jude et al (1961). Much more is now known about resuscitation physiology, and modifications to traditional resuscitation methods have been suggested in recent years, with more efficient methods of providing circulatory and ventilatory assistance (Jowett and Thompson, 1988b; Varon and Fromm, 1993).

When conventional CPR was first introduced, it was believed that the heart was emptied by being squeezed between the sternum and the thoracic spine. However, this 'cardiac pump' hypothesis assumes that the heart valves remain competent during external compression, which is not the case. Two-dimensional echocardiography has shown that the heart valves remain open, and there are no changes in left ventricular size, as might be expected were the heart acting as a pump (Rich et al, 1981). Although there is no difference in pressure within intrathoracic organs during compression, there is between intrathoracic and extrathoracic vessels. The current idea is that the whole of the chest acts as a pump during external compression, and blood is probably ejected by the production of an intermittent pressure gradient between the inside of the chest and the rest of the body (the 'thoracic pump' mechanism), with the heart and the great vessels constituting the pump. The mitral and aortic valves remain open, and partial closure of the pulmonary valve, with collapse of the great veins, helps to prevent retrograde blood flow (Rudikoff et al, 1980).

External chest compression only produces a cardiac output of about 25% of normal, which provides poor perfusion of the carotid and coronary arteries (Niemann, 1984), and hence methods to augment this have been sought. The term 'new CPR' has arisen following research into new techniques for improving blood flow during resuscitation (Varon and Fromm, 1993). These have included simultaneous chest compression and ventilation, abdominal compression with synchronised ventilation, interposed abdominal compression and continuous abdominal binding.

Abdominal binding or abdominal compression may help by raising intra-abdominal diastolic pressure within the aorta and promoting coronary and cerebral perfusion (Chandra et al, 1981). However, the central venous pressure is also elevated, and this may compromise coronary perfusion. Abdominal binding is preferred to abdominal compression, which may cause intra-abdominal trauma, including laceration of the liver. It must be remembered, though, that binding of the abdomen takes time, and abdominal compression requires a third resuscitator, which might delay implementation of normal resuscitative measures. However, a recent study has demonstrated that interposed abdominal compression may improve survival, and further trials need to be carried out (Sack et al, 1992).

Open chest cardiac massage has been practised since the 19th century and became the routine procedure until 1960, when closed chest compression was introduced. Access to the heart is via a left thoracotomy, which can be easily taught to and performed by those without formal surgical training. Despite open massage being probably more efficient, it is probably best reserved for cases with a recent sternotomy (following cardiac surgery), suspected cardiac tamponade or rigid chest walls, when external chest compression may be ineffective (Robertson and Holmberg, 1992).

Resuscitation guidelines

In the past, standards developed by the American Heart Association were generally followed, but in 1986, the Resuscitation Council of the United Kingdom was joined by a group representing five Nordic countries to produce guidelines more suited to European practice. The European Resuscitation Council was officially established in 1990 as a multidisciplinary group representing many countries, its primary aim being to save lives by improving standards of CPR. It also aimed to standardise and simplify many of the procedures. Drawing on recent research papers as well as the latest views on resuscitation expressed by the American Heart Association, new guidelines in Basic and Advanced Life support were put together in 1992 (European Resuscitation Council Basic Life Support Working Party, 1993a). These are much simpler, play down the emphasis on the many drugs hallowed by tradition, which have little scientific evidence for their efficacy (Gonzales, 1993; Jaffe, 1993), and finally, and most crucially, have given paramount importance to the speed with which the first defibrillatory shock is administered.

DEFINITIONS AND AETIOLOGY OF CARDIAC ARREST

Cardiac arrest is the cessation of effective cardiac contraction, with a consequent and lethal fall in cardiac output. In clinical practice, this implies either ventricular standstill (asystole) or ventricular fibrillation, although there may be virtual circulatory arrest with profound bradycardias or ventricular tachycardia. Electromechanical dissociation (EMD) describes a state in which normal electrical complexes continue to show on the electrocardiograph but there is no effective pulse or blood pressure. This may complicate many primary disorders, including cardiac rupture or tamponade, severe haemorrhage, pulmonary embolism and electrolyte imbalance.

The majority of cardiac arrests occur outside hospital, and 'sudden deaths' are usually due to ventricular dysrhythmias. Cardiac arrest may be due to problems arising within the heart (e.g. myocardial infarction) or elsewhere in the body (e.g. hypovolaemia, hypoxia or hyperkalaemia). Common precipitating causes are acute myocardial ischaemia, valvular heart disease (especially aortic stenosis), cardiomyopathy, chronic obstructive airways disease and drugs. In hospital, conditions commonly associated with cardiac arrest include myocardial infarction, pulmonary embolism, valvular heart disease, postoperative hypoxia and some investigative procedures.

Occasionally, there are warning signs preceding cardiac arrest, which experienced nurses on coronary care units can recognise, and certain rhythm disturbances, especially R-on-T ectopic beats, left ventricular ectopic beats and multifocal ectopic beats, have long been associated with the onset of ventricular fibrillation. Unfortunately, many cases of ventricular fibrillation occur with no warning.

There are two main phases of CPR:

- Basic life support (BLS)
- Advanced cardiac life support (ACLS)

BASIC LIFE SUPPORT

The main objective of CPR is to provide oxygen to the vital organs (brain, heart, kidneys) until spontaneous oxygenation returns or until definitive medical treatment (advanced cardiac life support) can be initiated. The lungs can withstand long periods of anoxia, although the heart and kidneys can only survive for 30 minutes before irreversible ischaemic changes result. Unfortunately, and perhaps crucially, the cerebral cortex can only withstand anoxia for about 5 minutes. The critical factor in basic life support, therefore, is speed. The most impressive reports showing success of CPR are in those cases in which resuscitation was initiated within 4 minutes of collapse, with advanced resuscitation techniques being commenced within 8 minutes (Cobb et al, 1980). This applies not only within hospital, but also in the community, where bystander resuscitation may be used to good effect (Myerburg et al, 1982).

Basic life support (BLS) is designed to:

● Prevent circulatory or respiratory arrest through recognition and intervention
● Support circulation and ventilation, if required, by CPR

The first ABC of basic life support

Basic life support has traditionally been taught by an ABC sequence of Airway, Breathing and Circulation (Evans, 1986). Our practice is to precede this with another ABC as follows:

A: Ascertain arrest

An assessment phase is critical and must start with the recognition and confirmation of cardiopulmonary arrest. The alternative term 'assess responsiveness' is sometimes used.

Recognition

During cardiac arrest, there is ineffective mechanical activity of the heart, a reduced cardiac output and cerebral hypoperfusion. Loss of consciousness, apnoea (or gasping respiration) and loss of pulses occur within seconds. Other signs, such as cyanosis and dilatation of the pupils, take much longer and should not be awaited. Speed in initiating CPR is essential, and any delay may be fatal; a false alarm is better than a dead patient. Cardiac arrest does not necessarily reflect serious myocardial damage, but the neurones of the cerebral cortex undergo irreversible changes after 3–5 minutes. If prompt and efficient CPR is not started within this time, permanent cerebral damage will occur. Hence, cardiac arrest must be assumed to have occurred with:

● Any sudden loss of consciousness
● Sudden onset of a seizure in a non-epileptic patient
● Sudden onset of cyanosis or respiratory distress

Other underlying causes (e.g. syncope, cerebrovascular accidents, haemorrhage or epilepsy) may be responsible, but where there is any doubt, CPR should be instituted immediately.

Confirmation

Immediate clinical assessment of a patient who has suffered a cardiac arrest will show:

● A rapidly deteriorating level of consciousness

- A change in skin colour: pallor or cyanosis
- Absence of a pulse (put an ear to the chest; time should not be wasted in trying to feel peripheral pulses)
- Absence of respiration (note that a spontaneous 'gasping' ineffective respiration may occur for a few minutes following circulatory arrest)

B: Bang on chest

The precordial thump is not included in the current recommendations for basic life support but is encouraged in the advanced cardiac life support recommendations. Since this manoeuvre takes only a few seconds, and is only of value very early on (within 30 seconds of arrest), it is probably more relevant for mention here so that it may be employed by more experienced rescuers, particularly on coronary care units, where it may be used whilst the defibrillator is charging.

Using a precordial thump for restoring sinus rhythm was reported in 1920 by Schott, who terminated a Stokes–Adams attack with a precordial blow. This method of restoring sinus rhythm was widely practised until it was suggested that such a manoeuvre might convert ventricular tachycardia to ventricular fibrillation. However, the potential benefit of the precordial thump to mechanically cardiovert ventricular fibrillation to sinus rhythm greatly outweighs its risks (Caldwell et al, 1985). About 40% of patients with ventricular tachycardia and 2% of patients with ventricular fibrillation will cardiovert into sinus rhythm. A similar mechanical stimulus may be given by raising the legs to promote venous return and may terminate ventricular tachycardia. Conscious patients with ventricular tachycardia may restore sinus rhythm by forceful coughing, and some patients can maintain cerebral circulation by repeated coughing (cough-CPR). Arterial pressures of 100 mmHg are achieved using the pressure changes in the chest produced by coughing and give support to the thoracic-pump theory of CPR (Criley et al, 1976).

C: Call for help

Once cardiac arrest is confirmed, help will be required for basic and advanced cardiac resuscitation: shout for immediate help and make sure that an 'arrest call' is put out.

The second ABC of basic life support

The second ABC refers to the basic resuscitation skills of Airway clearance, initiating artificial Breathing and Circulation.

A: Airway

Effective CPR requires the patient to be supine and on a flat, firm surface. The head must not be raised above the level of the thorax, or the brain will not be perfused. The patient should be placed on his back on a hard surface. If there is no board under the mattress, the patient is best pulled on to the floor. The rescuer should kneel at the patient's shoulders to allow access to both mouth and chest.

The most important initial action is to open the airway. In 90% of unconscious patients, the upper airway will be obstructed, usually by the tongue, which falls back into the pharynx when muscle tone is lost, allowing its supporting structure to relax. Since the tongue is attached to the lower jaw, moving the jaw forward will lift the tongue away from the back of the throat and open the airway. There are three ways of opening the airway (Figure 10.1):

● The head-tilt/chin-lift method
● The head-tilt/jaw-thrust method
● The head-tilt/neck-lift method

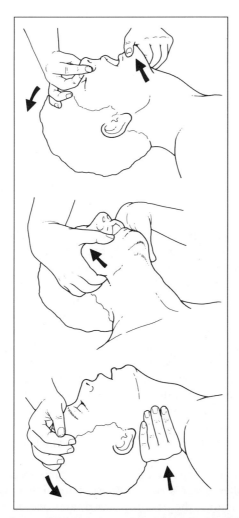

Fig. 10.1 Opening the airway: the head-tilt/chin-lift method, head-tilt/jaw-thrust method and head-tilt/neck-lift method

Since it may be a lay-person who is first on the scene, it is necessary for the manoeuvre to be simple, safe, easily learned and effective. The widely taught head-tilt/neck-lift method does not fulfil these criteria and is no longer recommended (European Resuscitation Council Basic Life Support Working Party, 1993b). The simplest method is the head-tilt/chin-lift method, although medical staff may find the head-tilt/jaw-thrust method more useful. It is technically more difficult and tiring, but is highly effective and especially useful if neck injury is suspected, since it may be used without hyperextending the neck.

Head-tilt/chin-lift manoeuvre

The head is tilted back by firm backward pressure on the patient's forehead with the palm of the hand. The fingers of the other hand are used to lift the chin forward so that the teeth almost close together. This supports the jaw and helps hold the head back.

Head-tilt/jaw-thrust

The mandible is pulled forward by grasping the angle of the jaw on both sides and tilting the head back. This may be made easier if the rescuer's elbows are allowed to rest on the floor close to the patient's head.

B: Breathing

The absence of respiration is deduced by the lack of chest movement and by listening and feeling for expired air from the mouth and nose ('look–listen–feel'). The presence of vomit or foreign bodies (e.g. dentures) should be suspected if the airway is not cleared after proper positioning of the head and neck. The mouth should be checked for obvious obstruction, but if none is found, the possibility of inhalation exists. The application of chest or abdominal thrusts is more efficient than traditional blows to the back for dislodging foreign bodies in the airway. Basic life support often needs to be instituted when equipment is not always to hand, and the use of mouth-to-mouth and mouth-to-nose respiration is of great emergency benefit. However, not only does the sight of vomit and blood usually deter the most hardened resuscitator, the theoretical risks of serum hepatitis and AIDS (the acquired immune deficiency syndrome) have now also to be contended with. Nevertheless, delay should not be allowed to occur, since there is still no evidence of disease transmission during mouth-to-mouth ventilation. Most cases of cardiac arrest occur at home, and the previous health of the victim is often known. Within hospital, the number of occasions upon which any individual is called to administer mouth-to-mouth ventilation are few, and again the health of the patient is usually known.

Mouth-to-mouth ventilation should be started immediately and may be made easier with an oropharyngeal airway. Whilst maintaining the airway using the head-tilt/chin-lift technique, the nose is pinched, and one or two slow breaths are delivered in succession (2 seconds each), with the lips sealed over the patient's mouth. Pre-oxygenation with up to four quick, full breaths without allowing the chest to deflate, previously recommended, should not be used. It is almost impossible to inflate the lungs in under a second, and attempts at faster inflation simply force air down the oesophagus, leading to gastric dilatation, which promotes vomiting and limits full expansion of the lungs. The chest should be observed for equal and satisfactory movements, and expiration of air should be heard when the chest falls. If these do not occur, the airway is obstructed and should be cleared. Subsequent inflation of the patient's lungs should be slow, to minimise pressure on the pharynx and hence reduce the risk of gastric dilatation (Melker, 1985). The expired volume should not be greater than 1200 ml, which is enough just to raise the chest visibly. The normal adult tidal volume is 400 ml, and the forced vital capacity is 4500 ml (3200 ml in women), so that it can be seen that a full, forced expiration is not required, but rather a slow exhalation, following a quick intake of breath. Each sequence of 10 breaths should take between 40 and 60 seconds, although timing is not important; it is best to wait for the chest to fall.

Mouth-to-nose respiration may be more effective than mouth-to-mouth ventilation and is associated with a lower incidence of regurgitation of gastric contents. It is, additionally, of great value in cases of oral trauma or trismus. The mouth is sealed around the patient's nose, and ventilation is carried out as previously described.

C: Circulation

Circulatory arrest should be assessed by palpation of the carotid artery, which lies in the groove between the trachea and the sternomastoid (strap) muscles in the neck. Peripheral pulses should not be used, as low-output states may masquerade as cardiac arrest. If there is no pulse, and the precordial thump is unsuccessful, external chest compression should be started.

External chest compression

The application of compressions over the lower half of the sternum has been used to effect artificial circulation for over 30 years (Kouwenhoven et al, 1960). The heel of the hand nearest the patient's head is placed over the lower half of the sternum, and the other hand is placed over the top, with the fingers either extended or interlocked (but not in contact with the chest). Pressure of the fingers on the ribs or lateral pressure increases the possibility of rib fractures or costochondral separation. The arms should be kept straight, with the elbows locked, so that pumping action is delivered in a straight line from the shoulders by pivoting at the hips to depress the sternum 4–5 cm in adults.

Compressions should be smooth, regular and uninterrupted, at a rate between 60 and 100 per minute. Whilst some studies have suggested using 'high-impulse CPR', with compression rates approaching 120 per minute, this is, in practice, very difficult to achieve or maintain (Maier et al, 1986).

At the end of each compression, relaxation must be complete, to allow adequate refilling of the thoracic pump, although the hands should not lose contact with the patient, in case the correct position is lost. Applying cardiac massage at the wrong site may lead to laceration of the liver, fractured ribs, pneumothorax or lung contusion. The optimal compression : relaxation ratio is between 50% : 50% and 60% : 40%, so that at least half the cycle is spent in the compression phase (Taylor et al, 1977). Coronary blood flow takes place during the relaxation phase, and cerebral blood flow in the compression phase, and thus such a ratio gives priority of blood flow where it is needed.

The ratio of ventilation : number of compressions depends upon whether there is one rescuer or two. With one rescuer, a ratio of 15 compressions to 2 breaths is used, whilst a ratio of 5 : 1 may be employed if there are two rescuers. As the chances of restoring cardiac rhythm without defibrillation are remote, time should not be wasted in trying to assess the pulse, **Resuscitation must be continuous, rhythmic and uninterrupted.** If, however, the patient tries to breath spontaneously, or moves, the pulse should be assessed; this should not take more than 5 seconds.

Changing the initial sequence of ventilation and compression (CAB rather than ABC) was taught by the Dutch Heart Association (Crul et al, 1985), since most patients with cardiac arrest are well oxygenated up until the time of cardiac standstill. Under these circumstances, the early application of a stimulus to the heart may lead to a return in spontaneous cardiac activity, as is the case with the precordial thump. However, whilst this line of argument makes sense within hospital in the case of a witnessed arrest, in most other cases the period of anoxia is not known and the lay bystander would be best to use the ABC approach to avoid applying cardiac massage inappropriately.

An algorithm for basic life support is shown in Figure 10.2.
The arrival of help should, ideally, lead to advanced resuscitative measures. These include:

- Securing an airway (preferably with an endotracheal tube)
- Augmentation of oxygenation with portable oxygen
- Recognition of cardiac rhythms with an ECG
- Treatment of dysrhythmias with drugs and electrical defibrillation
- Cardiovascular stabilisation to allow transport of the patient to a high-dependency unit

ADVANCED CARDIAC LIFE SUPPORT

Advanced cardiac life support (ACLS) combines basic life support with the use of specialist techniques and equipment for maintaining circulation and respiration. The key components are:

- Early defibrillation
- Ensuring an adequate airway
- Establishing intravenous access
- Electrocardiographic monitoring
- Pharmacological therapy

The design of basic life support does not require the use of equipment, although the highest priority must be given to early defibrillation. The use of other adjuncts is useful, although not so critical, and basic resuscitation should never be neglected because of the absence of medical aids. Once instituted, therapy should be continued until admission to a specialist unit or until a decision is made for life support to be terminated.

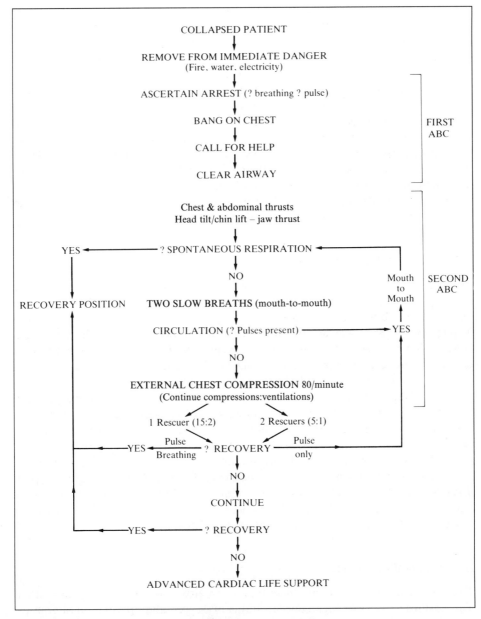

Fig. 10.2 An algorithm for basic life support

Airway management

The airway can be cleared in most patients by correct positioning of the head and neck and suction. There are many adjuncts that may be used to secure an airway and improve oxygenation. Expired air has a fractional inspired oxygen (FIO_2) of about 17%, so that enrichment with portable oxygen is highly desirable. All airways should use 100% oxygen wherever possible. Oropharyngeal airways should be used only in unconscious patients, as they may otherwise induce vomiting. Care and practice is required for correct insertion, or the tongue may be displaced backwards into the pharynx and obstruct the airway.

Self-inflating bag–valve–mask units can deliver higher oxygen concentrations providing an oxygen reservoir is used ($FIO_2 > 60\%$), but most people accept that successful application needs two people to be effective. One rescuer maintains the jaw-thrust position and ensures a tight seal between the mask and the patient's face, whilst the other inflates the lungs by squeezing the bag. Laerdal pocket masks are extremely effective for mouth-to-mask ventilation and should be carried by all would-be resuscitators. In hospital, where oxygen is readily available, an oxygen inlet nipple enables increased oxygen concentrations to be dispensed. There is no doubt that for a single rescuer, the pocket mask is superior to the bag–valve–mask unit in all but the most experienced hands (Maull, 1984).

The main disadvantage of mask ventilation is gastric distension, leading to diaphragmatic splinting and oesophageal regurgitation.

Alternatives to tracheal intubation

Because of the difficulties associated with laryngoscopy and intubation, simpler methods of securing an airway have been investigated. The introduction of the oesophageal obturator and oesophageal gastric tube airways (Jowett and Thompson, 1988b) have led to more promising devices, such as the pharyngo-tracheal lumen airway and laryngeal mask airway (LMA). Both have attracted enormous interest in Europe and America (Baskett, 1992). The latter device consists of a plain flexible tube with a distal inflatable silicone ring diagonally attached (Figure 10.3). The ring is designed to obliterate the hypopharynx and oesophageal isthmus, achieving a low-pressure seal between the tube and trachea and reducing the risk of gastric regurgitation and aspiration. The use of any ventilatory devices that imperfectly protect the patient's airway should be avoided wherever possible, and any preliminary steps should be converted to endotracheal intubation as soon as possible. Nevertheless, if junior hospital doctors, nurses and paramedics were taught the relatively simple procedure of placing the LMA, it might improve patient ventilation, particularly for cases of difficult intubation because of anatomical problems.

Endotracheal intubation

The best means of securing and maintaining an airway is endotracheal intubation. This ensures delivery of high concentrations of oxygen and provides an alternative route for drug administration. The procedure requires skill, which can only be

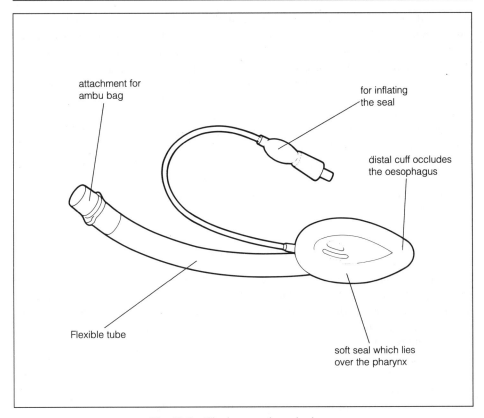

attachment for
ambu bag

for inflating
the seal

distal cuff occludes
the oesophagus

Flexible tube

soft seal which lies
over the pharynx

Fig. 10.3 The laryngeal mask airway

gained by practice; repeated attempts to intubate should not be made, and the maximum interruption in ventilation should be 30 seconds. Endotracheal tubes are labelled with the internal diameter in millimetres and should be cut to appropriate lengths. Female patients will require the 7.0–8.0 mm size, and male patients the 8.0–9.0 mm. Passage of the tube may sometimes be aided by external pressure on the cricoid cartilage (the Sellick manoeuvre), which occludes the upper part of the oesophagus and prevents aspiration of gastric contents (Sellick, 1961).

After intubation, the position of the tube should be verified by watching for equal expansion of both sides of the chest and listening over the lungs with a stethoscope. Ventilation should be about 12–15 inflations per minute and can be performed independently of chest compression.

Intravenous access

Intravenous access is essential for the administration of fluids and drugs. Peripheral lines are the simplest, since the veins are easily seen, despite their tendency to collapse following cardiac arrest. The site of choice is the antecubital fossa, since cannulation of the subclavian and neck veins needs practice and may require a temporary halt of CPR. Peripheral administration of drugs may cause significant delay (1–2 minutes) in arrival at the heart, even with optimal external cardiac massage (Doan, 1984), and a large volume of flushing solution is required or the passage of a long line through a peripheral cannula. An additional central line is often very useful, since the larger veins allow faster infusion of fluids and drugs into the central circulation. They may, additionally, be used for transvenous pacing, if required.

Regardless of the aetiology of the arrest, increased vascular permeability allows plasma proteins and water to pass into the extravascular spaces, leading to intravascular hypovolaemia (Safar, 1984). However, caution is advised in routinely administering large volumes, since cerebral and myocardial blood flow may be diminished. Expansion of circulating blood volume is, of course, critical in patients with severe acute blood loss, and cardiac arrest in these patients is often marked by electromechanical dissociation (see below).

Cardiac monitoring

Most sudden deaths are due to malignant ventricular dysrhythmias, especially in the early period following myocardial infarction, when rhythm disturbances are usually abrupt and without warning. Electrocardiographic monitoring should be established as soon as possible in all patients following myocardial infarction or sudden collapse (Jowett et al, 1985).

The three lethal dysrhythmias commonly associated with cardiac arrest are ventricular fibrillation, asystole and electromechanical dissociation, although there are other serious dysrhythmias that may be precursors of cardiac arrest or associated with a critical fall in cardiac output (e.g. profound bradycardia or ventricular tachycardia).

Arrest rhythms

Ventricular fibrillation

This is the most common arrest dysrhythmia. There is a total breakdown of ordered electrical activity within the heart, and contraction of individual myocardial fibres is random and independent. The generated work is counterproductive, and cardiac output falls dramatically. The ECG shows random waves, which will usually diminish into asystole if left untreated. Consciousness is lost within 20 seconds.

Ventricular tachycardia is another allied dysrhythmia, which in the context of acute myocardial infarction does not differ practically from ventricular fibrillation.

Asystole

Asystole is characterised by ventricular standstill due to suppression of the cardiac pacemakers by myocardial disease, anoxia, electrolyte imbalance or drugs. Strong cholinergic activity may depress the sinus and AV nodes following myocardial infarction or episodes of myocardial ischaemia.

Asystole may occur without warning, or may be preceded by various types of heart block, and is found in about 25% of hospital cardiac arrests (10% outside hospital). It often represents massive cardiac damage and sometimes appears as the last dying rhythm of the heart following prolonged ventricular fibrillation. Survival is less than 4%. The ECG shows a flat trace, which must be differentiated from fine ventricular fibrillation or, sometimes, from faulty connection of the leads and monitor.

Electromechanical dissociation

This is characterised by regular complexes on the ECG in the presence of circulatory failure; the ECG trace is an indication of the heart's electrical activity and not its contractile state. Electromechanical dissociation (EMD) may complicate anoxia, hypovolaemia, tension pneumothorax, severe acidosis or pulmonary embolism. The occurrence of EMD following myocardial infarction usually signifies a terminal event, such as rupture of the heart or cardiac tamponade.

EMD is rare outside hospital practice, but occurs in about 5% of hospital cardiac arrests. The prognosis is very poor.

Treatment of cardiac arrest

Effective myocardial function depends on the coordinated contraction of myocardial fibres. Ventricular fibrillation is the extreme example of disorganisation, which will result in death due to total abolition of cardiac output. Prompt therapy is mandatory. There are essentially two methods of restoring normal cardiac rhythm: electrical and pharmacological. Defibrillation is the cornerstone of advanced resuscitation (Zoll et al, 1956), and the earlier this is performed, the more likely sinus rhythm is to result. Any delay allows further myocardial ischaemia, anoxia and acidaemia, which will inhibit the restoration of normal rhythm. Defibrillation should, therefore, be carried out with or without ECG confirmation of ventricular fibrillation.

Defibrillation

The defibrillator basically consists of a large capacitor for storing electrical energy and two conductive paddles for delivering this energy to the heart. The energy delivered is usually measured in joules (volts × amps × time) and is displayed on a meter. Older models are usually calibrated from 0 to 400 J as energy 'stored', but recent machines are calibrated for energy 'delivered' (0–360 J). The pulse width is usually fixed at 3 ms and is not variable. The shock is delivered by the two handheld paddles, which are well insulated. Two buttons are usually built into the handles of the paddles for delivery of the defibrillating shock; both must be pressed to prevent inadvertent defibrillation. In many machines, these paddles can act simultaneously as electrodes for ECG monitoring and, when not transmitting electricity to the patient, can convey the heart's electrical activity back to a conventional oscilloscope to show the cardiac rhythm ('quick-look paddles').

Conductive electrocardiographic paste should be sparingly applied to the conducting surfaces, or a solid conducting gel should be placed directly on to the skin. The latter is preferable, being quicker and less messy, aiding electrode contact and preventing 'jelly-bridging'. The paddle position is important, to maximise the energy delivered to the heart. Standard placement requires one paddle to be placed to the right of the upper sternum inferior to the clavicle (2nd–3rd intercostal space), with the other in the anterior axillary line, just lateral to the left nipple (Figure 10.4a). The paddles should be placed firmly against the skin with at least 25 lb pressure, to prevent loss of current, flying sparks and skin burns. Obese patients have increased transthoracic resistance, and the chest-to-back method may be more useful for elective cardioversion (Figure 10.4b). Here, the patient is rolled into the right lateral position and one electrode is placed over the left precordium at the base of the sternum, with the other posteriorly, slightly to the left of the spine (which would otherwise prevent good skin contact). Transthoracic resistance can also be overcome by using higher energies or multiple discharges or by shortening the intervals between shocks (Kerber et al, 1981).

The amount of energy required to restore sinus rhythm without producing myocardial damage is very difficult to calculate and depends upon such variables as paddle size and position, blood pH and drugs. The sequence of energies is now conventional (200 J, 200 J and 360 J). The rationale for starting at lower energies was originally based upon the slow charging speed of older equipment. This is now no longer a problem with modern equipment, and all units must have defibrillators that can recharge rapidly; they must be capable of delivering these first three shocks within 30–45 seconds. Starting the sequence at a lower energy level is retained in current CPR guidelines, since a balance between successful defibrillation and myocardial damage may be important. A defibrillation algorithm is shown in Figure 10.5. The operator should stand well clear of the patient and bed and ensure that colleagues do, too. This especially applies to the anaesthetist, who may be hand-ventilating the patient and will not thank the operator for delivering the current to him.

Automatic and semi-automatic defibrillators

These were designed and developed for paramedical staff but have been shown to be useful in other circumstances (Cummins et al, 1986). For example, using a defibrillator in semi-automatic mode may be more rapid than a fully manual machine. Rather than using traditional 'paddles', large adhesive chest pads are applied, which can both monitor heart rhythm and, additionally, conduct a defibrillatory shock to the patient. A computer decides whether or not a shock should be delivered, based upon the recorded cardiac rhythm. This is delivered either automatically or semi-automatically, when it is up to the operator whether to discharge the defibrillator. Energy levels are usually preset, and warning buzzers sound to make sure that no one is in contact with the patient at the time of defibrillation. A manual override facility is required in case the machine misinterprets dysrhythmias such as ventricular flutter, allowing operator-instituted defibrillation.

Following introduction of automatic defibrillators in Scottish front-line ambulances, it has become clear that this system can be easily and effectively introduced for out-of-hospital cardiac arrest (Cobbe et al, 1991). They may also have a hospital role for 'showing' the decision-making process to help the confidence of new resuscitators.

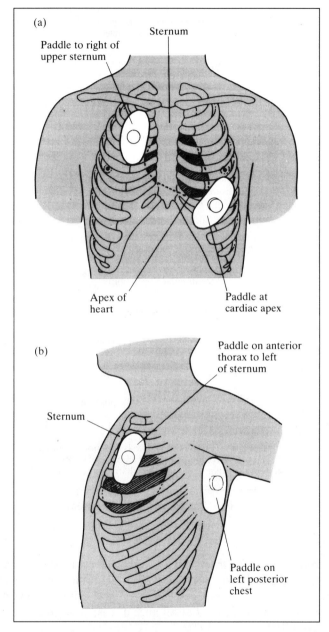

Fig. 10.4 Positioning of defibrillation paddles for (a) a normal weight patient and (b) an obese patient (From Jowett and Thompson, 1988b. Reproduced by kind permission of Churchill Livingstone)

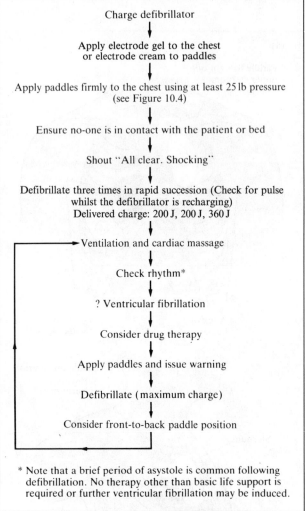

Fig. 10.5   Procedure for defibrillation

Drug therapy

The value of drug therapy for treatment of cardiac arrest is probably minimal, and the importance of basic life support with early defibrillation cannot be stressed enough. In recent years, numerous controversies have arisen about whether pharmacological intervention is required at all and, if it is, about the optimal route for delivery (Gonzales; 1993; Jaffe, 1993).

Pharmacological intervention may be used during cardiac arrests to:

- Correct hypoxia and acidosis
- Accelerate or reduce the heart rate
- Suppress ectopic activity
- Stimulate the strength of myocardial contraction

Because of the haemodynamic changes during CPR, the administration of drugs into the central circulation is preferable, although gaining access is often difficult and should not be allowed to hinder basic life support or defibrillation.

Adrenaline

Adrenaline has strong alpha- and beta-adrenergic agonist activity, with a powerful vasoconstrictor action. Administration will result in peripheral vasoconstriction, which augments the effect of chest compression, leading to increased cerebral and coronary perfusion (Waller and Robertson, 1991). The beta-agonist properties (positive chronotropic and inotropic effects) certainly help myocardial stimulation following attainment of sinus rhythm.

Adrenaline is the first drug given for all types of cardiac arrest. The recommended dose in adults is 1 mg (10 ml of a 1:10 000 solution), which may be repeated every 2–3 minutes. In asystolic arrests, a single dose of adrenaline 5 mg should be considered if initial smaller doses have not helped. However, its value is unproven.

Atropine

Atropine lowers vagal tone, although its value after the first few minutes following cardiac arrest is unclear, since significant vagotonia is unlikely to be present. However, a single dose of 3 mg is still recommended in asystolic and bradycardiac arrest, to ensure that vagal block tone is fully blocked, in order to relieve cholinergic overactivity on the conducting tissues (Brown et al, 1979). Repeat doses should be avoided, since they may reduce the electrical stability of the heart, making ventricular fibrillation more likely (Cooper and Abinader, 1979).

Sodium bicarbonate

A major consideration in managing cardiac arrest is to combat the metabolic acidosis that inevitably accompanies poor tissue perfusion, with a build-up of lactic acid and increased levels of carbon dioxide. This acidosis depresses myocardial contractility, produces vasodilatation and capillary leakage, inhibits catecholamine activity and increases the likelihood of dysrhythmias.

Intravenous sodium bicarbonate has been widely used in the past for correcting the metabolic acidosis that follows cardiac arrest, but there is little evidence that this therapy improves outcome. Indeed, the guidelines from the National Conference on Cardiopulmonary Resuscitation and Emergency Cardiac Care (1986) ceased recommending its use, because of the frequent occurrence of deleterious side-effects, including increasing carbon dioxide levels, hypernatraemia, inactivation of concurrently-administered catecholamines and tissue necrosis if accidentally given extravascularly.

Critically-ill patients in hospital may warrant early therapy with sodium bicarbonate if there is developing hyperkalaemia or acidosis that might precede a cardiac arrest, but these occasions are now the exception rather than the rule.

The principal method of correcting acidosis is by establishing adequate alveolar ventilation. Hyperventilation corrects respiratory acidosis by removing carbon dioxide, which freely diffuses across cellular membranes. Optimal oxygenation, ventilation and airway control are, therefore, vital.

Calcium chloride and calcium-channel blockers

The critical role of calcium ions in myocardial contraction and impulse formation is well established. However, the routine administration of calcium salts during cardiopulmonary resuscitation is questionable (Dembo, 1984). Calcium may cause coronary and cerebral vasospasm, as well as increasing ventricular irritability in patients taking digoxin. Doses of 2–4 mg/kg (2 ml 10% calcium chloride solution) may be useful for cardiac arrest complicated by:

- Hypocalcaemia
- Hyperkalaemia
- Electromechanical dissociation

or for patients on high doses of calcium-channel blocking agents (e.g. nifedipine, verapamil and nicardipine).

The therapeutic role of calcium-channel blockers for the relief of vasospasm is of interest. Although no value has been shown during cardiac arrest, they may be useful in post-resuscitation care for relieving cerebral vasospasm in the post-anoxic state.

Lignocaine

Lignocaine has been used for many years for the control of ventricular dysrhythmias complicating cardiac arrest and myocardial infarction. Its major action during cardiac arrest is to inhibit the initiation of re-entry dysrhythmias in the ischaemic myocardium, but it use makes defibrillation more difficult (Chamberlain, 1991). Its routine use is, therefore, to be discouraged, although consideration after prolonged arrest may be entertained, when bolus therapy may be used every 8–10 minutes (0.5 mg/kg). Reduced hepatic circulation may make lignocaine toxicity more likely, and no more than 3 mg/kg should be administered.

Bretylium and amiodarone

Bretylium tosylate (400 mg iv) or amiodarone (300 mg) can be used in ventricular fibrillation refractory to defibrillation and lignocaine. The effect of these drugs does not appear immediately, and it may be necessary to continue CPR for up to 30 minutes.

Intracardiac and transbronchial administration of drugs

Adrenaline can be given intravenously or directly into the heart. It can also be given transbronchially via the endotracheal tube in two to three times the intravenous dose, diluted with 5–10 ml of water. Lignocaine can also be given in this way. Its onset of action is as rapid as an intravenous bolus, and its effect is twice

as long. Other agents that can be given transbronchially are atropine and naloxone. Bicarbonate, calcium carbonate and noradrenaline must not be given via the
endotracheal tube as they are very irritant to the tissues. Drug absorption from the
bronchial tree is erratic and impaired by pulmonary oedema, atelectasis and,
perhaps, the drugs themselves; for example, adrenaline causes local vasoconstriction. After instillation, five inflations should be given to aid distribution and
absorption.

The use of intracardiac adrenaline is controversial. Direct ventricular puncture is
performed via the 4th intercostal space on the left or via the subxiphisternal route.
Aspiration of blood confirms cardiac puncture. However, since major complications may occur, including coronary laceration, pericardial effusion and tamponade, this approach should only be used as a last resort.

The treatment of ventricular fibrillation (Figure 10.6)

Since spontaneous reversion from ventricular fibrillation is rare, immediate defibrillation gives the best chance of restoring normal rhythm. The speed with
which this is done is critical, and it should be given highest priority. Whilst
successful defibrillation can take place for several minutes following cardiac arrest,

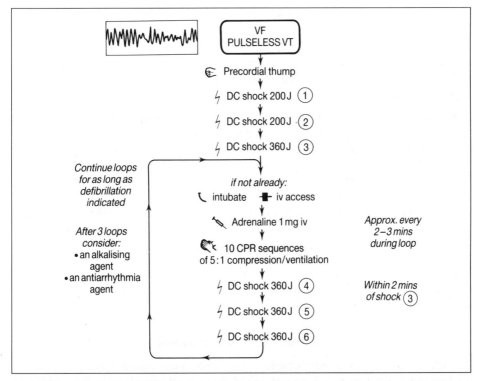

Fig. 10.6 Ventricular Fibrillation (VF). Adapted from Guidelines for Advanced Life
Support, *Resuscitation* **24** (1992). Elsevier Scientific Publications Ireland Ltd.

the chances of success and favourable outcome are considerably reduced if the first shock is delayed by as little as 90 seconds (Cobbe et al, 1991). The precordial thump is advised in witnessed arrests, or in monitored ventricular fibrillation, and should be used rather than basic life support. Basic life support should be instituted if the defibrillator arrival is delayed or if the defibrillator is not charging fast enough (Jowett and Thompson, 1988a).

The three initial shocks (200 J, 200 J, and 360 J) are now conventional and should be given in rapid succession, since this will lower transthoracic resistance and hence maximise energy delivery to the heart. It should be possible, with modern equipment, to deliver these within 30–45 seconds, and basic life support between shocks is not necessary. These shocks may, therefore, be given without removing the paddles from the chest. The pulse and/or ECG rhythm should be checked between shocks, but it is better to rely on feeling the pulse, because delay may occur in waiting for the ECG tracing to return.

At this point, a brief attempt to intubate the patient and obtain intravenous access should be made. Neither procedure should interfere with basic life support or further defibrillation shocks; 15–20 seconds is perhaps the maximum time allowable.

If normal rhythm has not returned after the initial shocks, the chances of recovery are very much reduced, although not hopeless. If appropriate, continuing resuscitation must change priorities to preserving cerebral and myocardial perfusion. This is best done by administration of adrenaline, combined with basic life support. The ventricular fibrillation algorithm, therefore, enters a loop (see Figure 10.6), which includes administration of 1 mg adrenaline, 10 sequences of 5:1 compressions:ventilations and three further shocks (all now at 360 J). Palpation of the pulse is restricted to the start of each loop, i.e. after every third defibrillation.

After every three loops, consideration may be given to alkalising or antidysrhythmic agents:

● Sodium bicarbonate (50 mmol) by injection (not infusion) may be useful, since acidosis can complicate the arrest despite adequate basic life support. Ideally, knowledge of the arterial or central pH and base deficit is required
● Lignocaine (1 mg/kg), procainamide (100 mg), bretylium (5–10 mg/kg) and amiodarone (300 mg) may be used in this now-desperate situation, and phenytoin (150–300 mg) may be of value if the patient has been taking digoxin. There is little to support the use of calcium, magnesium or potassium

Treatment of ventricular tachycardia

Ventricular tachycardia may respond to the precordial thump or other mechanical methods, such as coughing or raising the legs. The treatment of pulseless VT is the same as for ventricular fibrillation.

Treatment of torsade de pointes

Torsade de pointes is a polymorphic ventricular tachycardia associated with a prolonged QT interval and is characterised by gradual alteration in the amplitude and direction of the electrical activity. It is often caused by antidysrhythmic drugs,

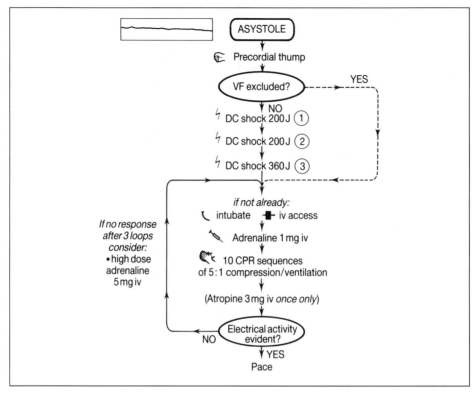

Fig. 10.7 Treatment of asystole. Adapted from Guidelines for Advanced Life Support, *Resuscitation* **24** (1992). Elsevier Scientific Publications Ireland Ltd.

many of which prolong the QT interval. Treatment is as for ventricular fibrillation if the patient is compromised, and intravenous magnesium sulphate may be useful. Atrial pacing or isoprenaline infusion may also be used.

Treatment of asystole (Figure 10.7)

Fine ventricular fibrillation may often appear as asystole, so that a defibrillatory shock is always worth while. If an additional monitor lead is connected, the rhythm can be checked, and if 'quick-look' paddles are being used, they should be rotated through 90° to confirm the rhythm. Adrenaline (1 mg intravenously every 2–3 minutes) is recommended for first-line drug therapy. Atropine 3 mg is recommended as a single intravenous dose at the end of the first CPR cycle.

Pacing is perhaps a more logical approach to treating asystole if there is evidence of atrial activity, which may indicate trifascicular block. The occasional QRS complex may also give some hope of the successful use of pacing, which may be carried out transoesophageally, transvenously or transthoracically. Pacing is usually ineffective if the arrest is due to extensive myocardial damage.

If there is no sign of activity after initial resuscitation, further loops may be considered, but recovery is very rare. High dose adrenaline (5 mg) could be given after three loops, but its value is unproven.

Treatment of electromechanical dissociation (Figure 10.8)

The prognosis of EMD is grave, and an aggressive search for possible underlying causes should be made. These include severe acidosis, hypoxia, hypovolaemia, tension pneumothorax, cardiac tamponade and pulmonary embolus.

Treatment is with adrenaline (1 mg) in the first instance, combined with the usual CPR. Calcium may help, especially if the QRS complex is widened to greater than 0.12 second (Camm, 1986). Sodium bicarbonate may be needed to correct severe acidosis. High dose adrenaline (5 mg) should be considered.

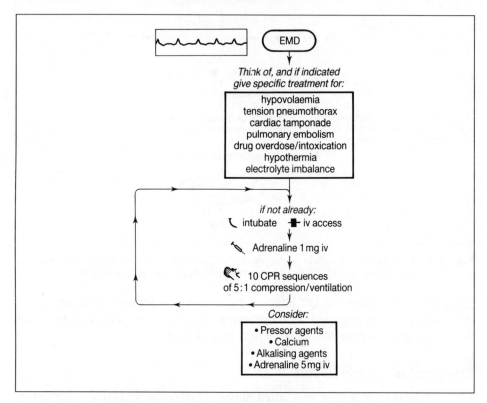

Fig. 10.8 Electromechanical dissociation (EMD). Adapted Guidelines for Advanced Life Support, from *Resuscitation* **24** (1992). Elsevier Scientific Publications Ireland Ltd.

CHANCES OF SUCCESS WITH CPR

The likelihood of survival following cardiac arrest is dependent on many variables, the most important of which are:

- Where the arrest takes place
- The patient's overall physical fitness
- The underlying pathology
- The patient's condition after arrest

The development of out-of-hospital resuscitation has been shown to be of bene-fit in reports from the USA, the UK and Sweden (Geddes, 1986), with immediate bystander CPR doubling the percentage of survivors. The improved prognosis noted in these speedily-resuscitated patients may be because early CPR limits the extent of myocardial damage by establishing early reperfusion.

Most patients who arrest in hospital have recently sustained a myocardial infarc-tion, hence the importance of coronary care units and special observation of these patients, especially those with hypotension and heart failure. Ventricular fibrilla-tion will not always be preceded by warning dysrhythmias. 'Step-down' coronary units, between the coronary care unit and the ward, have been advocated for high-risk patients.

The prognosis of patients resuscitated within hospital is often governed by where the arrest takes place. The time between collapse and initiation of resuscita-tion is critical. Long-term survival in ward patients is only 2–3% (Hershey and Fisher, 1982), probably reflecting the increased time spent in confirmation of diag-nosis and initiation of definitive therapy. Initial success rates in all cases of adult resuscitation may be as low as 30%, falling to 10% in the long term (Peatfield et al, 1977). Nevertheless, these poor results should not discourage attempts at resuscitation, since there are many full cardiac arrests that can be averted in the early stages when warning dysrhythmias or pure respiratory arrest have occurred. The best results may be obtained if resuscitation equipment is readily available and the nursing staff are able to defibrillate on their own initiative. The resuscita-tion rate then approaches 75%, 50% of all arrest cases being discharged from hospital (Mackintosh et al, 1979).

POST-ARREST MANAGEMENT

The treatment of a patient following resuscitation depends on the initial outcome of CPR. Full recovery from cardiac arrest is rarely immediate and can only be said to have occurred when the patient is fully conscious, with full cardiac, cere-bral and renal function. These will be more likely if prompt CPR and defibrilla-tion are carried out and if the underlying dysrhythmia is ventricular fibrillation. After stabilisation, all standard care should be given (preferably in an intensive care environment), although the amount of care patients require following a cardiac arrest varies enormously (Table 10.1). Because of the temporary systemic fibrinolytic state induced by thrombolytic agents, thrombolytic therapy is not recommended after prolonged or traumatic CPR. However, because of the enor-mous benefits that may be conferred by thrombolysis, resuscitation should not be an absolute contraindication (Cross et al, 1991). Indeed, one might argue that those experiencing primary ventricular fibrillation have had larger infarcts and stand to gain most by thrombolysis. If the patient has already received throm-bolytic treatment, haemorrhagic complications are much more common and should be anticipated.

Following successful resuscitation, the patient's condition may be broadly classi-fied into four groups:

Table 10.1 First steps after resuscitation

1. Check ventilation is adequate:
   - Endotracheal tube is correctly placed
   - 100% oxygen
   - Air entry is going to all areas of the chest
2. Obtain blood gases and potassium
3. Insert urinary catheter
   - Measure hourly output
4. Insert nasogastric tube
   - Aspirate gas and fluid
5. Obtain ECG and chest X-ray
6. Consider need for:
   - Low-dose dopamine infusion
   - Lignocaine infusion

- Immediate recovery with no sequelae
- Unconscious for a few hours. These patients may well be amnesic but some suffer anxiety, confusion, delusions and difficulty in concentrating for several months
- Unconscious for more than 24 hours. These patients often exhibit signs of spasticity, stroke or incoordination. The prognosis is variable
- Decerebrate. Death is usual within a few days.

The patient should be examined to assess haemodynamic status and to look for complications of the resuscitation procedure, such as bleeding (thrombolysed patients), aspiration of gastric contents or pneumothorax (secondary to rib fracture or central venous catheterisation). An underlying cause for the arrest, such anoxia or drug toxicity, should be considered. Elective ventilation and prophylactic drug therapy may be required. The routine use of lignocaine remains controversial; the property of negative inotropy should be weighed against the presence or intended suppression of ventricular dysrhythmias. It must be remembered, however, that there will be impaired renal and hepatic flow, and drug pharmacokinetics will alter.

Special attention should be given to the following:

Cardiovascular system

A full ECG and chest X-ray should be obtained. Blood should be sent for analysis of blood gases and electrolytes. An adequate blood pressure and cardiac output must be obtained to allow renal, coronary and cerebral perfusion. Formal haemodynamic monitoring with a Swan–Ganz catheter and arterial lines may be needed (Stokes and Jowett, 1985). Low-dose dopamine is often of value in promoting renal perfusion to avert acute renal failure. It is important, to maintain an adequate and stable blood pressure at a level as close to the patient's norm as possible. Cerebral autoregulation will be impaired, and both cerebral hypoperfusion and oedema need to be avoided.

Respiratory system

Ventilation/perfusion defects are common in both lungs following resuscitation, and oxygen therapy should always be given. Arterial blood gases should be measured, and artificial ventilation may be required. Hyperventilation to lower the P_{CO_2} may be useful in reducing cerebral oedema acutely.

Renal system

Adequate renal perfusion must be obtained as a priority, and an adequate blood pressure should produce 40–50 ml of urine per hour. Catheterisation of the bladder will usually be required, with urine output measured at hourly intervals to detect early signs of renal failure. Some authorities advocate the use of frusemide or mannitol to prevent renal shut-down or cerebral oedema. Low-dose dopamine may also be considered. Renal failure should be treated along conventional lines. Careful consideration must be given to the use of drugs excreted by the kidneys and those with potential nephrotoxic side-effects.

Central nervous system

Primary cerebral damage may be caused by hypoxia during the arrest. Secondary damage may also occur after circulation is restored if the injured brain becomes oedematous. A flat trace on the electroencephalogram (EEG) is seen within 10 seconds of loss of cerebral circulation, and cerebral glucose is depleted within 1 minute. Microthrombi may form in the small cerebral vessels when blood flow ceases, which compromises cerebral perfusion when circulation is restored. Micro-emboli may also be ejected from the heart and great vessels during cardiac massage. The continuing widespread use of calcium during cardiac arrest is questionable (other than for electromechanical dissociation), since it promotes vasospasm in the cerebral vessels. Calcium antagonists given after the arrest may, theoretically, be of value to relieve this. Adequate arterial oxygenation is of great importance, if necessary using mechanical ventilation. Cerebral oedema may be reduced by the use of intravenous mannitol (200 ml of 20% solution) and dexamathasone (10 mg intravenously, followed by 4 mg orally every 6 hours). Limitation of intravenous fluids and elevation of the head to 30° to increase venous drainage may also help. An EEG may be of prognostic importance.

Convulsions increase cerebral metabolic requirements and intracranial pressures, contributing to brain damage. They should be controlled in the usual way.

Acid–base status

The acid–base balance must be assessed urgently, and plasma potassium must be measured immediately and frequently after the arrest. Both should be corrected as required. Care is required in administration of sodium bicarbonate, since it can lead to a rapid fall in plasma potassium levels and a rise in P_{CO_2} (thereby worsening cerebral oedema).

WHEN TO STOP

The decision to terminate resuscitation is a medical one and should be made by the most senior physician present. This decision should follow an assessment of the patient's cerebral and cardiovascular status, as well as prognosis (Baskett, 1986). Prolonged resuscitation is seldom justified; the mortality following an arrest of over 15 minutes is 90% (Bedell et al, 1983). Deep coma, dilated pupils and absence of spontaneous respirations usually indicate death.

All patients who die suddenly should be considered as potential organ donors, and visceral perfusion and oxygenation should be maintained until a decision is made.

It is appropriate for all team members to be thanked for their efforts by the team leader. All tubes, lines and leads should be removed prior to the patient being 'laid out'. A senior doctor should discuss the death with relatives as soon as possible, and the presence of an experienced nurse is of great value.

AUDIT

Open discussion by all members of an arrest team (preferably immediately after an arrest) is of value, to identify weaknesses and allay anxieties. Misplaced confidence may be unmasked, and whilst regular attendance at cardiac arrests increases confidence, it is not necessarily matched by increased competence (Wynne et al, 1987; Marteau et al, 1990). There is no substitute for training, retraining and feedback via the audit process (Berden et al, 1993).

DEFIBRILLATION AND CARDIOVERSION

The use of an electric current to terminate ventricular fibrillation in man was first reported in 1947 by Beck et al, who applied 120 V directly to the ventricles. Later an alternating current (AC) defibrillator was developed for terminating ventricular fibrillation by passing a current across the chest at 720 V (Zoll et al, 1956). The modern direct current (DC) defibrillator was developed by Lown in 1962, with the advantages of being smaller, chargeable with batteries and (because smaller currents were being employed) less likely to cause myocardial damage or precipitate dysrhythmias.

Electrical defibrillation depolarises myocardial tissue ahead of the intrinsic depolarisation wave, making it refractory to conduction. The whole myocardium is thus suddenly depolarised and awaits intrinsic pacemaker function to return, hopefully from the SA node. It follows that, if an insufficient current is applied, not all the myocardium will be depolarised, and defibrillation will not be successful. Following its application to ventricular fibrillation, the defibrillator was applied to other dysrhythmias with marked success. Electrical treatment of cardiac dysrhythmias has marked advantages over drugs, in that it is free from pharmacological side-effects (especially depression of myocardial contractility), and it is useful against a wide variety of tachydysrhythmias, especially those originating from the ventricles (VT and VF). An early complication of this procedure was ventricular fibrillation, which was believed to occur following delivery of the shock to the heart at a time coincident with the vulnerable 30 ms preceding the apex of the T wave of the cardiac cycle (R-on-T). Synchronised defibrillators have thus been developed, which trigger the shock just after the R wave.

Indications for cardioversion

Many cardiologists prefer to treat tachydysrhythmias with drugs, provided there is no contraindication, such as profound hypotension or heart failure. There is obviously no choice if the dysrhythmia is causing circulatory collapse.

Elective synchronised cardioversion is useful for the treatment of both supraventricular and ventricular dysrhythmias. Typical indications include atrial flutter (which is very sensitive to low energies), ventricular tachycardia and supraventricular tachycardia unresponsive to drug therapy. Atrial fibrillation is usually initially treated with drugs, but cardioversion may be employed for recent-onset atrial fibrillation (especially peri-infarction), after therapy for heart failure has reduced cardiac size or after cardiac surgery. Anticoagulants should not be necessary for recent-onset atrial fibrillation, but other cases should be given warfarin for 2–6 weeks before cardioversion and possibly up to a month after.

Metabolic and drug considerations

Patients with hypoxaemia and acidaemia are difficult to defibrillate. For successful defibrillation, attention needs to be directed to these metabolic upsets. Careful attention should also be paid to electrolyte levels, particularly those of potassium. Drugs may also influence the heart's response to cardioversion. Digoxin reduces the energy threshold required for defibrillation, and much smaller currents should be delivered. In contrast, quinidine, lignocaine and phenytoin all increase the threshold, and higher energies will be needed to restore sinus rhythm.

Technique

The procedure should be explained to the patient and consent obtained. The patient should be fasted for 6–8 hours. A standard 12-lead ECG should be recorded before and after cardioversion, and a rhythm strip should be recorded during the procedure. An anaesthetist should be in attendance to administer a short-acting anaesthetic, and resuscitation equipment must be on hand. It is usual to pre-oxygenate the patient, and oxygen should be delivered throughout the procedure and during recovery.

There are two main methods of paddle placement, although there appears to be no superiority in either method:

● *Pre-cordial*. One paddle is applied close to the sternum over the right 2nd–3rd intercostal space and the other just below the apex of the heart

● *Chest-to-back*. One paddle is placed to the left of the base of the sternum and the other between the scapulae, slightly to the left of the spine (which would otherwise prevent good skin contact)

The technique is the same as used for defibrillation, as in the first part of Figure 10.5 (p.272).

It is best to ensure that the ECG is set so that the QRS complex displays the most upright R wave, to aid synchronised discharge of the defibrillator. The discharge will not necessarily occur as soon as the button is pressed, and the operator must not be tempted to release pressure on the paddles until after the shock has been delivered. Because myocardial damage increases with the amount of energy applied, the shock should be 'titrated' against the type of dysrhythmia; typical energy levels required are:

● Atrial fibrillation – start at 100 J
● Atrial flutter, supraventricular tachycardias – start at 50 J
● Ventricular tachycardia – start no lower than 100 J
● Ventricular fibrillation – normal rapid sequence (200 J, 200 J, 360 J)

If the shock causes a stable rhythm to deteriorate into ventricular fibrillation, an immediate unsynchronised shock of at least 200 J should be delivered.

Antidysrhythmic drugs are occasionally needed between shocks, to help to restore sinus rhythm, and these are always worth trying if the first two or three attempts fail. Administration of a suitable antidysrhythmic agent (e.g. lignocaine) is particularly recommended if multiple ventricular ectopic beats develop after an unsuccessful shock.

After restoration of sinus rhythm, a further 12-lead ECG should be obtained, vital signs recorded and arrangements made for monitoring for at least 8 hours.

Complications

Dysrhythmias may occur after cardioversion, either because the underlying problem that precipitated the original dysrhythmia is still present or as a direct consequence of cardioversion.

Bradydysrhythmias frequently occur immediately following cardioversion and are self-limiting. Sinus bradycardias, wandering pacemakers and junctional rhythms are not serious and can be treated with atropine if they persist. A few ventricular ectopic beats may also be seen and, again, are usually self-limiting. However, runs of ectopics, ventricular tachycardia and fibrillation need treating along usual lines. Because these complications may develop up to 8 hours after cardioversion, prolonged monitoring is indicated. This is particularly the case if antidysrhythmic drugs have also been used or if hypokalaemia is present. The risk of ventricular fibrillation and ventricular tachycardia is increased if the patient has been taking digoxin, and although many discontinue the drug prior to cardioversion, this is not required, and the procedure is well tolerated, providing there are no signs of digoxin toxicity (Dalzell et al, 1990). Injury to the myocardium may occur, especially with multiple shocks (Dahl et al, 1974), and makes subsequent dysrhythmias more likely. It is, therefore, advisable to start defibrillation at lower energies and allow 2–3 minutes to elapse before the next shock is given. Clinical signs of myocardial injury are not usually evident, even after multiple shocks. ST/ T wave changes may be seen on the ECG but CK-MB levels are only rarely elevated (Jakabsson et al, 1990).

Thromboembolic complications occur in about 2% of cases restored to sinus rhythm. Those at risk are patients with long-standing dysrhythmias (classically atrial fibrillation), dyskinetic ventricular walls or dilated hearts. The risk may be minimised by prior anticoagulation for a few weeks before and after cardioversion. Paddle burns are uncommon if careful attention is paid to application of the electrodes. Any inflammation will quickly respond to topical steroid cream such as 1% hydrocortisone.

Cardioversion in a patient with a pacemaker

Modern pacemakers and implanted defibrillators have circuitry to protect against external defibrillation, although reports of pacemaker damage have been reported. It is, therefore, a good idea routinely to assess pacemaker function prior to discharge from hospital. External defibrillation pads should be placed away from the pulse generator, and it may be necessary to use the anteroposterior paddle positions if the generator is in the right infraclavicular area.

References

Aarons E J and Beeching N J (1991) Survey of "do not resuscitate" orders in a district general hospital. *British Medical Journal*, **303:** 1504–1506.
Advanced Life Support Working Party of the European Resuscitation Council (1992) Guidelines for Advanced Life Support. *Resuscitation*, **24:** 111–121.
Basic Life Support Working Party of the European Resuscitation Council (1992) Guidelines for Basic Life Support. *Resuscitation*, **24:** 103–110.
Baskett P J F (1986) The ethics of resuscitation. *British Medical Journal*, **293:** 189–190.
Baskett P J F (1992) Advances in cardiopulmonary resuscitation. *British Journal of Anaesthesia*, **69:** 182–193.
Beck C S, Prilchard W H and Feil H S (1947) Ventricular fibrillation of long duration abolished by electric shock. *Journal of the American Medical Association*, **135:** 985–986.
Bedell S E, Delbanco T L, Cook E F and Epstein F H (1983) Survival after cardiopulmonary resuscitation in hospital. *New England Journal of Medicine*, **10:** 569–576.
Berden H J J M, Willems F F, Hendrick J M A, Pijls N H J and Knape J T A (1993) How frequently should basic CPR training be repeated to maintain adequate skills? *British Medical Journal*, **306:** 1576–1577.
Brown D C, Lewis A J and Criley J M (1979) Asystole and its treatment: the possible role of the parasympathetic nervous system in cardiac arrest. *Journal of the American College of Emergency Physicians*, **8:** 448–452.
Caldwell G, Millar G, Quinn E, Vincent R and Chamberlain D A (1985) Simple mechanical methods for cardioversion: defence of the precordial thump and cough version. *British Medical Journal*, **291:** 627–630.
Camm A J (1986) ABC of resuscitation: asystole and electromechanical dissociation. *British Medical Journal*, **292:** 1123–1124.
Casey W F (1984) Cardiopulmonary resuscitation: a survey of standards among junior hospital doctors. *Journal of the Royal Society of Medicine*, **77:** 921–924.
Chamberlain D A (1991) Lignocaine and bretylium as adjuncts to electrical defibrillation. *Resuscitation*, **22:** 153–157.

Chandra N, Snyder L and Weisfeldt M L (1981) Abdominal binding during CPR in man. *Journal of the American Medical Association*, **246:** 351–353.

Cobb L A, Werner J A and Trobaugh G B (1980) Sudden cardiac death: parts 1 and 2. *Modern Concepts in Cardiovascular Disease*, **49:** 31–42.

Cobbe S M, Redmond M J, Watson J M, Hollingworth J and Carrington D (1991) "Heartstart Scotland" – initial experience of a national scheme for out-of-hospital defibrillation. *British Medical Journal*, **303:** 1517–1520.

Cooper M J and Abinader E G (1979) Atropine-induced ventricular fibrillation: case report and review of the literature. *American Heart Journal*, **99:** 225–228.

Criley J M, Blaufuss A H and Kissel G L (1976) Cough-induced cardiac compression. *Journal of the American Medical Association*, **236:** 1246–1250.

Cross S J, Lee H S, Rawles J M and Jennings K (1991) Safety of thrombolysis in association with cardiopulmonary resuscitation. *British Medical Journal*, **303:** 1242.

Crul J F, Neursing B T and Zimmerman A H (1985) The ABC sequence of cardiopulmonary resuscitation (CPR). *Journal of the World Association of Emergency and Disaster Medicine*, **1**(supplement 4): 236–245.

Cummins R O, Eisenberg M S and Shultz K R (1986) Automatic external defibrillators: clinical issues in cardiology. *Circulation*, **73:** 381–385.

Dahl C F, Ewy G A and Warner E D (1974) Myocardial necrosis from direct current countershock: effect of paddle electrode size and time interval between discharge. *Circulation*, **50:** 956–961.

Dalzell G W, Anderson J and Adgey A A (1990) Factors determining success and energy requirements for cardioversion in atrial fibrillation. *Quarterly Journal of Medicine*, **76:** 903–913.

David J and Prior-Willeard P F S (1993) Resuscitation skills of MRCP candidates. *British Medical Journal*, **306:** 1578–1579.

Dembo D H (1984) The role of calcium chloride in cardiac arrest. *Journal of the American Medical Association*, **250:** 3327–3329.

Doan L A (1984) Peripheral versus central venous delivery of medications during CPR. *Annals of Emergency Medicine*, **13:** 784–786.

Doyal L and Wilsher D (1993) Withholding cardiopulmonary resuscitation: proposals for formal guidelines. *British Medical Journal*, **306:** 1593–1596.

Elam J O and Greene D G (1961) Mission accomplished. Successful mouth to mouth resuscitation. *Anesthesia and Analgesia (Current Research)*, **40:** 440–442, 578–580, 672–676.

European Resuscitation Council Basic Life Support Working Party (1993a) Guidelines for Basic Life Support. *British Medical Journal*, **306:** 1587–1589.

European Resuscitation Council Basic Life Support Working Party (1993b) Adult advanced cardiac life support: the European Resuscitation Council Guidelines 1992 (abridged). *British Medical Journal*, **306:** 1589–1593.

Evans T R (1986) *ABC of Resuscitation*, Evans T R (ed.). London: British Medical Association.

Florin D (1993) Do not resuscitate orders: the need for a policy. *Journal of the Royal College of Physicians of London*, **27:** 135–138.

Gass E A and Curry L (1983) Physicians' and nurses' retention of knowledge and skills after training in CPR. *Canadian Medical Association Journal*, **128:** 550–551.

Geddes J S (1986) Twenty years of prehospital coronary care. *British Heart Journal*, **56:** 491–495.

Gonzales E R (1993) Pharmacological controversies in CPR. *Annals of Internal Medicine*, **22:** 317–323.

Hershey C O and Fisher L (1982) Why outcome of CPR in general wards is poor. *Lancet*, **i:** 31–34.

Jaffe A S (1993) The use of anti-arrhythmics in advanced cardiopulmonary resuscitation. *Annals of Emergency Medicine*, **22:** 307–316.

Jakabsson J, Odmansson I and Norlander R (1990) Enzyme release after elective cardioversion. *European Heart Journal*, **11:** 749–752.

Jones A, Peckett W, Clark E, Sharpe C, Krimholtz S and Russell M (1993) Nurses' knowledge of the resuscitation status of patients and action in the event of cardiorespiratory arrest. *British Medical Journal*, **306:** 1577–1578.

Jowett N I and Thompson D R (1988a) Basic life support. The forgotten skills? *Intensive Care Nursing*, **4:** 9–17.

Jowett N I and Thompson D R (1988b) Advanced cardiac life support: current perspectives. *Intensive Care Nursing*, **4:** 71–81.

Jowett N I, Thompson D R and Bailey S W (1985) Electrocardiographic monitoring. I. Static monitoring. *Intensive Care Nursing*, **2:** 71–76.

Jude J R, Kouwenhoven W B and Knickerbocker G G (1961) Cardiac arrest. Report of application of external cardiac massage in 118 patients. *Journal of the American Medical Association*, **178:** 1063–1070.

Kaye W and Mancini M E (1986) Retention of cardiopulmonary resuscitation skills by physicians, registered nurses and the general public. *Critical Care Medicine*, **14:** 621–623.

Kerber R E, Grayzel J and Hoyt R (1981) Transthoracic resistance of human defibrillation: influence of body weight, chest size, serial shocks, paddle size and paddle contact pressure. *Circulation*, **63:** 676–682.

Kouwenhoven W B, Jude J R and Knickerbocker G G (1960) Closed chest cardiac massage. *Journal of the American Medical Association*, **173:** 1064–1067.

Mackintosh A F, Crabb M E, Brennan H, Williams J H and Chamberlain D A (1979) Hospital resuscitation from ventricular fibrillation in Brighton. *British Medical Journal*, **i:** 511–513.

Maier G W, Newton J R, Wolfe J A, Tyson G S, Olsen G O, Glower D D, Spratt J A, Davis J W, Feneley M P and Rankin J S (1986) The influence of manual chest compression rate on hemodynamic support during cardiac arrest: high impulse cardiopulmonary resuscitation. *Circulation*, **74**(supplement IV): 51–59.

Marteau T M, Wynne G, Kaye W and Evans T R (1990) Resuscitation: experience without feedback increases confidence but not skills. *British Medical Journal*, **300:** 849–850.

Maull K I (1984) Pocket-mask ventilation: a critical appraisal. *Archives of Emergency Medicine*, **1:** 161–163.

Melker R J (1985) Recommendations for ventilation during cardiopulmonary resuscitation: time for a change? *Critical Care Medicine*, **13:** 882–883.

Myerburg R J, Kessler K M, Zarman L, Conde C A and Castellanos A (1982) Survivors of prehospital cardiac arrest. *Journal of the American Medical Association*, **247:** 1485–1490.

National Conference on Cardiopulmonary Resuscitation and Emergency Cardiac Care (1986) Standards and guidelines for cardiopulmonary resuscitation and emergency cardiac care. *Journal of the American Medical Association*, **255:** 2905–2984.

Niemann J T (1984) Differences in cerebral and myocardial perfusion in closed chest resuscitation. *Annals of Emergency Medicine*, **13:** 849–853.

Peatfield R C, Sillett R W, Taylor D and McNicol M W (1977) Survival after cardiac arrest in hospital. *Lancet*, **i:** 1223–1225.

Resuscitation Council (1984) *Resuscitation for Citizens*. London: Resuscitation Council.

Rich S, Wix H L and Shapiro E P (1981) Clinical assessment of heart chamber size and valve motion during cardiopulmonary resuscitation by two-dimensional echocardiography. *American Heart Journal*, **102:** 367–373.

Robertson C and Holmberg S (1992) Compression techniques and blood flow during cardiopulmonary resuscitation. *Resuscitation*, **24:** 123–132.

Royal College of Physicians (1987) Resuscitation from cardiopulmonary arrest. Training and organisation. *Journal of the Royal College of Physicians*, **21:** 175–182.

Rudikoff M T, Maughan W L, Effron M, Freund P and Weisfeldt M L (1980) Mechanisms of blood flow during cardiopulmonary resuscitation. *Circulation*, **61:** 345–352.

Sack J B, Kesselbrenner M B and Bregman D (1992) Survival from in-hospital cardiac arrest with interposed abdominal counterpulsation during CPR. *Journal of the American Medical Association*, **267:** 379–385.

Safar P (1984) Cardiopulmonary–cerebral resuscitation. In *Textbook of Critical Care*, Shoemaker W C, Thompson W C and Holbrook P R (eds), p. 15. Philadelphia: W B Saunders.

Safar P, Escarra L and Elam J (1958) A comparison of the mouth to mouth and mouth to airway methods of artificial respiration with the chest pressure arm-lift method. *New England Journal of Medicine*, **258:** 671–677.

Sellick B A (1961) Cricoid pressure to control regurgitation of stomach contents during induction of anaesthesia. *Lancet*, **ii:** 404–406.

Skinner D V (1985) Cardiopulmonary skills of pre-registration house officers. *British Medical Journal*, **290** 1549–1550.

Stokes P H and Jowett N I (1985) Haemodynamic monitoring using the Swan–Ganz catheter. *Intensive Care Nursing*, **1:** 9–17.

Sullivan M J J and Guyatt G H (1986) Simulated cardiac arrests for monitoring quality of in-hospital resuscitation. *Lancet*, **ii:** 618–620.

Taylor G J, Tucker W M, Green M T and Weisfeldt M L (1977) Importance of prolonged compression during cardiopulmonary resuscitation in man. *New England Journal of Medicine*, **296:** 1515–1517.

Tunstall-Pedoe H, Bailey L, Chamberlain D A, Marsden A K, Ward M E and Zideman D A (1992) Survey of 3765 cardiopulmonary resuscitations in British Hospitals (the BRESUS study); methods and overall results. *British Medical Journal*, **304:** 1347–1351.

Varon J and Fromm R E (1993) Cardiopulmonary resuscitation. New and controversial techniques. *Postgraduate Medical Journal*, **93**(8): 235–239.

Waller D G and Robertson C E (1991) Role of sympathomimetic amines during CPR. *Resuscitation*, **22:** 181–190.

Williams R (1993) The "Do not resuscitate" decision; guidelines for policy in the adult. *Journal of the Royal College of Physicians of London*, **27:** 139–140.

Wynne G, Marteau T M, Johnston M, Whiteley C A and Evans T R (1987) Inability of trained nurses to perform basic life support. *British Medical Journal*, **294:** 1198–1199.

Zoll P M, Linenthal A J, Gibson W, Paul M and Normal L (1956) Termination of ventricular fibrillation in man by externally applied counter shock. *New England Journal of Medicine*, **254:** 727–732.

11

Cardiac Pacing

Control over the electrical activity of the heart is frequently made by means of an artificial pacemaker. If pacing is for a short time only, an external power source is used to deliver electricity to the heart, either endocardially, via the skin (transcutaneous pacing) or via the oesophagus (oesophageal pacing). Temporary cardiac pacing is often used in coronary care and intensive care units to treat transient conduction problems. However, when long-term control is required, a permanent pacemaker is implanted. The first implant was reported in 1958, and now over 200 000 permanent pacemakers are implanted worldwide every year.

INDICATIONS FOR PACING

Indications for pacing vary widely both nationally and internationally. A summary of some of the indications is shown in Tables 11.1 and 11.2.

Stokes–Adams attacks

Stokes–Adams attacks are frequently associated with second- and third-degree heart block and require pacing without the need for further investigation. Less frequently, the aetiology is the sick sinus syndrome or paroxysmal tachycardias, which should usually be further evaluated by electrophysiological testing.

Low-output states associated with bradycardia

Raising the heart rate to between 70 and 80 beats per minute by inserting a temporary pacemaker can dramatically improve cardiac failure or other symptoms, if these have been associated with bradycardia. Raising the rate of the heart above 80–90 beats per minute, however, may be detrimental and result in a fall of the cardiac output. In these circumstances, it is preferable to insert an atrial pacing wire and synchronise atrial and ventricular emptying in physiological sequence. Such procedures are not without risk, and the extra benefits obtained may be minimal.

Conduction defects following acute myocardial infarction

Inferior myocardial infarction

Pacing is usually indicated if the heart rate falls below 60 beats per minute (unresponsive to atropine), where there are symptoms or signs attributable to low-output cardiac failure. Observation only is needed in the remaining cases.

Table 11.1   Some indications for temporary pacing

Acute myocardial infarction
(i)   Anterior myocardial infarction accompanied by:
         Complete heart block
         Second-degree heart block
         First-degree heart block with bifascicular block
         Newly-acquired left bundle branch block

(ii) Inferior myocardial infarction accompanied by:

      Any of the above accompanied by actual or threatened haemodynamic decompensation

Prior to permanent pacing
When patients are symptomatic and immediate permanent pacing facilities are not available

Prophylactic perioperatively
(i)   During general anaesthesia or cardiac catheterisation in patients with:
         Intermittent heart block
         Bifascicular block with first-degree heart block

(ii) During cardiac surgery
         Especially for aortic and tricuspid surgery
         Septal defect closure

Treatment of Tachycardias
Overdrive pacing (rare)

Table 11.2   Some indications for permanent pacing

General agreement
Acquired symptomatic complete heart block
Symptomatic second-degree heart block
Symptomatic sinus bradycardia
Sinus node dysfunction
Carotid sinus syndrome

Frequent indications
Asymptomatic complete heart block
Asymptomatic second-degree heart block
Transient Mobitz type II heart block following acute myocardial infarction
Bi-fascicular block in patients with syncope
Overdrive pacing for recurrent ventricular tachycardia

Generally not indicated
Syncope of unknown cause
Asymptomatic bradycardia
Sinus bradycardia with non-specific symptoms
Asymptomatic sinus arrest
Nocturnal bradycardia

Anterior myocardial infarction

The prognosis for conduction defects following anterior myocardial infarction is poor, and the indications for pacing are controversial (Klein et al, 1984). Certainly complete heart block needs pacing, but whether bifascicular, first-degree and second-degree heart block need insertion of a prophylactic pacing wire is not clear.

Refractory tachycardias

Where tachydysrhythmias are not controlled by medical therapy, permanent pacing may have a beneficial role. Ectopic foci can be suppressed by ventricular pacing at a higher rate than sinus rhythm (*overpacing*). Alternatively, fixed-rate pacing in short bursts either slower (*underdrive*) or faster (*overdrive*) than sinus rate may be effective in preventing dysrhythmias. In the 'brady–tachy' syndrome, where the patient has both fast and slow dysrhythmias, drugs such as beta-adrenergic blocking agents and digoxin can be given to control the faster rates, using a pacemaker to prevent very slow heart rates.

Perioperative heart block

Patients with sino-atrial disease or incomplete heart block may be at risk of developing complete heart block during drug therapy or surgery. General anaesthesia with fluorinated hydrocarbons (e.g. halothane) may adversely affect atrioventricular conduction. A pacing wire may, therefore, need to be inserted perioperatively for prophylactic reasons.

Miscellaneous

Temporary pacing may be required in cases of permanent pacemaker failure or for extreme bradycardias caused by drugs (e.g. digoxin or beta-adrenergic blocking agents) or electrolyte disturbances. Pacemakers are also sometimes used to aid diagnosis in complex conduction disorders or during electrophysiological testing procedures (Cobbe, 1986).

TEMPORARY CARDIAC PACING

Temporary endocardial pacing has been used since the early 1960s to maintain cardiac output during episodes of extreme bradycardia, heart block and asystole, particularly in association with acute myocardial infarction. Before the advent of cardiac pacemakers, the combination of acute myocardial infarction and complete heart block was usually fatal (Cohen et al, 1958). Although it is of some value, the use of isoprenaline has now virtually disappeared, other than in places where pacing facilities do not exist (Christiansen et al, 1973). Pacing electrodes can now be rapidly passed percutaneously into the right ventricle under local anaesthesia, and, in experienced hands, this is a safe and simple procedure.

There is little doubt that pacing may be life-saving acutely, but long-term value is a little more difficult to assess. Prognosis is influenced not only by complications of the procedure (dysrhythmias, cardiac perforation and septicaemia), but also by the degree of underlying myocardial damage that originally led to the conduction defect. Many patients effectively treated acutely by temporary pacing die later, whilst still in hospital, from heart failure due to extensive myocardial infarction (Norris et al, 1972). The principal determinant of prognosis is the site of the infarct. Anterior infarction may have necrosed the bundle branches, as well as a greater part of the left ventricular myocardium, which leads to pump failure. Inferior infarcts, on the other hand, do not usually involve so much critical myocardium and normally result only in reversible ischaemia and oedema in the region of the atrioventricular node. In patients who have not suffered an acute myocardial infarction, temporary pacing is most often required in cases of chronic atrioventricular block and sick-sinus syndrome. The underlying disease in most of these cases is *Lenegre's disease* (AV fibrosis), and only a small number are due to ischaemic damage. As such, left ventricular function is usually greater, and the outcome following pacing is much better (Hayward, 1981). Patients found to have the sick-sinus syndrome, however, may have a coexisting cardiomyopathy, which could adversely influence the prognosis.

Acute myocardial infarction, heart block and pacing

Pathophysiology (Table 11.3)

Inferior myocardial infarction is usually caused by acute occlusion of the right coronary artery, which supplies the inferior wall of the heart. The AV node is

Table 11.3 Characteristics of complete heart block complicating inferior and anterior myocardial infarction

	Anterior infarction	Inferior infarction
Incidence	25–40%	60–75%
Pathology	Septal necrosis and infarction of the AV node and bundle branches	Ischaemia of the bundle branches
Timing	Usually sudden, following sinus rhythm or second-degree heart block	Normally slow, following first- and second-degree heart block
Ventricular response	30–40 unstable	40–60 stable
QRS morphology	Widened	Narrow
Risk of asystole	High	Low
Mortality	60–75%	25–40%
Prognosis	Often permanent	Most reverse within 14 days

supplied by the right coronary artery in 90% of cases and by the circumflex artery in the remainder. As a result, conduction disturbances commonly occur following acute inferior myocardial infarction and are usually caused by ischaemia or oedema of the conducting system. These effects will be worsened if there is pre-existing damage to the conducting tissues, such as ischaemia or fibrosis of the AV node and bundle branches. Fortunately, for unknown reasons, ischaemic injury to the AV node following inferior myocardial infarction is rarely permanent. Complete heart block usually develops slowly, and the escape rhythm is usually high junctional at 40–60 beats per minute. This is generally haemodynamically stable, and pacing is not usually necessary, providing blood pressure and renal perfusion are maintained. Conduction disturbances can occur at any time in the first 2 weeks but are usually transient, with normal conduction returning in hours or days.

Anterior myocardial infarction is caused by occlusion of the left anterior descending coronary artery, which additionally provides the major blood supply to the bundle of His and bundle branches. Proximal occlusion of the left coronary artery leads to extensive myocardial damage, often resulting in heart failure and cardiogenic shock. Heart block is a sinister and sudden complication and is due to ischaemic destruction of the conducting tissues below the AV node. Emergent ventricular escape rhythms are unreliable, slow and irregular; there is a marked tendency to develop asystole. The insertion of a temporary pacing wire under these circumstances probably has little influence on the outcome, although it is usual practice. Mortality is high, and late deaths are common (Mullins and Atkins, 1976).

Complete heart block (CHB) complicates 9–33% of acute myocardial infarctions and is associated with a high mortality (Kostuk and Beanlands, 1970). The lower incidence may reflect the difficulty of recognising CHB electrocardiographically. Atrioventricular dissociation is often confused with complete heart block and is usually not associated with severe myocardial damage. Other episodes of CHB that appear to have a good prognosis could be first-degree heart block with accelerated junctional rhythm.

Hypertension, pre-existing diabetes mellitus and high blood glucose concentrations on admission to hospital are common risk factors for those requiring temporary pacing following acute myocardial infarction. Disorders of atrioventricular and intraventricular conduction are significantly more common in diabetic patients with acute myocardial infarction than in those who are not diabetic (Czyzyk et al, 1980), and this may be due to pre-existing micro-angiopathic damage of the conducting system (Blandford and Burden, 1984). The higher incidence of previous myocardial infarctions and hypertension in those patients requiring pacing is probably an indication of a greater degree of underlying myocardial damage.

The prognosis in patients with complete heart block appears to be related to factors other than conduction abnormality, especially following anterior myocardial infarction, where mortality is higher than in those with inferior infarction (Lassers and Julian, 1968; Norris, 1969). Although restoration of stable haemodynamics will affect immediate morbidity and mortality due to bradycardia and asystole, it will not help those with extensive myocardial damage, who often have mechanical heart failure and cardiogenic shock.

The benefits of routine pacing for inferior myocardial infarction are also in doubt. Mortality has been reported as 37% without pacing (Cohen et al, 1958), and is almost as high in those who are paced. Insertion of wires for heart block complicating inferior infarction is often routine on many coronary care units, even in the absence of haemodynamic decompensation. However, the majority of cases do not deteriorate, and insertion of a temporary wire is usually not necessary (Jowett et al, 1989).

Prophylactic pacing

The potential complications of temporary pacing (especially bleeding following thrombolysis) should be considered before prophylactic wires are inserted following acute myocardial infarction. The more important indications are bifascicular block with AV block or left bundle branch block acquired during the infarct.

Temporary pacemakers

There are three main forms of temporary pacing:

- Transcutaneous
- Transoesophageal
- Transvenous

Transcutaneous pacing

External temporary cardiac pacing was first introduced in 1952 and was used widely as a temporary measure for the treatment of profound bradycardia and asystole until superseded by transvenous pacing in 1959. Nevertheless, the availability of external transthoracic pacing on coronary care may be vital in buying extra time in an emergency until arrangements can be made for insertion of a temporary wire. Because it is simple to institute following minimal training, it can be safely and quickly applied by those with no experience of transvenous pacing, nurses and paramedics.

With the advent of thrombolysis, there may be certain occasions on which invasive techniques are particularly hazardous, and having such equipment on stand-by is of use when prophylactic temporary pacing would normally be considered.

Two large pad electrodes are attached to the chest (preferably in the antero-posterior position). The positive electrode is located beneath the left scapula and the negative electrode under the left breast. The output from the unit is then increased, until the pacing impulse 'captures' the heart. Modern units use a longer pulse duration, allowing a lower pulse amplitude, so that pacing is usually well tolerated, with little more than slight cutaneous discomfort (tingling or tapping) and occasional muscle twitching (Zoll and Zoll, 1985). Transcutaneous pacing is not a substitute for transvenous pacing, which should be established as soon as possible.

Transoesophageal pacing

The technique of transoesophageal pacing was originally described in the late 1960s in New York (Burack and Furman, 1969). Although transvenous cardiac pacing is the treatment of choice, the transoesophageal route can often act as a holding measure until a percutaneous wire can be inserted. The electrode is passed transnasally into the oesophagus (rather like a nasogastric tube) and the current switched on, initially at about 30 V. When the diaphragm is reached (producing diaphragmatic twitching), the electrode is slowly withdrawn, until ventricular capture is seen on the ECG monitor, and the threshold is then determined. Unfortunately, the method is not very reliable.

Transvenous pacing

Transvenous endocardial pacing is the most common pacing method employed and involves the passage of a bipolar electrode, which is activated by an external impulse generator, into the apex of the right ventricle. The wire is best positioned with the aid of fluoroscopy but may be located 'blindly' using a balloon-tipped 'flotation' pacing wire in patients who cannot be screened. Wires positioned in this way are often unstable, and transthoracic (external) pacing is probably a better emergency alternative (see above).

It is usual for a special room to be set aside for pacing, so that there are facilities for sterility, fluoroscopy and resuscitation (Fitzpatrick and Sutton, 1992). The use of fluoroscopy is governed by a European Economic Community Directive (EEC, 1988). Those operating such equipment are required to be certified for proficiency, with an awareness of the safety aspects of radiation to the patient, the operator and others present.

Choice of route for insertion of temporary pacing wires

The choice of site of insertion depends upon the expertise of the operator and the problems with the wire in the chosen location. Of the usual insertion sites (internal jugular, subclavian, supraclavicular, femoral, brachial and external jugular), the least skill is required for the femoral and brachial approaches, whilst the subclavian route is the most hazardous, largely because of the dangers of pneumothorax and subclavian arterial puncture. The last is, however, much more stable, is the most comfortable for the patient and does not inhibit mobility.

The right internal jugular approach is the most direct to the right ventricle if there is difficulty entering the heart, particularly if a flotation catheter is used. The British Cardiac Society recommend this route, particularly for those with limited experience of central venous catheterisation.

All central venous cannulation may become less hazardous with the advent of ultrasound guides, although these are expensive (presently about £5 000).

Methods of catheterisation

- Percutaneous needle and sheath techniques
- Percutaneous Seldinger technique, using a guide wire
- Cut-down, suitable for the arm veins

The method of choice is probably the Seldinger technique, although, once again, experience of the technique is desirable. The advantage is that a long cannula is passed into the superior vena cava, which helps the passage of the pacing wire into the heart. In addition, unlike shorter cannulae, it will not become displaced if external cardiac massage is required during the insertion procedure. If there is a cardiac arrest, it can be occluded and pacing resumed following resuscitation. The cannula can also be conveniently used for infusing drugs and other fluids as required.

The pacing wire becomes more pliable as it warms to body temperature, so should be inserted as quickly as possible. Sometimes, there is difficulty in passing the electrode into the superior vena cava, which may be made easier by moving the patient's shoulders or rotating the arm across the body. Passage through the heart requires experience and the ability to judge position from the fluoroscopic image. Traversing the tricuspid valve is a frequent problem, particularly if the heart rate is fast or if the myocardium is irritable. Gentle manipulation or looping in the right atrium may help. Passage into the right ventricle can be confirmed by observing the characteristic 'bucking' of the catheter by the tricuspid valve about 5 cm from the tip. Wedging the electrode is sometimes made easier by passing it directly into the pulmonary artery (especially if a balloon flotation-type catheter has been used) and then letting it fall back into the apex. This can be seen just medial to the apex on the cardiac silhouette, and the tip of the electrode should point slightly inferiorly. Once wedged, verification of pacing and threshold measurements are necessary. The former is judged from the appearance of a pacing 'spike' preceding the QRS complex on the ECG. Each spike should capture a QRS complex (Figure 11.1). The pacing threshold is obtained by determining the lowest pacing voltage that produces a paced beat. This threshold should be less than 1 V and preferably below 0.5 V. The wire can then be fixed to the skin with a suture. The pacing mode is then selected (usually 'demand') and the voltage set at about twice the threshold.

Problems during transvenous pacing

Pacing and thrombolysis

The presence of complete heart block following acute myocardial infarction should not contraindicate thrombolysis, for fear that pacing would not be possible. As for other cases of myocardial infarction, thrombolysis (preferably TPA) should be

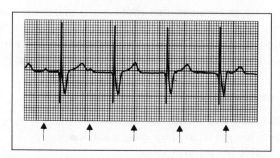

Fig. 11.1 ECG: trace obtained when the cardiac pacing wire is correctly positioned. The pacing spike can be seen preceding each QRS complex. Independent atrial P waves are indicated

given immediately, providing there are no contraindications, along with atropine. In the majority of cases (which will be due to inferior myocardial infarction), AV conduction improves, and many cases of complete heart block may be tolerated without the need to insert a temporary pacemaker (Jowett et al, 1989). Anterior myocardial infarction complicated by complete heart block always warrants temporary pacing, but thrombolysis should still be given first.

Because of the inherent dangers of central cannulation following thrombolysis, particularly if the arterial circulation is entered, temporary pacing should be avoided if possible, and trials of atropine, isoprenaline or external pacing should be considered.

If transvenous pacing is unquestionably required, an insertion site that may be easily compressed should be chose, and thus the femoral, brachial or external jugular routes are preferred. The femoral route is often the best, since access to the apex of the right ventricle from below is fairly easy, although the internal jugular should be considered.

Dysrhythmias

The major complications of temporary pacing are ventricular tachycardia and fibrillation, which are probably produced by mechanical irritation of the endocardium. The appearance of ventricular ectopics is usually a good sign that the catheter has entered the right ventricle, but the wire should be moved if these are frequent or occur in runs. This complication may also be caused electrically if the 'fixed' rather than 'demand' mode is selected on the pacing box or if an inappropriately high pacing threshold is used. Standard resuscitation is required during ventricular fibrillation, although overpacing can sometimes be used to restore a more stable rhythm in ventricular tachycardia.

Patients with temporary wires should have the wire disconnected during the defibrillatory shock, to prevent damage to the external generator.

Perforation of the heart or septum

This may be an early or late complication, and may be indicated by:

- Failure to pace despite good radiological position
- Signs of pericarditis or tamponade
- Diaphragmatic twitching

A change of the ECG pacing pattern from the usual left bundle branch block to right bundle branch block indicates that the wire has perforated the septum. This is usually insignificant, but the wire should be moved.

Failure to pace

Pacing failure may be evident from absence of a pacing spike (implying failure of pulse generation) or the spikes failing to capture (implying a displaced electrode or change in threshold). The box or the wire will then need replacing or repositioning.

Pacemaker dependence

Pacing wires not infrequently need repositioning, because they have moved, because of a rapidly increasing pacing threshold or because of dysrhythmias. Unfortunately, pre-existing rhythms are often abolished after pacing for a while, leaving complete asystole as the underlying rhythm (seen if the pacing box is momentarily turned off). Movement of the wire or transient rises in the threshold may then be associated with Stokes–Adams attacks, because the heart has become 'pacemaker dependent'. This problem may need the passage of a second pacing wire, to take over whilst the other is relocated or removed.

When to stop temporary pacing

Following acute myocardial infarction, it is usual to leave pacing wires *in situ* for 24–48 hours after reliable atrioventricular conduction has recovered.

Patients with inferior myocardial infarction usually develop AV nodal dysfunction because of oedema rather than necrosis, and may be mediated by adenosine (Shah et al, 1987). The recovery period is usually short but may be up to 14 days. Those with anterior infarcts, however, usually have infarcted conduction tissue and often need permanent pacing. Because these patients often have severe left ventricular damage, consideration needs giving to dual chamber pacing to maximise cardiac output.

Care of patients with temporary pacing wires

Patients often feel much better following temporary pacing, and are in a much better physical and psychological state for discussion about the pacemaker and its implications. Mobility will necessarily be restricted, but if the subclavian approach has been used, this will be minimal. However, the wire should be secured to the body to prevent accidental pulling. Many pacing boxes are now small and portable, thus enabling early mobilisation of the patient. There is usually not much pain at the site of wire insertion, but this should be routinely observed for signs of bleeding and infection. Routine checks are also required on the equipment, with attention to connections and performance. The threshold and underlying rhythm need charting on a twice-daily basis and settings discussed for the following 12-hour period. This should be documented in the patient's notes and the nursing notes, as well as on the charts beside the bed. Although many pacing units are protected, it is advisable to turn off the pacemaker to prevent electrical damage if the patient needs defibrillation.

Removal of the pacing wire is a simple and straightforward procedure carried out at the patient's bedside. The unit should be turned off and the dressing and retaining sutures removed. Whilst observing the ECG monitor for ectopic activity, the wire should be slowly withdrawn and a sterile pad held firmly over the puncture site for a few minutes, to prevent bleeding. It may be advisable to remove the tip of the disposable pacing wire aseptically, for sending to the bacteriology laboratory, particularly if the patient is pyrexial. Special care is required to ensure that the end is not being detached from a reusable pacing wire!

PERMANENT PACEMAKERS

The development of implantable cardiac pacemakers and other cardiostimulatory devices has made the selection of the correct unit required for permanent pacing very difficult, and recommendations are rapidly changing. The ever-increasing demand for specialist patient assessment and pacemaker implantation may soon lead to cardiac pacing being established as a subspecialty. About 200 new pacemakers are inserted annually for every million people in Britain, and this number is expected to increase substantially in the coming years.

The indications for pacing are based upon careful evaluation of symptoms, ECGs, Holter tapes and intracardiac electrophysiological tests. Additionally, long-term prognosis and general medical and psychological health need to be taken into account before any decision is made to implant a permanent pacemaker.

The permanent pacemaker

The modern pacemaker is a small metal box weighing 30–130 g, and powered by a lithium battery that lasts up to 15 years. Two types of pulse generator are currently available for permanent implantation: single-chamber pacemakers (the electrode placed in either the atrium or the ventricle) and dual-chamber pacemakers (electrodes situated in both chambers). Although non-programmable pacemakers are still in use, programmable models are increasingly being used (Table 11.4). These enable greater flexibility in pacemaker function (e.g. rate, output, sensitivity and inhibitory functions), which can be altered to meet the specific requirements of the individual patient.

These specific requirements change in about 20% of patients following implantation of a permanent pacemaker and can be altered without need for a second operation or implantation of a different pacemaker.

Table 11.4 Programmable functions of cardiac pacemakers

Rate
    Beats per minute
    Upper rate limit
    Lower rate limit

Energy output
    Milliamps
    Volts
    Pulse duration

Refractory period

Sensitivity of the sensing electrode(s)

Atrioventricular delay between atrial sensing and ventricular pacing

Mode of function
    DDD
    DVI, etc.

Indications for permanent pacing (Table 11.2 above)

Pacing may be considered for either symptomatic benefit or to improve prognosis. For example, untreated complete heart block has a poor prognosis, with a mortality of up to 30% per year, even in asymptomatic patients. Treatment by cardiac pacing restores normal life expectancy.

The British Pacing and Electrophysiology Group (BPEG) Working Party (1991) and the North American Task Force (ACC/AHA, 1991) have produced similar recommendations for the selection of pacemakers for particular patients. The main points are that the ventricle should be paced if there is threatened or actual AV block, and the atrium should be sensed or paced unless contraindicated. Wherever possible, a paced mode that produces the best equivalent of sinus rhythm should be adopted, and, with the exception of atrial fibrillation, this is best produced by dual-chamber systems (Petch, 1993).

Single- and dual-chamber pacing

The original permanent pacemakers were single-chamber pacemakers (VVI units), the electrode being located in the right ventricular apex. However, ventricular pacing results in the reduction of about 20% of the cardiac output because of the loss of the haemodynamic contribution of atrial systole. This may be critical in patients with poor left ventricular function, who would benefit from synchronised sequential atrioventricular activity. Atrial pacemakers will obviously overcome this problem, provided there is no AV nodal conduction block. These simple pacemakers are useful for those patients with symptomatic sino-atrial disease and require a single electrode in the right atrial appendage. A second, and often distressing, problem with ventricular pacemakers is the *pacemaker syndrome,* again caused by impairment of cardiac output (Kenny and Sutton, 1986). Although the pacemaker may be functioning correctly, the patient continues to complain of dizzy spells, syncope, exercise limitation and postural hypotension. This is a consequence of episodic mechanical atrioventricular dissociation, when the atria contract during ventricular systole. Retrograde conduction from the ventricles to the atria causes them to contract against closed AV valves, resulting in raised left and right atrial pressures. A fall in cardiac output and systemic blood pressure then follows, which is often symptomatic. Drugs. Such as flecainide and disopyramide can be used to prevent this abnormal conduction, often with complete resolution of these distressing symptoms. However, what is required (and preferred) is sequential AV contraction, as occurs physiologically. This has led to the introduction of dual-chamber pacemakers.

Dual-chamber pacemakers have separate electrodes. One is situated in the right atrium and the other in the right ventricle, and both can pace and sense. Most patients with complete heart block will have variable atrial rates (depending on, for example, physical activity), and thus the usual arrangement is for ventricular pacing to occur whenever atrial activity is sensed by the atrial electrode. For this reason, dual chamber pacemakers are not a good idea for patients with recurrent supraventricular tachycardias. If there is coexistent sino-atrial disease with a slow atrial rate, the electrodes can be fired sequentially, mimicking normal atrioventricular myocardial contraction.

Over the past 10 years, pacing of the atrium to improve symptoms and exercise tolerance has become routine. Restoring atrial transport improves cardiac output and reduces the risk of atrial fibrillation and thrombus. In addition, symptoms attributable to the pacemaker syndrome are abolished (Traville and Sutton, 1992). In 1992, 25% of the 10 000 permanent pacemakers that were implanted were dual-chamber devices, with obvious cost implications; simple ventricular systems cost about one third the price of dual-chamber systems, which cost over £2000.

An international identification code, universally referred to as the 'NBG code', has been produced jointly by the British Pacing and Electrophysiology Group (BPEG) and the North American Society for Pacing and Electrophysiology (NASPE). The five-letter code provides a standardised means of identifying the functional operation of a cardiac pacemaker, regardless of its trade mark or model. The minimum code length is three letters, 0 being used if a function is not present. Code letters IV and V are often omitted if they would be represented by 0. The current system of nomenclature is shown in Table 11.5. The first two positions indicate the chambers in which the pacemaker operates, position I representing the chamber paced and position II indicating the chamber sensed. If the pacemaker can sense and pace in the same chamber, it is designated D (dual).

Code position III describes the mode of response of the pacemaker, such as I for 'inhibited' (when the presence of sensed electrical activity from the heart inhibits the pacemaker) or T for pacemakers that are 'triggered' by spontaneous cardiac electrical activity. D in position III indicates a double response: an atrial-triggered and ventricular-inhibited pacemaker. Reverse pulse generators (R) come into action only during abnormally fast rates, to terminate the dysrhythmia.

Position IV describes the programmable features, such as rate and/or output, which may be altered non-invasively. In its simplest form, programming is achieved by a magnet applied over the unit. By certain movements, the programming may be altered. More commonly, the programming is transmitted using strings of electronic impulses from a programming head. An increasing number of pacemakers incorpo-

Table 11.5 Code of pacing modes and functions

Position of letter				
I Chambers paced	II Chambers sensed	III Mode of response	IV Programmable functions	V Tachyarrhythmia functions
V Ventricle	V Ventricle	T Triggered	P Programmable (rate and/or output only)	B Bursts
A Atrium	A Atrium	I Inhibited	M Multiprogrammable	N Normal rate competition
D Dual	D Dual	D Dual	C Communicating	S Scanning
		0 None	R Rate responsive	
	0 None	R Reverse	0 None	E Externally controlled

rate some kind of sensor, which can be programmed to modify the pacing rate in response to exercise or emotion, thus improving functional capacity. These sensors may detect physical activity, changes in respiratory rate or oxygen saturation, or right ventricular and central venous pressure and modify the pacing rate accordingly (rate responsive or rate adaptive systems). Position IV may be used to identify the presence of adaptive rate pacing, denoted by the letter 'R'.

The letter 'C' in position IV indicates a communicating pacemaker. These units may be 'interrogated', allowing information such as pacemaker type, clinical function and performance to be extracted from the unit. Any physician can access the data from the implanted pacemaker to determine unit programming, battery life, patient medication and physiological ·data, such as ectopic activity, heart rate variability, conduction patterns and other parameters.

Position V is used to indicate antidysrhythmic function, the pacemaker being employed to prevent or terminate tachydysrhythmias by inducing changes in heart rate and rhythm using single or multiple stimuli. These pacemakers must be able to differentiate simple physiological sinus tachycardias from abnormal rhythms. The unit is designed to break the re-entrant circuit by making any myocardial cells in the path of the circuit refractory.

The most sophisticated pacemaker system is the DDD ('universal'), where both atria and ventricles can sense and pace. Hence, they can pace atria on demand in patients with sinus bradycardia and intact AV nodes, ventricles in response to sensed atrial activity, and atria and ventricles sequentially in patients with sinus bradycardia and AV block.

Permanent pacing following acute myocardial infarction

Permanent pacing is seldom required following inferior myocardial infarction; those patients who do not regain normal conduction usually do not survive the acute infarct, often dying in cardiogenic shock. The prognosis in terms of conduction is excellent for those who survive. However, following acute anterior myocardial infarction, the mortality in patients who develop heart block is very high, and conduction defects are often permanent in those who survive. It is likely that all these patients are at risk of further symptomatic rhythm disturbances, although indications for permanent pacing in this group are controversial (Frye et al, 1984: Klein et al, 1984). Possible indications for permanent pacing in this group are shown in Table 11.6.

Table 11.6 Possible indications for permanent pacing in patients recovering from acute myocardial infarction with AV block

Infarct/block	Pace?
Inferior with transient AV block	No
Inferior with permanent second-/third-degree block	Yes
Anterior with fascicular block	No?
Anterior with transient second-/third-degree block	Yes?
Anterior with permanent second-/third-degree block	Yes

For those who recover normal AV conduction, exercise testing and 24-hour Holter monitoring are useful for post-infarction assessment. Electrophysiological testing, if available, may give early indication of impaired infranodal conduction, allowing consideration for permanent pacing before problems arise (Cobbe, 1986).

References

ACC/AHA Task Force (1991) Guidelines for implantation of cardiac pacemakers and antiarrhythmia devices. *Journal of the American College of Cardiology*, **18:** 1–13.

Blandford R L and Burden A C (1984) Abnormalities of cardiac conduction in diabetics. *British Medical Journal*, **289:** 1659.

British Pacing and Electrophysiology Group (1991) Recommendations for pacemaker prescriptions for symptomatic bradycardia. Report of a Working Party. *British Heart Journal*, **66:** 185–191.

Burack B and Furman S (1969) Trans-oesophageal cardiac pacing. *American Journal of Cardiology*, **23:** 469–472.

Christiansen I, Haghfelt T and Amtorp O (1973) Complete heart block in acute myocardial infarction: drug therapy. *American Heart Journal*, **85:** 162–166.

Cobbe S M (1986) Electrophysiological testing after acute myocardial infarction. *British Medical Journal*, **292:** 1290–1291.

Cohen D B, Doctor L and Pick A (1958) The significance of atrioventricular block complicating myocardial infarction. *American Heart Journal*, **55:** 215–219.

Czyzyk A, Krolewski A S, Szablowska S, Alot A and Kopczynski J (1980) Clinical course of myocardial infarction amongst diabetic patients. *Diabetes Care*, **4:** 526–529.

EEC (1988) *Ionising Radiation Regulations*. Brussels: EEC.

Fitzpatrick A and Sutton R (1992) A guide to temporary pacing. *British Medical Journal*, **304:** 365–369.

Frye R L, Colins J J, DeSanctis R W, Dodge H T, Dreifus L S, Gillette P C and Fisch C (1984) Guidelines for permanent cardiac pacemaker implantation. *Circulation*, **70:** 331A–339A.

Hayward R (1981) Who do we pace? *British Journal of Hospital Medicine*, **25:** 466–474.

Jowett N I, Thompson D R and Pohl J E (1989) Temporary transvenous endocardial pacing: six years experience in one coronary care unit. *Postgraduate Medical Journal*, **65:** 211–215.

Kenny R A and Sutton R (1986) Pacemaker syndrome. *British Medical Journal*, **293:** 902–903.

Klein R C, Vera Z and Mason T (1984) Intraventricular conduction defects in acute myocardial infarction: incidence, prognosis and therapy. *American Heart Journal*, **108:** 1107–1113.

Kostuk W J and Beanlands D S (1970) Complete heart block associated with myocardial infarction. *American Journal of Cardiology*, **26:** 380–384.

Lassers B W and Julian D G (1968) Artificial pacing in the management of complete heart block complicating acute myocardial infarction. *British Medical Journal*, **ii:** 142–146.

Mullins C B and Atkins J M (1976) Prognosis and management of ventricular conduction blocks in acute myocardial infarction. *Modern Concepts in Cardiovascular Disease*, **45:** 129–133.

Norris R M (1969) Heart block in posterior and anterior myocardial infarction. *British Heart Journal*, **31:** 352–356.

Norris R M, Mercer C J and Croxson M A (1972) Conduction disturbances due to anteroseptal myocardial infarction and their treatment by endocardial pacing. *American Heart Journal*, **84:** 560–566.

Petch M C (1993) Who needs dual chamber pacing? *British Medical Journal*, **307:** 215–216.

Shah P K, Nalos P and Peter T (1987) Atropine resistant post-infarction complete AV block: possible role of adenosine and improvement with aminophylline. *American Heart Journal*, **113:** 194–195.

Traville C M and Sutton M (1992) Pacemaker syndrome: an iatrogenic condition. *British Heart Journal*, **68:** 163–166.

Zoll P M and Zoll R H (1985) Non-invasive temporary cardiac stimulation. *Critical Care Medicine*, **13:** 925–926.

12

Rehabilitation after
Myocardial Infarction

Cardiac rehabilitation is the process by which patients with coronary heart disease are enabled to achieve their optimal physical, emotional, social, vocational and economic status. Rehabilitation cannot be regarded as an isolated form of therapy but must be integrated with the whole treatment, of which it forms only one facet (World Health Organization, 1993). It is a multidisciplinary approach to improve short-term recovery and to promote long-term changes in life-style, which correct adverse risk factors (Horgan et al, 1992). Myocardial infarction often causes distress and impairment of quality of life for patients and for their relatives, especially their partners; for a substantial minority of families, such consequences are greater and more persistent than can be physically justified (Mayou et al, 1978; Thompson et al, 1987).

In the past, strict and prolonged bed-rest played a central role in the early management of acute myocardial infarction. However, it soon became clear that prolonged immobilisation had undesirable and sometimes dangerous side-effects, including deep vein thrombosis and pulmonary embolism. Other effects included impaired respiratory function, with a tendency to chest infections, negative nitrogen balance and a decrease in skeletal muscle mass and muscular contractile strength. Prolonged immobilisation also resulted in marked physical weakness and a reduced ability to exercise. This was, in part, due to a reduction in left ventricular stroke volume, and resumption of activity often resulted in tachycardia and orthostatic hypotension.

Cardiac rehabilitation can be traced back to New York in the early 1940s, when assessing and improving exercise capacity played a prominent role in 'work classification units'. Rehabilitation, however, should not be equated with exercise training alone; no observation or trial has shown that exercise alone reduces morbidity and mortality following myocardial infarction.

In the early 1970s, the World Health Organization set up a study into rehabilitation and secondary prevention following myocardial infarction, and the results have shown that patients who are involved in formal rehabilitation programmes have a decreased mortality and an earlier return to work (Dorossiev, 1983). However, too much emphasis should not be placed on these endpoints alone, and it is preferable to concentrate, particularly in the early months following the illness, on improving the quality of life. The following are major areas for rehabilitation:

- Medical therapy
- Psychological adjustment and motivation
- Self-care

- Financial matters and income
- Housing
- Transport
- Occupation
- Recreation
- Sexual activity

The major components of rehabilitation are early ambulation, health education and counselling of the patient and family. In theory, the rehabilitation process should begin the moment the patient enters the hospital and continue after discharge; in practice it rarely does. Many patients leave hospital unaware that they have even had a heart attack, let alone what this means and what to do about it once they get home.

In the UK, there has been progress in early mobilisation and discharge from hospital, but interest in other aspects of cardiac rehabilitation are only just emerging. This is not the case in other countries such as Germany, where over 80% of patients are admitted to 'heart groups' following myocardial infarction (Scheuermann et al, 1985).

Cardiac rehabilitation involves the use of a wide range of skills from different health professionals, including the nurse, doctor, physiotherapist, occupational therapist, clinical psychologist, dietitian and social worker. The nurse assumes a central role by being responsible, directly or indirectly, for controlling the many factors that influence the patient's recovery (Runions, 1985). She is in most frequent contact with the patient and family and is responsible for planning and coordinating the amount of activity the patient is expected to undertake. The nurse can assist the patient and family to understand, accept and adapt to the illness and may be able to stimulate them to take an active part in recovery and rehabilitation. In addition, she can assist them in making realistic plans for the future. In order to achieve this, attainable goals need to be defined, plans being jointly agreed by the patient, the family and other members of the health-care team. An attitude of optimism should be adopted by staff, remembering that most patients who are going to die from acute myocardial infarction do so before reaching hospital.

From early convalescence in hospital, the patient and partner should realise that a return to normality within a matter of a few weeks is not only expected, but is also safe and beneficial, given that the patient's condition warrants it. It is the success of coping and support that often ultimately determines the outcome of the patient's illness; the heart may recover more rapidly than the patient's often depressed mental state.

REHABILITATION PROGRAMMES

Cardiac rehabilitation services should include exercise training, risk factor modification, education and attention to the psychological sequelae of ischaemic heart disease for both the patient and family, especially the partner. The principal justification for rehabilitation is the encouragement of return to expected levels of activities and a reduction in the well-documented convalescent problems of lack of confidence, anxiety, depression, poor sleep, sexual problems, fatigue and worry about non-specific physical symptoms, together with excessive caution about everyday activities (Horgan et al, 1992).

Recent pooled data from several studies suggest that cardiac rehabilitation results in a reduction of around 25% in overall and cardiovascular mortality (Oldridge et al, 1988; O'Connor et al, 1989). All the programmes reviewed included some degree of risk factor modification, at least 6 weeks physical exercise supervision and a follow-up period of at least 24 months. Studies of risk factor intervention and psychological support alone (Houston-Miller et al, 1990; Blumenthal and Wei, 1993) have produced less dramatic, but still impressive, effects, not only for the patient, but also the spouse (Thompson, 1990). Numerous studies have shown that comprehensive rehabilitation programmes can produce worthwhile improvements in quality of life, and it has been recommended that they should be routinely offered to all patients with ischaemic heart disease (Horgan et al, 1992).

Although the efficacy and importance of cardiac rehabilitation is now well recognised (Greenland and Chu, 1988; Bertie et al, 1992; Horgan et al, 1992; Bittner and Oberman, 1993), the nature of existing services in the UK, be they in hospital or in the community, varies considerably at local, district and regional levels. Despite the large numbers of appropriate candidates, it is not known how many are offered, or participate in, cardiac rehabilitation. In the USA, fewer than 15% of eligible patients undergo supervised cardiac rehabilitation, and the proportion is undoubtedly lower in the UK. The need to develop rehabilitation programmes that begin with the cardiac event itself, and that emphasise that long-term changes in life-style must be promoted, is well recognised. Whilst exercise and risk factor control are undoubtedly essential components of a rehabilitation programme, the psychosocial aspects are often neglected (Frasure-Smith, 1992), despite evidence that long-term quality of life following myocardial infarction may depend as much on psychological reactions and how they are managed as on medical care (Ebbesen et al, 1990; Mayou and Bryant, 1993). A number of approaches, for example cognitive–behavioural techniques (Frasure-Smith and Price, 1989) and self-help packages (Lewin et al, 1992), merit further development and evaluation. For example, a home-based self-help rehabilitation programme has been shown to reduce psychological distress by roughly 50% and to lead to fewer readmissions to hospital and visits to the general practitioner (Lewin et al, 1992). There is a need to assess objectively the physical, psychosocial and economic benefits of these programmes and to develop and evaluate comprehensive, multidisciplinary programmes that include graded exercise, education and support and secondary prevention measures. Certain client groups, such as elderly people (Siddiuqi, 1992), women (McGee and Horgan, 1992) and ethnic groups, warrant special attention.

Fewer than half the health districts in the UK have established cardiac rehabilitation programmes, and there is considerable variability in the services provided. It is evident that services are inadequate, poorly coordinated with medical care and excessively rigid and hospital based (Horgan et al, 1992). Few of the programmes that exist have been subjected to careful audit, and there is little information available about, for example, the type of service offered, the client group characteristics, the use and training needs of health professionals involved, the resources and funds used and the outcome measures. This is despite a significant increase in investment and interest by purchasers in the effectiveness of cardiac rehabilitation services, an increase in the proportion of health professionals' time spent on hospital and community cardiac rehabilitation and an increase in expectations of the client population.

The prevalence of coronary heart disease varies considerably across the UK, but for a district population of 200 000, this will usually mean that between 200 and 600 patients a year are suitable for cardiac rehabilitation. These figures justify the maintainence of a viable programme.

Successful rehabilitation should not be viewed narrowly in terms of economic or vocational outcomes, but rather as the achievement of a life-style that enables the patient and his family to enjoy a full and active life (with some allowance for physical limitations), in which he can usefully contribute to his family and society.

Cardiac rehabilitation programmes consist of patient education (often coupled with counselling) and exercise.

The *education and counselling* components involve teaching patients and their families better to understand the illness and its management (including the factors that may have caused it) and to enable them to assume a large degree of responsibility for their care.

The *exercise* component involves a graduated programme, beginning with passive and low-level activities and aiming for a full return to normal activities.

Patient education

Information provided to patients and their partners about their stay in hospital is frequently lacking. Although patient teaching is increasingly being recognised as an important nursing function, there is little evidence to show that it is being effectively and consistently accomplished. It is the responsibility of the health-care team to ensure that the patient and his family understand the illness, the purpose of treatment and how to cope both within and outside the hospital. The nurse is in an ideal position to teach, because she frequently becomes the most familiar person to the patient and is thus often in the best position to communicate with the patient and family.

Teaching programmes during the patient's stay in hospital are designed to decrease the patient's feeling of helplessness, to help restore self-esteem and to bolster the patient's confidence in terms of a successful outcome. Patients who understand the cause and significance of their illness and its management are likely to have improved motivation to comply with therapy and cope with the consequences of their illness (Thompson, 1990). Patients particularly need information about potential events that may occur after their return home, when professional help is not immediately available.

Teaching and learning is a two-way process, and the individual patient's requirements will vary with his general educational background and intellectual capabilities.

Assessment should include:

● Demographic variables, such as family composition, ethnic and religious background and educational level
● Pre-existing knowledge and misconceptions of coronary heart disease
● Life-style and habits
● Readiness to learn

Simple language should always be used, and it should be remembered that earlier statements are remembered better than later ones. Repetition increases recall, as does specific rather than general advice.

Contemporary approaches to patient teaching are numerous and varied, but information should be tailored to individual needs and given in a consistent and structured fashion. The comprehension of new information will be at its best when the patient is motivated and when the information is presented clearly, concisely and in small doses (Redman, 1984). There is no substitute for personal advice, and its value depends heavily upon the attending medical and nursing staff adopting an informed, committed and uniform approach. Similar education of the patient's family is equally important, and giving this at the bedside (when the patient is surrounded by high technology and obvious intensive care) may reinforce the importance of such advice.

Instructional aids (physical, printed and audiovisual) are very useful as part of the educational process. Vocabulary, sentence length, illustrations, type size and style, as well as readability and accuracy of the information presented, should be carefully considered. Visual information is usually assimilated better than the spoken word, so illustrations, pamphlets and models are a helpful and useful adjunct. A plastic model of the heart can be used to demonstrate cardiac anatomy and the coronary arteries and explain about the blood supply to the heart. This helps to correct the common myth that the heart receives its nourishment by blood flowing through the chambers. The atherosclerotic process may then be described, including plaque formation, progressive narrowing and obstruction of the coronary arteries and myocardial infarction. The discussion should include an explanation of other symptoms that the patient may have experienced, such as sweating and palpitations. The role of coronary artery spasm can be discussed if the patient has a history of variant angina. The healing process of the heart and the meanings of ECG and laboratory findings should also be briefly explained. It is important to stress that there is no cure for ischaemic heart disease but that some medical intervention and modification of life-style may be necessary to alleviate symptoms and reduce the risk of further problems.

Structured teaching seems to improve patients' knowledge about their myocardial infarction, particularly if booklets and discharge information sheets are given (Gregor, 1981). However, some researchers have found only limited effects with inpatient or outpatient teaching and counselling (Sivarajan et al, 1983). There may be various reasons for this: there may be lack of individual attention or the patient may have indirectly (and incorrectly) obtained information from other patients while in hospital (Thompson 1990).

Nurses, doctors and patients generally agree upon certain topics that should be included for discussion, including the recognition of signs and symptoms of myocardial infarction, the names, dosages and side-effects of medications and knowledge of personal risk factors and how to modify them (Casey et al, 1984). Other aspects that need to be covered are the nature of the disease, emergency treatment, resumption of activities and physical, psychosocial and financial problems encountered on return to home and work. Aspects frequently neglected include how to take the pulse, sexual activity and instruction on the normal convalescence (Moynihan, 1984). It is important to try to avoid presenting information in a standardised fashion, and the nurse needs to find out what the patient's needs are (Runions, 1985).

Providing information may be made more effective by employing the 'IIFAC scheme' outlined by Nichols (1985):

I   *Initial information check.* What do the patient and spouse know, and are they suitable candidates for receiving further information?

I   *Information exchange.* An exchange of essential knowledge and information in acceptable terms.

FAC *Final accuracy check.* Do the patient and spouse accurately and fully understand the information, or do they require further teaching?

Questionnaires may be useful for evaluating the patient's needs and level of comprehension. However, when assessing the efficacy of the education programme, it is important to differentiate between what the patient learns and what he is actually going to do about it; the acquisition of new information does not necessarily result in a change of behaviour.

Involvement of the patient's family

The family can have a direct influence on the rehabilitation process by understanding the illness and helping the patient adapt to it. They can also help in modification of the patient's life-style. They should, therefore, be included in most, if not all, teaching, so that they are equipped with the necessary information. Partner involvement has been minimal in rehabilitation, despite the widespread opinion that success generally depends upon their support. A programme that involves both patients and partners provides an ideal opportunity for giving information, instilling hope and redefining health (Dracup et al, 1984). The rest of the family also needs information to feel useful to the patient, and to understand that he is receiving appropriate care (Gaglione, 1984).

Information on the coronary care unit and the ward

Education initiated on the coronary care unit helps the patient to understand what has happened, what is immediately being done and what is likely to happen over the ensuing days. Teaching needs to be relevant to the individuals concerned; vagueness and ambiguity will only result in increased fear and anxiety (Geissler et al, 1985). A programme centred around these principles is likely to improve the patient's attitudes, behaviour and understanding of the illness and improve his recovery.

At an early stage, brief explanations of the staff, equipment, procedures and routines of the coronary care unit will reduce anxiety and misunderstanding. The nurse should avoid bombarding patients with too much information during the early phase, as they invariably retain very few facts during this acute stage. Capacity for learning is impaired by fear, anxiety, pain and fatigue. Patients will, however, benefit from answers to specific questions, and answers should be clear, simple and repeated frequently.

If the patient has to undergo a painful or invasive procedure, information on the patient's likely experiences and sensations will be more effective in alleviating anxiety than will details about the procedure alone (Johnson, 1980). When the patient's mental and physical condition permits the assimilation of more detailed and complex information, the nurse can provide information about his condition, its limitations, possible problems and outcome.

Physical activity

Early studies on the role of exercise in the prevention of coronary heart disease in the 1940s and 1950s showed that roughly half the number of coronary deaths occurred in those with physically-active jobs, as opposed to those with sedentary occupations (for example, bus conductors and postmen had lower mortality rates than bus drivers and telephone operators). Since then, favourable associations have been reported between the taking of vigorous physical activity and a reduced risk of coronary heart disease (Morris et al, 1980). Physical fitness also leads to improvements in coronary risk factors; exercise increases HDL cholesterol concentrations and reduces weight and often blood pressure, too (Paffenbarger and Hyde, 1980).

Emphasising physical exercise following acute myocardial infarction usually represents a major change to the typical patient's sedentary life-style, involving the car, labour-saving devices and long hours in front of the television. However, exercise improves mood and morale, and physical fitness allows an earlier return to normal life-style and work. Regular exercise also helps cardiovascular performance, keeps the body supple and helps to control body weight. Coronary rehabilitation programmes are to be encouraged to this end.

Regular moderate exercise (30–45 minutes three or four times per week) at a level of 75–85% of maximal capacity is an ideal way of achieving physical fitness. Vigorous physical activity may be employed later and is recognised as an important factor in protection against the development of coronary heart disease (Morris et al, 1980); the greater the energy expenditure, the lower the incidence of coronary heart disease seems to be Paffenbarger and Hyde (1980) estimate that the risk of myocardial infarction is reduced by 5% for each hour spent per week in vigorous activity. However, care is required in those with pre-existing heart disease; exercise is not without hazard, and low-level activities are preferable in older and less fit patients.

Formal exercise programmes are very useful following acute myocardial infarction. Early graduated physical activity, starting with gentle passive exertion, has been designed to avert or minimise the risk of venous stasis and its complications (deep vein thrombosis and pulmonary emboli). When the patient is first allowed out of bed, he is often shocked at the tremendous feeling of physical weakness, which is usually not expected or easily explicable in terms of the short period of bed-rest and inactivity. The patient will need reassuring and encouragement gradually to increase the level of activity. Any restrictions thought necessary should be carefully explained in a positive fashion, so that the patient does not become frustrated.

Information regarding physical activity will depend on the stage of recovery the patient has reached. Initially, the reasons for temporary restriction of activity will need to be explained, and that the resumption of activity will be gradual to allow the myocardium to heal.

Activity planning

The functional classification of the New York Heart Association provides a crude guide for determining appropriate activities as well as expected symptoms in patients following acute myocardial infarction (Table 12.1). Advice about specific activities should be individualised and take into account the extent and severity of the myocardial infarction, the patient's previous level of activity, the extent of recovery and the stability of the current condition.

Progress in early rehabilitation has been greatly assisted by the use of *metabolic equivalents* (METs) for prescribing specific physical activities (Table 12.2). One MET is defined as the oxygen consumption by the patient at rest and is roughly equivalent to 3.5 ml of oxygen per minute (1.4 calories per minute).

Table 12.1 Functional classification of patients with heart disease (New York Heart Association Criteria Committee, 1964)

Class I:	Heart disease with no limitation on ordinary physical activity
Class II:	Slight limitation. Ordinary physical activity (e.g. walking) produces symptoms
Class III:	Marked limitation. Unable to walk on the level without disability. Less than ordinary activity produces symptoms
Class IV:	Dyspnoea at rest. Inability to carry out any physical activity

Table 12.2 Approximate energy requirements for selected activities

Category	METs	Examples
Very light	<3	Washing, dressing, driving car, working at desk, washing up dishes, walking at 2 mph
Light	3–5	Light shopping, dancing, golf, tennis (doubles), walking at 3–4 mph, cycling on flat (7 mph)
Moderate	5–7	Stairs, digging soft soil, tennis (singles), walking 4–5 mph, cycling (10 mph), swimming
Heavy	7–9	Jogging (5 mph), non-competitive squash, cycling (12 mph)
Very heavy	>9	Shovelling snow, running >6 mph, cycling >13 mph (or steep hills), competitive sport

Three months or more after an uncomplicated myocardial infarction, the average post-infarction patient is capable of performing at a level of up to 9 METs. This is equivalent to running at about 5 miles per hour, cycling at 12 miles per hour or playing 'non-competitive' squash. If less than ordinary activity produces symptoms, it may be necessary for a more suitable activity level to be planned. Patients who have had congestive heart failure, for example, are often limited to 3–5 METs at 3 months.

Physical activity on the coronary care unit

Early ambulation in the uncomplicated myocardial infarction is essential to avert or minimise the deleterious effects of prolonged bed-rest, including decreased physical work capacity. It also reduces the anxiety and depression that often follow acute myocardial infarction.

In some coronary care units, patients are encouraged to sit out of bed on the day of admission, provided they are free from pain and significant dysrhythmias. If there has been a prolonged period of bed-rest, resumption of activity often results in a moderate tachycardia and orthostatic hypotension. Physical activities should, therefore, be at a low level of intensity (1–2 METs), such as eating, dressing and undressing, washing of the hands and face, use of a bedside commode, simple arm and leg exercises or sitting in a bedside chair. Observation of the patient as he performs these activities is useful to ensure that he can cope and that an inappropriate tachycardia is not provoked. Early rehabilitation should not be associated with chest pain, dyspnoea, sweating, palpitations or excessive fatigue. Dysrhythmias and ST segment displacement on the cardiac monitor should not occur, and systolic blood pressure should not fall more than 10–15 mmHg.

The patient is usually the best judge of how much he can do, but he should be warned of the feelings of weakness that may accompany increases in activity.

Physical activity on the ward

Once the patient leaves the coronary care unit, the aim is for him to attain a level of activity that permits personal care and independence (or at least semi-independence) by the time of discharge from hospital. In these days of early discharge following uncomplicated myocardial infarction, patients usually return home after 5–7 days.

The ward activity plan should consist of 'warm-up' isotonic (dynamic) exercises, which allow the heart rate to increase proportionally to the intensity of the activity. The systolic blood pressure increases slowly, and the diastolic blood pressure remains unchanged or decreases slightly. Isometric exercises should be avoided. These result in a minimal increase in heart rate but a significant and steep increase in the systolic blood pressure. This causes a sudden increase in cardiac afterload, which may be poorly tolerated by an ischaemic left ventricle, resulting in angina or malignant tachydysrhythmias (Nutter et al, 1972).

Table 12.3 In-hospital exercise plan

Day	METs	Examples
1	1	Self-feeding, washing with help, passive movement of limbs, commode
1–2	2	Active movement of limbs, sitting out of bed for 20 minutes twice daily
2–3	3	Sitting out for an hour twice daily, walking to bathroom
4–5	4	Walking up to 50 yards, short flight of stairs

Walking with a gradual and progressive increase in speed and distance should be the major component of the activity plan (Table 12.3). It is advisable for most patients who will have to climb stairs at home to try stairs in hospital under supervision. This results in increased confidence and reduced worry for the patient and family. At the time of discharge from hospital, patients should be able to perform activities at peak levels of 3.5–4.0 METs for short periods, to simulate usual activities at home.

Exercise stress testing

The current practice of early ambulation and exercise training soon after myocardial infarction has resulted in the more widespread use of exercise testing earlier in the course of the illness and often before discharge home. A normal response to an early exercise test reliably identifies patients at low risk of future cardiac events. It is beneficial for spouses to observe and even participate in stress testing, to gain more confidence in the patient's physical and cardiac capability (Taylor et al, 1985).

Physical activity during convalescence

When the patient returns home, progressive increases in physical activity are used to achieve a level of activity that allows normal daily activities and will later permit a return to work. The activity plan within hospital will usually have helped to allay the patient's and family's fears of a further heart attack or sudden death resulting from physical exertion. Patients should be encouraged to exercise daily, and it should be stressed that a lack of exercise may be harmful rather than beneficial. The best form of exercise is walking, but golf, swimming, jogging and cycling can be encouraged when the patient feels well enough. Exercises that use less than half of the patient's working capacity will not help to increase fitness.

The benefits of exercise, including weight control, improvement of respiratory function and a general feeling of well-being, should be stressed. Practical advice is helpful too, for example only exercising in warm environments and not after heavy meals by the fire-side in winter, or in the midday sun in summer. Competitive sports are not advisable in the early months following infarction, for obvious reasons.

Table 12.4 Exercise targets following acute myocardial infarction

Weeks	METs
1–2	2–4
3–8	5–7
>8	7 and over

The levels of activity performed at the end of the hospital stay should be maintained and gradually increased (Table 12.4). Walking speed and distance should be increased, so that by the end of 4–6 weeks the patient may walk up to 5 miles per day (Oberman, 1984). The patient and family will usually gain confidence, and the patient more independence, when he accomplishes each objective.

Formal exercise programmes for outpatients

The main emphasis for rehabilitation has been early programmes of hospital-based exercise training, but it is now widely accepted that there is need for a wider and more flexible range of methods, greater individual prescription of care and closer cooperation with on-going medical care. Exercise is popular with many patients and appears effective in the early stages in improving exercise capacity, reducing anxiety and encouraging a rapid return to activities, but it is difficult to demonstrate continuing advantages after 1 year (Oldridge et al, 1991). Both light and heavy exercise have been shown to be of benefit in improving physical conditioning (Goble et al, 1991), and, although these can easily be provided in a hospital gym, they can just as successfully be provided in the community (Bethell and Mullee, 1990).

Although there is some debate about the benefits derived from formal exercise programmes, there are some indications that they may be of value (Shephard, 1986). Most studies claim that patients who have participated in these programmes show increased physical fitness, a better understanding of their illness and treatment and fewer psychological problems, with an earlier and larger number returning to work (Prosser et al, 1978; Mayou et al, 1981). In particular, fewer fatal reinfarctions have been found to occur in those who have been involved in such programmes (Shephard, 1983).

During exercise sessions, direct observation, including ECG monitoring by telemetry, is recommended. A warm-up period of 5 minutes is needed, gradually to increase the pulse rate and blood pressure and to help joint flexibility. Maintaining a target heart rate is a useful guide for achieving the correct intensity of exertion. The level of activity is altered until the desired heart rate is achieved, and the exercise is maintained for the duration of the session (continuous training) or interspersed with brief rest periods (intermittent training). The exercise devices used include the treadmill, arm/leg ergometer, rowing machine and wall pulleys. The ECG is observed for dysrhythmias or ST segment displacement. Heart rate and adverse signs or symptoms need to be recorded. At the conclusion of the exercise session, it is important to taper the activity down gradually (a 'cool down'), rather than to stop it abruptly.

Home-based exercise programmes are probably as effective as group training (Miller et al, 1984), although a rehabilitation programme that is community based may be more beneficial in terms of social contact and support (Bethell et al, 1983).

PREPARATION FOR DISCHARGE

Exercise sessions may usefully be combined with education and counselling of the patient and family and providing information for convalescence.

It is not uncommon for the patient and family to be left to cope by themselves with only vague instructions about discharge and rehabilitation, which results in uncertainty, distress and failure to adjust. A well-planned programme is desirable, to anticipate the patient's homecoming and return to work. Patients and spouses often have specific questions about convalescence, medication, diet, drinking, driving and smoking, as well as resumption of leisure, and sexual and work activities (Cay, 1982).

Group discussions after the exercise session provide a means of asking questions, sharing feelings and concerns and learning from others who have similar problems. Patients and partners who participate in group counselling seem to suffer less anxiety, depression and anger, as well as having improved compliance with advice about treatment (Dracup, 1985). There is good evidence that beneficial effects occur where patients provide each other with information, advice and support (Ibrahim et al, 1974; Rahe et al, 1979). Counselling also reduces depression and promotes independence and sociability (Stern et al, 1983).

General health recommendations to all coronary patients and their families should include:

● A varied diet with appropriate calorific intake to achieve or maintain an ideal body weight
● The cessation of smoking
● A programme of regular and vigorous physical activity
● A regular health examination, including testing of the urine for sugar and protein, measurement of blood pressure and assessment of plasma lipids

Psychological aspects

Many patients are confronted by fear and uncertainty when they arrive back home, which, when combined with minor physical symptoms, result in increased anxiety and depression. Considerable psychological distress and a low level of understanding have been found to occur in many post-coronary patients and their spouses (Mayou et al, 1976, 1978a). Such reactions may impair the recovery of a group of patients in whom psychological factors are stronger determinants of readjustment to normal life than is their physical status (Wiklund et al, 1984).

Predischarge counselling is useful in improving morale and aiding a successful return to home and work. Preparation should include discussions of potential problems, such as anxiety, depression, poor concentration, irritability, sleeplessness and fear of complications (especially death), that may occur on the return home. The partner often experiences a greater degree of anxiety than the patient and may need careful and supportive counselling (Thompson and Cordle, 1988; Thompson, 1990). The family particularly needs to be cautioned against overprotectiveness towards the patient.

Only a few well-controlled studies of in-hospital psychological interventions have been reported in patients following acute myocardial infarction. These have varied from individual daily supportive psychotherapy (Gruen, 1975) to stress management and relaxation techniques (Langosch et al, 1982) or combinations of these (Oldenburg et al, 1985). Such interventions have generally shown significant improvements in psychosocial and physical functioning for at least a year after the infarct (Thompson, 1990). Whether these improvements can be sustained over a longer period remains to be seen.

Because the transition from hospital to home is frequently a traumatic and neglected aspect of post-myocardial infarction management, it may be appropriate to make arrangements that will ensure continuity of care. Periodic checks (e.g. telephoning the patient and partner or home visits) may be useful, in some instances, to bridge this gap, and this is probably best achieved by close liaison between hospital and community nurses. The community nurse can play an important role in teaching, counselling and evaluating the care that has been initiated within the hospital. She is also ideally placed for informing the patient and partner about community resources, including counselling services, home helps and rehabilitation facilities. She may also liaise with the patient's family doctor.

The multidisciplinary health team approach is advantageous as it combines the skills of different professionals, provides continuity between hospital and community care and thus maximises the resources available to the patient and family. Nevertheless, it is important to avoid encouraging patient and family dependence; ultimately, each individual is responsible for his or her own health and must be encouraged to assume overall responsibility and control.

Impressive benefits for mood have been claimed for a self-help behavioural programme (especially suitable for low-risk patients) (Lewin et al, 1992). It is estimated (Lewin et al, 1992) that up to 30% of subjects might benefit from individually-planned extra help in later convalescence (even if they have attended early rehabilitation programmes).

Sexual counselling

If the patient is to be properly rehabilitated, his sexual needs cannot be ignored. Although discussion of this intimate aspect of the patient's life is difficult for both patient and medical staff, sexual counselling should be viewed as an integral part of the cardiac rehabilitation programme (Thompson, 1983). It is recommended that the subject of sex should be approached as a matter of routine in the rehabilitation of all coronary patients and their partners.

The energy expenditure during intercourse is not as great as popularly believed, being equivalent to that of climbing about two flights of stairs (4 METs). Experimental data have demonstrated that peak heart rates occur during orgasm, and adequate foreplay will allow the pulse rate to increase gradually from resting levels to a transient peak of about 180 beats per minute. Blood pressure also rises gradually, to peak just before or during orgasm, with increases of 20–100 mmHg systolic and 20–40 mmHg diastolic. Hyperventilation occurs, with respiratory rates recorded of up to 60 per minute. These physiological variables rapidly return to precoital levels after orgasm. Extramarital and other illicit encounters may, however, expend much more energy, and are often associated with faster heart rates, higher blood pressures and an increased risk of sudden death.

Sexual problems

Patients recovering from acute myocardial infarction often suffer from a depressed libido, which may result in sexual disharmony. Interestingly, impotence is rarely a problem. The partner is often more concerned than the patient and may be frightened of resuming sexual activity because of precipitating a heart attack or sudden death (Thompson, 1983). The severity of the infarct and the extent of cardiac decompensation are much less important causes of sexual debility than is the psychological condition of the patient.

The PLISSIT model (Annon, 1976) provides a useful framework for those involved in dealing with sexual counselling of coronary patients and their partners. This model provides four levels of approach (Thompson and Cordle, 1986).

Permission

This is permission to discuss and ask questions about sex. For instance, the counsellor can introduce the topic by saying, 'Many people are worried about when they can resume normal sexual relations. I wonder whether there are any questions or concerns that either of you may have regarding your sex life?'

Limited information

This means providing the couple with factual information directly relevant to their particular situation or sexual concern. Many patients lack sufficient information, which results in unnecessary worry. For instance, the most common fear is that of reinfarction or death occurring during intercourse. This is, in fact, a rare occurrence, accounting for about 0.6% of cases of cardiac deaths (Ueno, 1963). Most of these fatalities occur during extramarital sex. Fear of resuming sexual activity is more harmful than the actual activity, and sexual frustration should be avoided at all costs. In general, most patients can resume sexual intercourse about 2–4 weeks after discharge home. Typical advice may be, 'If you can make it up the stairs to the bedroom in one go, you can resume sexual activity'. Good sex need not be an athletic feat.

If these two stages are insufficient to resolve sexual concerns, two options are available.

Specific suggestions

This stage involves careful and detailed assessment of the couple's specific problems. There may be a need to advise patients on how to minimise symptoms that may accompany intercourse. A warm bedroom and warm sheets are desirable. If chest pain, breathlessness or palpitations occur during or after sexual activity, the couple should stop and seek medical advice. Often, all that is required is for prophylactic GTN to be taken immediately before coitus, as the patient might do before any form of physical activity. Beta-blockers are also very useful for limiting heart rate and myocardial work. It should be noted that patients using cutaneous nitrates may deposit some of their medication on their partner, imparting typical nitrate side-effects of them ('Not now, I've got a head-ache!').

If psychological problems remain unresolved, it may be necessary to refer the patient for intensive counselling.

Intensive therapy

Specialised sexual counselling by a clinical psychologist, often within a sexual dysfunction clinic, may be indicated for intensive therapy in resistant cases.

Medication

Compliance with drug therapy varies from patient to patient but often remains unacceptably poor. Difficulty in understanding and complying with drug therapy may occur for a variety of reasons, including fear of dependency or of side-effects. The more complex the drug regimen, the less likely compliance seems to be, and careful review of the patient's medication is necessary before discharge. Many patients will not have taken tablets before their heart attack, and the habit of taking regular medication may be unfamiliar.

Information should include correct identification of the drug, what it is for, the dosage and other special instructions (for example the storage and limited life of GTN). Reissue of prescriptions needs to be covered: patients often stop what is intended to be continuous therapy when they have finished 'the course'. In addition, they should be warned that they should not allow themselves to run out of tablets or go away on holiday with insufficient supplies. Sudden withdrawal of certain drugs (e.g. beta-blockers) may be associated with sudden cardiac events, including unstable angina, myocardial infarction and sudden death. Patients should enquire about whether or not it would be cheaper to obtain an annual prescription 'season ticket', rather than paying for individual medications.

It may be useful to issue a small record card listing the patient's medications, with dose, time to be taken, action and possible side-effects written on the card. This may be kept with the medication at home, thus serving as a reminder and providing important information about the drugs. The cards are also useful to summarise therapy when prescriptions are being reissued by the patient's family doctor, and they can be taken to hospital appointments so that all concerned know what medication is actually being taken.

Family participation in teaching about drugs may exert a strong influence on the patient's understanding and thus improve compliance with therapy.

Driving

Patients can usually resume driving 4 weeks after an uncomplicated myocardial infarction. However, they should initially avoid rush-hour traffic and long journeys, as well as aggressive or competitive driving. Patients may be precluded from holding licences to drive large goods (LGV) or passenger carrying vehicles (PCV) after they have had a myocardial infarction. If recovery is satisfactory, driving may be permitted without notifying the licensing authority (the DVLA at Swansea). However, motor insurance companies normally require formal notification about changes in health circumstances.

Flying

Patients are usually safe to travel by air as soon as the period of convalescence is over, although long flights are probably initially inadvisable.

Return to work

The return to work usually gives the patient increased self-satisfaction, restored self-respect and relief from financial worries. Many consider return to work to be the goal of cardiac rehabilitation, although in the current gloomy employment climate, it is increasingly difficult to use the return to work as a valid outcome of post-infarction rehabilitation.

At about 6 weeks after acute myocardial infarction, the greater part of the affected heart muscle should be healed by the formation of a firm scar, and any collateral circulation should also be well developed. As a consequence, most patients should be ready to resume work, provided it is not physically or mentally too demanding. It is important that the myocardial infarction is not seen as an absolute deterrent to returning to work.

In general, the rates of return to work for post-infarction patients are not as good as might be anticipated (Mayberry et al, 1983). Only about one half to three-quarters of patients return to their former employment. By 1 month, most of these are back at work, although only about half work as well as they had done before their coronary (Cay, 1982). About 25 million working days are lost annually from coronary heart disease in the UK. Several factors influence the return to work, including:

- The severity of myocardial infarction
- Post-coronary complications and symptoms (especially breathlessness and angina)
- Advanced working age
- Stressful work environment
- A sporadic pre-coronary work record
- Family instability

It can be seen from these factors that non-cardiac causes of invalidity are just as important as cardiac causes in failure to return to work (Cay et al, 1973).

Discouragement by the family is a major cause of the patient not returning to work (Mayou, 1979). This may be because of shared fear of further cardiac problems, although possible early retirement and Social Security payments may sometimes create a disincentive to return. Ill-considered advice from the patient's medical advisor to 'lay off work and take things easy for a few months' will not help, and some employers seem to believe that coronary patients cannot or should not work at all.

Those patients likely to do best are those given encouragement from the start of the illness, particularly from their family. It is likely that the better the patient perceives his health to be, the more likely he is to return to work. A multidisciplinary approach is often required, involving the social worker, disability employment advisor and employer. Initially, the patient may be advised to return to work on a part-time basis, occasionally with lighter work. A few patients involved in heavy manual work may need to change their occupation, although this is not always acceptable or practical. When the patient does return to work, his level of activity may need to be closely monitored. Many manual workers continue to try to carry out heavy duties, which may be harmful. The patient may dispute this and feel fully capable or not wish to show weakness.

The daily workload of the female patient who is a housewife also needs careful consideration. She has often played a central role in home life and feels a tremendous responsibility to her family, both while she is in hospital and on her return home. Such patients often feel that the house has been neglected, shopping for essential items has been forgotten and the house has not been cleaned adequately. They worry about being unable to look after their family, including cleaning, shopping and cooking. The family will need careful counselling about the psychological stresses on such women and must provide both moral and physical support. Patients should not initially be left at home alone and will need help in performing the household chores, particularly physically taxing jobs such as making the beds and hanging out the washing.

Sickness benefit

Many patients and partners are anxious about how and when to claim sickness benefit. It is helpful to provide them with brief details.

In the UK, sickness benefit is paid by the employer, providing that sufficient NI contributions have been paid during the relevant tax year. Sickness benefit will be paid for up to 28 weeks, and thereafter an invalidity benefit may be paid. Supplementary benefit (for items such as the mortgage) may additionally be payable from the Department of Social Security. The old age pension is payable at the age of 65 years for men and 60 for women, the amount being dependent on the length of working life and the contributions paid.

THE DEVELOPMENT OF REHABILITATION PROGRAMMES

Cardiac rehabilitation programmes seem justified in terms of cost-effectiveness (Levin et al, 1991; Oldridge, 1991; Oldridge et al, 1993). The running cost of a cardiac rehabilitation session is estimated to be only £4–15 per patient (Horgan et al, 1992). The 'Heart Manual' programme (Lewin et al, 1992) costs £20 per patient (including staff training). The financial benefits gained in terms of productivity and maintaining an occupational income by returning to work are clear, and rehabilitation may result in lower rehospitalisation costs (Ades et al, 1992).

An experienced coronary care nurse is probably the best person to take responsibility for coordinating the programme (Todd et al, 1992). Contact should be established with other health and social support services where appropriate. Simple, in-hospital counselling by a coronary care nurse should be an integral part of routine care, as this can have a significant impact on recovery for both the patient and partner, with effects being sustained up to 6 months after the heart attack (Thompson and Meddis, 1990a, 1990b).

Locally- or nationally-agreed evaluation and audit mechanisms need to be developed (Thompson 1994). Outcome measures in cardiac rehabilitation (Hoskins Michel, 1992) could include:

- *Risk factor reduction outcomes*: blood pressure, cholesterol, smoking, weight and physical activity
- *Physical outcomes*: mortality, reinfarction, cardiac arrest, ventricular function, myocardial ischaemia, physical working capacity, symptom limitations and task and activity performance
- *Psychosocial outcomes*: well-being, quality of life and return to work
- *Other outcomes*: adverse events, non-compliance and readmission

Given current information, it is reasonable to conclude that cardiac rehabilitation is safe and effective and should be made available to all who would benefit. It requires considerable commitment and the effective use of local resources. With such support, the patient and family are likely to achieve a markedly improved quality of life. Individual programmes should evaluate their outcome, and a standard format of audit is necessary to allow comparison. Nationally-agreed guidelines, along the lines of those produced in the USA (American Association of Cardiovascular and Pulmonary Rehabilitation, 1995) are urgently needed.

References

Ades P A, Huang D and Weaver S O (1992) Cardiac rehabilitation participation predicts lower rehabilitation costs. *American Heart Journal*, **123**: 916–921.

American Association of Cardiovascular and Pulmonary Rehabilitation (1995) *Guidelines for Cardiac Rehabilitation Programs*, 2nd edn. Champaign, Illinois: Human Kinetics.

Annon J S (1976) *The Behavioural Treatment of Sexual Problems: Brief Therapy*. New York: Harper and Row.

Bertie J, King A, Reed N, Marshall A J and Ricketts C (1992) Benefits and weaknesses of a cardiac rehabilitation programme. *Journal of the Royal College of Physicians of London*, **26**: 147–152.

Bethell H J N and Mullee M A (1990) A controlled trial of community based coronary rehabilitation. *British Heart Journal*, **64**: 370–375.

Bethell H J N, Larvan A and Turner S C (1983) Coronary rehabilitation in the community. *Journal of the Royal College of General Practitioners*, **33**: 285–291.

Bittner V and Oberman A (1993) Efficacy studies in coronary rehabilitation. *Cardiology Clinics*, **11**: 333–347.

Blumenthal J A and Wei J (1993) Psychobehavioral treatment in cardiac rehabilitation. *Cardiology Clinics*, **11**: 323–331.

Casey E, O'Conell J K and Price J H (1984) Perceptions of educational needs for patients after myocardial infarction. *Patient Education and Counselling*, **6:** 77–82.

Cay E L (1982) Psychological problems in patients after a myocardial infarction. *Advances in Cardiology*, **29:** 108–112.

Cay E L, Vetter N J, Philip A E and Dugard P (1973) Return to work after a heart attack. *Journal of Psychosomatic Research*, **17:** 231–243.

Dorossiev D (1983) *Rehabilitation and Comprehensive Secondary Prevention after Acute Myocardial Infarction: Report on a Study*. EURO Reports and Studies No. 84. Copenhagen: WHO Regional Office for Europe.

Dracup K (1985) A controlled trial of couples group counselling in cardiac rehabilitation. *Journal of Cardiopulmonary Rehabilitation*, **5:** 436–442.

Dracup K, Meleis A I, Clark S, Clyburn A, Shields L and Stanley M (1984) Group counselling in cardiac rehabilitation: effect on patient compliance. *Patient Education and Counselling*, **6:** 169–177.

Ebbesen L S, Guyatt G H, McCartney N and Oldridge N B (1990) Measuring quality of life in cardiac spouses. *Journal of Clinical Epidemiology*, **43:** 481–487.

Frasure-Smith N (1992) In-hospital symptoms of psychological stress as predictors of long-term outcome after acute myocardial infarction in men. *American Journal of Cardiology*, **67:** 121–127.

Frasure-Smith N and Price R (1989) Long-term follow-up of the Ischaemic Heart Disease Life Stress Monitoring Program. *Psychosomatic Medicine*, **5:** 485–513.

Gaglione K M (1984) Assessing and intervening with families of coronary care patients. *Nursing Clinics of North America*, **19:** 427–432.

Garrow J S (1981) *Treating Obesity Seriously*. Edinburgh: Churchill Livingstone.

Geissler W, Cay E and Dorossiev D (1985) Educational programmes after myocardial infarction. In *Rehabilitation after Myocardial Infarction. The European Experience*, Kallio V and Cay E (eds), pp. 89–102. Copenhagen: World Health Organisation.

Goble A J, Hare D L, Macdonald P S, Oliver R G, Reid M A and Worcester M C (1991) Effect of early programmes of high and low intensity exercise on physical performance after transmural acute myocardial infarction. *British Heart Journal*, **65:** 126–131.

Greenland P and Chu J S (1988) Efficacy of cardiac rehabilitation services. *Annals of Internal Medicine*, **109:** 650–663.

Gregor F M (1981) Teaching the patient with ischaemic heart disease: a systematic approach to instructional design. *Patient Counselling and Health Education*, **3:** 57–62.

Gruen W (1975) Effects of brief psychotherapy during the hospitalization period on the recovery process in heart attacks. *Journal of Consulting and Clinical Psychology*, **43:** 223–232.

Horgan J, Bethell H, Carson P, Davidson C, Julian D, Mayou R A and Nagle R (1992) Working party report on cardiac rehabilitation. *British Heart Journal*, **67:** 412–418.

Houston-Miller N, Taylor C B, Davidson D M, Hill M N and Krantz D S (1990) The efficacy of risk factor intervention and psychological aspects of cardiac rehabilitation. *Journal of Cardiopulmonary Rehabilitation*, **10:** 198–209.

Ibrahim M A, Feldman J G, Sultz H A, Staiman M G, Young L J and Dean D (1974) Management after myocardial infarction: a controlled trial of the effect of group psychotherapy. *International Journal of Psychiatry in Medicine*, **5:** 253–268.

Johnson J E (1980) Preparing patients to cope with stress while hospitalized. In *Patient Teaching*, Wilson-Barnett J (ed), pp. 19–33. Edinburgh: Churchill Livingstone.

Langosch W, Seer P, Brodner G, Kallinke D, Kulick B and Heim F (1982) Behaviour therapy with coronary heart disease patients: results of a comparative study. *Journal of Psychosomatic Research*, **26:** 475–484.

Levin L A, Perk J and Hedback B (1991) Cardiac rehabilitation – cost analysis. *Journal of Internal Medicine*, **230:** 427–434.

Lewin B, Robertson I H, Cay E L, Irving J B and Campbell M (1992) Effects of self-help post-myocardial-infarction rehabilitation on psychological adjustment and use of health services. *Lancet*, **339:** 1036–1040.

McGee H M and Horgan J H (1992) Cardiac rehabilitation programmes: are women less likely to attend? *British Medical Journal*, **305:** 283–284.

Mayberry J F, Kent S V, Jenkins B and Colbourne G (1983) Employment of men after myocardial infarction. *British Medical Journal*, **287**: 1262–1263.

Mayou R (1979) The course and determinants of reactions to myocardial infarction. *British Journal of Psychiatry*, **134**: 588–594.

Mayou R and Bryant B (1993) Quality of life in cardiovascular disease. *British Heart Journal*, **69**: 460–466.

Mayou R, Williamson B and Foster A (1976) Attitudes and advice after myocardial infarction. *British Medical Journal*, **i**: 1577–1579.

Mayou R, Foster A and Williamson B (1978) The psychological and social effects of myocardial infarction on wives. *British Medical Journal*, **i**: 699–701.

Mayou R, McMahon D, Sleight P and Florencio M J (1981) Early rehabilitation after myocardial infarction. *Lancet*, **ii**: 1399–1401.

Michel T H (1992) Outcome assessment in cardiac rehabilitation. *International Journal of Technology Assessment in Health Care*, **8**: 76–84.

Miller N H, Haskell W L, Berra K and DeBusk R F (1984) Home versus group exercise training for increasing functional capacity after myocardial infarction. *Circulation*, **70**: 645–649.

Morris J N, Everitt M G, Pollard R, Chave S P W and Semmence A M (1980) Vigorous exercise in leisure time: protection against coronary heart disease. *Lancet*, **ii**: 1207–1210.

Moynihan M (1984) Assessing the educational needs of post myocardial infarction patients. *Nursing Clinics of North America*, **19**: 441–447.

New York Heart Association Criteria Committee (1964) *Diseases of the Heart and Blood Vessels; Nomenclature and Criteria for Diagnosis*, 6th edn. Boston: Little, Brown.

Nichols K A (1985) Psychological care by nurses, paramedical and medical staff: essential developments for general hospitals. *British Journal of Medical Psychology*, **58**: 231–240.

Nutter D O, Schlant R S and Hurst J W (1972) Isometric exercises and the cardiovascular system. *Modern Concepts in Cardiovascular Disease*, **41**: 11–15.

Oberman A (1984) Rehabilitation of patients with coronary artery disease. In *Heart Disease*, Braunwald E (ed.), pp. 1384–1398. Philadelphia: W B Saunders.

O'Connor G T, Buring J E, Yusuf S, Goldhaber S Z, Olmstead E M, Paffenbarger R S and Hennekens C H (1989) An overview of randomized trials of rehabilitation with exercise after myocardial infarction. *Circulation*, **80**: 234–244.

Oldenburg B, Perkins R J and Andrews G (1985) Controlled trial of psychological intervention in myocardial infarction. *Journal of Consulting and Clinical Psychology*, **53**: 852–859.

Oldridge N B (1991) Cardiac rehabilitation services: what are they and are they worth it? *Comprehensive Therapy*, **17**: 59–66.

Oldridge N B, Guyatt G H, Fischer M E and Rimm A A (1988) Cardiac rehabilitation after myocardial infarction: combined experience of randomized clinical trials. *Journal of the American Medical Association*, **260**: 945–950.

Oldridge N, Guyatt G, Jones N, Crowe J, Singer J, Feeny D, McKelvie R, Runions J, Streiner D and Torrance G (1991) Effects on quality of life with comprehensive rehabilitation after acute myocardial infarction. *American Journal of Cardiology*, **67**: 1084–1089.

Oldridge N, Furlong W, Feeny D et al (1993) Economic evaluation of cardiac rehabilitation soon after acute myocardial infarction. *American Journal of Cardiology*, **72**: 154–161.

Paffenbarger R S and Hyde R T (1980) Exercise as protection against heart attack. *New England Journal of Medicine*, **302**: 1026–1027.

Prosser G, Carson P, Gelson A, Tucker H, Neophytou M, Philips R and Simpson T (1978) Assessing the psychological effects of an exercise training programme for patients following myocardial infarction: a pilot study. *British Journal of Medical Psychology*, **51**: 95–102.

Rahe R H, Ward H W and Hayes V (1979) Brief group therapy in myocardial infarction rehabilitation: three to four year follow-up of a controlled trial. *Psychosomatic Medicine*, **41**: 229–242.

Redman B K (1984) *The Process of Patient Education*. St Louis: C V Mosby.

Runions J (1985) A program for psychological and social enhancement during rehabilitation after myocardial infarction. *Heart and Lung*, **14**: 117–125.

Scheuermann W, Scheidt R, Nussel E and Deckert E (1985) Multicentre study on heart groups. In *Proceedings of the International Conference on Preventive Cardiology*, Moscow, June 1985. Abstract 123.

Shephard R J (1983) The value of exercise in ischaemic heart disease – a cumulative analysis. *Journal of Cardiac Rehabilitation*, **3**: 294–298.

Shephard R J (1986) Cardiac rehabilitation in prospect. In *Heart Disease and Rehabilitation*, Pollock M L and Schmidt D (eds), pp. 713–740. New York: John Wiley & Sons.

Siddiuqi M A (1992) Cardiac rehabilitation in elderly patients. *Age and Ageing*, **21**: 157–159.

Sivarajan E S, Newton K M, Almes M J, Kempf T M, Mansfield L W and Bruce R A (1983) Limited effects of outpatient teaching and counseling after myocardial infarction: a controlled study. *Heart and Lung*, **12**: 65–73.

Stern M J, Gorman P A and Kaslow L (1983) The group counselling versus exercise therapy study: a controlled intervention with subjects following myocardial infarction. *Archives of Internal Medicine*, **143**: 1719–1725.

Taylor C B, Bandura A, Ewart C K, Miller N H and DeBusk R F (1985) Exercise testing to enhance wives' confidence in their husbands' cardiac capability soon after clinically uncomplicated acute myocardial infarction. *American Journal of Cardiology*, **55**: 635–638.

Thompson D R (1983) Sexual counselling and cardiac patients. *British Journal of Sexual Medicine*, **10**: 16–18.

Thompson D R (1990) *Counselling the Coronary Patient and Partner*. London: Scutari Press.

Thompson D R (1994) Cardiac rehabilitation services: the need to develop guidelines. *Quality in Health Care*, **3**: 169–172.

Thompson D R and Cordle C J (1986) Sexual counselling following myocardial infarction. *British Journal of Sexual Medicine*, **13**: 16–17.

Thompson D R and Cordle C J (1988) Support of wives of myocardial infarction patients. *Journal of Advanced Nursing*, **13**: 223–228.

Thompson D R and Meddis R (1990a) A prospective evaluation of in-hospital counselling for first time myocardial infarction men. *Journal of Psychosomatic Research*, **34**: 237–248.

Thompson D R and Meddis R (1990b) Wives' responses to counselling early after myocardial infarction. *Journal of Psychosomatic Research*, **34**: 249–258.

Thompson D R, Webster R A, Cordle C J and Sutton T W (1987) Specific sources and patterns of anxiety in male patients with first myocardial infarction. *British Journal of Medical Psychology*, **60**: 343–348.

Todd I C, Wosornu D, Stewart I and Wild T (1992) Cardiac rehabilitation following myocardial infarction. *Sports Medicine*, **14**: 243–259.

Ueno M (1963) The so-called coition death. *Japanese Journal of Legal Medicine*, **17**: 330–340.

Wiklund I, Sanne H, Vedin A and Wilhelmsson C (1984) Psychosocial outcome one year after a first myocardial infarction. *Journal of Psychosomatic Research*, **28**: 309–321.

World Health Organization (1993) *Needs and Action Priorities in Cardiac Rehabilitation and Secondary Prevention in Patients with Coronary Heart Disease*. Copenhagen: World Health Organization Regional Office for Europe.

13

Reducing Risk and Assessing Prognosis after Myocardial Infarction

The early approaches towards the prevention of coronary heart disease concentrated on modifying one risk factor, so that an effect could be defined for each factor. However, this style of intervention did not provide consistent answers, mainly because, as we now know, the atheromatous process is multifactorial and addressing single risk factors has little or no effect. Nevertheless, these early observations were useful in demonstrating and confirming aetiological factors. More recently, a multifactorial approach has been taken, and the results of the various clinical trials offer strong support for intensified interventions in the prevention of coronary heart disease and the rehabilitation of patients following acute myocardial infarction (Neaton and Wentworth, 1992). These usually involve some modification of or major changes in the patient's life-style (European Atherosclerosis Society, 1992).

Secondary prevention of myocardial infarction describes any intervention that will prevent a recurrence of heart trouble. The rehabilitation programme should include changes relevant to the patient, particularly those that may result in a reduced risk of further cardiovascular events. It is important to explain that changing any life-long habit, whether it be smoking, diet or exercise, will never guarantee that patients will remain free from heart disease, or from any other ailment for that matter, in the future. What are being considered are *relative* risks, and it is important that this is appreciated by all concerned.

Counselling patients on risk factors presumes that the person will change on being informed about the risks involved in the manifestations of coronary heart disease. However, life-style modification is not easy. Life-long habits are hard to change, and denial very often has to be overcome, with belief that changing behaviour will help. Time to consider and reappraise the situation is essential for the patient, so that variations may be introduced gradually, with cooperation. Modifying behaviour is often a difficult and long-term process.

Although the hospital setting provides an ideal environment for discussion and motivation towards a healthier way of life, educational opportunities are often constrained by the acute illness and its associated anxiety. Nevertheless, counselling during the latter part of the patient's stay in hospital provides an ideal foundation for patient and family education.

ASSESSING OVERALL RISK

It is important to synthesise an informed judgement of the patient's overall risk of developing or worsening cardiovascular disease or its complications before deciding upon risk factor intervention. The severity, as well as the presence or absence of the major risk factors, is important; patients at highest risk are those with current evidence of coronary heart disease, two or more major risk factors or a single, but severe, risk factor. A risk factor profile has been developed, based upon the results of the United Kingdom Heart Disease Prevention Project, and has led to the development of the Dundee risk-disk (Tunstall-Pedoe, 1991). This small manual computer provides a valid means of assessing and monitoring modifiable risk factors. It is likely that similar information from clinical trials will lead to the development of computer programs or hand-held calculators for use in cardiac clinics and on the coronary care unit.

DIETARY ADVICE

Apart from providing essential nutrients to the body, eating and drinking are pleasurable experiences, a fact that often seems to be forgotten by those giving advice. Misconceptions regarding diet litter the popular press and bookstalls, and the problem is compounded by conflicting and unsubstantiated information given by friends, relatives and even some health professionals. Dietary modifications often require major change in the patient's normal eating habits, and, to be successful in achieving compliance, it is important that factual information is presented objectively, consistently and in a way that can be easily and readily understood by the patient and his family. In this respect, the recent World Health Organization guidelines (1990) have been welcomed as a policy for prevention of cardiovascular disease in the future. For most patients, it is better to emphasise an alteration in general eating habits rather than the necessity of adhering to a specific dietary plan; patients are not going to change the habits of a life-time based on a 10-minute chat with a doctor, nurse or dietitian. Involvement of the patient's family is also helpful; eating is usually a family or communal activity, and the women of the household are normally the ones who are responsible for shopping and the preparation of the meals. It is important both to educate those who buy and prepare the food and to enlist their help and cooperation in any dietary manipulation.

General advice includes eating a wide variety of foods and in the right amounts to prevent obesity. Fat and sugar should be avoided, and foods high in starch and fibre are to be encouraged. Where specific dietary restrictions are necessary (e.g. for diabetes or hyperlipidaemia), dietary modifications must be realistic and understood by the patient and family, if they are going to be adhered to. Spoken advice should be supplemented with leaflets, which can be referred to at home. Referral to a state-registered dietitian is advisable when detailed advice is required regarding more complex dietary changes. It is worth remembering that, without effective dieting, diabetes, hyperlipidaemia and hypertension are relatively resistant to drug therapy.

Weight control

The single most important dietary intervention is weight control. Being overweight is associated with elevated plasma lipids, glucose intolerance and hypertension, and it is desirable for most cardiac patients to achieve their correct body mass index. Body weight is essentially controlled by food intake, and it is always possible to lose weight by eating less food than the body requires, despite what our obese patients tell us. Long-established Western dietary habits are hard to break, and we

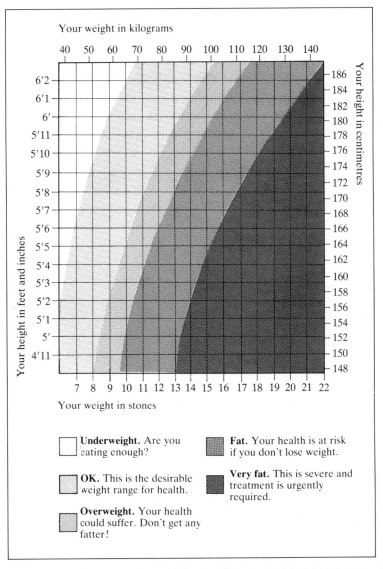

Fig. 13.1 Desirable body weight (From Garrow, 1981. Reproduced by kind permission of Churchill Livingstone, with acknowledgement to the Health Education Council and E Fullard, Oxford)

are generally encouraged to eat and drink more than is good for us, particularly saturated fats, simple sugars and alcohol.

A mutually-agreed goal for weight reduction should be established, and a record should be kept (e.g. with a graph) that gives a quick visual indication of how the patient is progressing. Practical advice should include explanation of calorific intake versus expenditure, the regular and slow eating of smaller amounts of food and the participation in regular physical activity. The ultimate goal is to achieve a body weight appropriate for age, height and sex (Figure 13.1). Attending 'Weight Watchers' or other slimming clubs may be helpful. It must be noted that it will be more difficult to influence the patient if family members and those counselling the patient are overweight.

Dietary fats

There are two main categories of fat in the diet: saturated fats (which tend to raise serum cholesterol levels) and unsaturated fats (which tend to lower blood cholesterol). The major dietary sources of fats are the spreading fats (butter and margarine), cooking fats, meat and dairy produce. In addition, much of our fat intake is hidden in foods such as cakes and biscuits. Offal (liver, kidney and pâté), shellfish and eggs all contain large amounts of cholesterol, although, contrary to popular belief, these foods will only have a small effect on serum cholesterol. Similarly, foods advertised as 'low cholesterol' are not necessarily healthy. Dietary saturated fats increase serum LDL and triglyceride levels, whilst polyunsaturated fats have the opposite effect.

There should be an overall reduction of saturated fat intake, with substitution of vegetable fats where possible; total fat intake needs to be no more than 30% of the total food energy intake, with two-thirds of this as vegetable fat (Bingham, 1991). Not all vegetable fats are acceptable; palm and coconut oil, for example, are high in saturated fat. Olive oil (a monounsaturated fat) may be a better source of vegetable fat. Unlike polyunsaturated fats, it does not reduce HDL-cholesterol levels, which may explain the negative correlation between olive oil consumption and coronary deaths. Fish oils have notable antithrombotic activity and reduce fibrinogen levels, as well as blood pressure. Oily fish consumption has, therefore, been emphasised in cardioprotective diets. Prospective trials in which fish was recommended and consumed at least twice weekly reported that the rates of coronary heart disease were reduced by a half in comparison to those who ate no fish. Interestingly, most of the fish consumed was not oily!

Dietary fibre

An increased fibre intake is usually recommended. Viscous fibre (e.g. guar or pectin) will help to lower plasma lipid and glucose levels. High consumption of bread and cereal products, particularly oats, may help to reduce cholesterol levels and has been associated with a reduced rate of coronary death.

Fresh vegetables and fruit provide excellent sources of pectin, vitamins and minerals.

Salt

The association of dietary salt and hypertension is a controversial issue, but the level of salt ingested in Western countries is greatly in excess of requirement. A reduction can be made by not adding it to food after cooking and by avoiding obviously salty foods (e.g. crisps, peanuts and Marmite), especially by those with high or borderline blood pressure.

Sugar

Countries with a high per capita intake of sugar have high rates of coronary heart disease (Keys, 1980). However, there is a close link between sugar and fat intake in the poorer countries, and it is unlikely that sugar is an independent risk factor. A reduction in simple sugars and other refined carbohydrates is, however, helpful in preventing obesity, treating glucose intolerance and reducing the incidence of dental caries.

Alcohol

The relationship of alcohol and coronary heart disease is complex, mainly due to the concomitant smoking and overeating that often accompany alcohol intake. Alcohol may directly damage the myocardium (leading to a dilated cardiomyopathy), as well as aggravating hypertension and hyperlipidaemia. Despite this, moderate intake of alcohol is probably protective against coronary heart disease, and even light drinkers have more cardioprotection than teetotalers. The Framingham study found that coronary risk was diminished by one third in those who consumed more than 30 g of alcohol per month. This effect probably derives from the beneficial influence on coagulation factors (fibrinogen and plasminogen activator) and platelets and from the increase in HDL cholesterol.

Garlic

Garlic has been used for hundreds of years for its medicinal purposes and may have a beneficial action on many cardiovascular risk factors (reduced blood pressure, increased HDL, reduced LDL and triglycerides), as well as advantageous effects on coagulation factors and platelets. The active ingredients, allicin and ajoene, may be destroyed by cooking or processing. Carefully dried slices may retain their active ingredients, but a daily intake of 1 g or more is probably needed for the most beneficial effect.

Electrolytes and trace elements

The myocardium is more susceptible to damage, dysrhythmias and digoxin in the presence of hypokalaemia. Most cases of chronic hypokalaemia are due to use of diuretics, and an increased intake of potassium in the diet is desirable for those on diuretic therapy. Fresh fruit and vegetables are excellent sources of potassium (one inch of banana = 1 mmol potassium). Magnesium depletion (due to thiazide diuretics, diabetes or diarrhoea) usually accompanies hypokalaemia and hypocalcaemia.

Vegetarian and Mediterranean diets

Communities in which vegetarianism is common have generally lower rates of cardiovascular disease, and individuals seem to live longer. This probably derives from avoidance of obesity and a higher intake of unsaturated fats, fresh fruit and vegetables which are often rich in vitamins A and C (antioxidant vitamins), and which prevent oxidation of LDL to a more atherogenic form. The diet of the Mediterranean countries have all these benefits, plus a higher intake of olive oil, lots of garlic and regular moderate alcohol (Ulbricht and Southgate, 1991).

The potential benefits from a 'healthy' diet

Modifying the diet is probably helpful in the treatment of hyperlipidaemia, hypertension and congestive heart failure and in the prevention of hypertension and atherosclerosis. Diets that are fat-modified, high in fibre and low in salt help to reduce serum cholesterol and blood pressure. Thrombogenicity may also decrease, via the reduced effect of fatty acids on platelet function. In addition, high-fibre diets are associated with a lower incidence of constipation, bowel cancer, diverticular disease, appendicitis, gallstones and haemorrhoids. Glucose tolerance may be improved, and high-carbohydrate, high-fibre, low-refined-sugar diets are recommended for patients with diabetes mellitus.

Many dietary recommendations have been advanced on the basis that they will prevent or minimise the risk of heart disease, and detailed and complicated dietary modifications are to be found in abundance in the medical literature and popular press (Thompson, 1983; Oliver, 1986). It should be appreciated that dietary modification alone has not been shown to prevent heart disease. Many patients become distressed when they make alterations to their diet and life-style only to find that they have heart disease.

HYPERLIPIDAEMIA

There is a strong, positive, graded relationship between serum cholesterol and death from coronary heart disease (Neaton et al, 1992). The main aim of treatment of hyperlipidaemia is to reduce this risk of developing premature vascular disease (primary intervention) or diminish the occurrence of further vascular events in those with current cardiovascular disease (secondary prevention). The potential for secondary prevention is substantially higher than for primary prevention, since the absolute coronary risk conferred by raised serum cholesterol is much higher in those with pre-existing coronary disease. Even a modest reduction of total cholesterol of around 10% (a target easily achievable by dietary intervention) may produce a reduction of between 20 and 50% risk of coronary heart disease events within 5 years (Law et al, 1994). Regression trials such as the St Thomas' Atherosclerosis Regression Study (STARS) have shown considerable success with diet and drugs in slowing the progress of atheromatous lesions or delaying their appearance (Watts et al, 1992).

The therapeutic goals defined by the British Hyperlipidaemia Association (1993) are:

- For patients with established coronary heart disease:
  Total cholesterol < 5.2 mmol/l (LDL < 3.4 mmol/l)

- For patients without established coronary heart disease:
  Total cholesterol < 6.0 mmol/l (LDL < 4.1 mmol/l)

It must be emphasised that treatment should be part of an overall plan to reduce cardiovascular risk, and hyperlipidaemia should not be viewed in isolation.

Dietary advice

Dietary modification must be the first-line of treatment of all types of hyperlipid-aemia, although the response will depend on both the underlying lipoprotein abnormality and its severity. The main influence upon plasma cholesterol levels is diet, and the elevating effect comes mostly from the ingestion of saturated fats. Eating cholesterol is generally less influential, but there appears to be individual sensitivity. Fat intake should be reduced to below one third of total requirements, and the proportion ingested as unsaturated fat should be increased from the typical 25% found in Western diets to about 75%. This action alone will reduce cholesterol levels and increase the HDL:LDL ratio, as well as making the fat-depleted diet more tolerable. The calorific deficit can be replaced by unrefined, high-fibre carbohydrates, although replacement should not be complete in the overweight. This applies particularly to those patients with predominantly raised triglyceride levels, as attainment of correct body weight will often be the only therapy required. Alcohol excess may also produce hyper-triglyceridaemia, but, unfortunately, 'excess' will vary from patient to patient, and abstention may sometimes be the only way of reducing triglyceride levels.

A typical cholesterol-lowering diet is shown in Table 13.1.

Table 13.1 A typical cholesterol-lowering diet

Food type	% Total calories
Total fat	< 30
(Roughly 10% each of saturated, monounsaturated and polyunsaturated fats)	
Carbohydrate	> 50
Protein	10–20
Fibre	> 35 mg/day
Cholesterol	< 300 mg day*

*The average British diet only contains about 500 mg of cholesterol; low cholesterol diets, per se, can only have a small effect on serum cholesterol.

Drug therapy

The decision to use drugs for hyperlipidaemia should be based on the clinical assessment of the patient's likelihood to develop coronary heart disease; the cholesterol concentration alone is seldom a reason for intervention (Jowett and Galton, 1987). Drug therapy should be used only after a careful trial of diet, employing the most rigorous diet achievable by the individual. Other risk factors will also need identifying and treating. Treatment with drugs is rarely justified at cholesterol levels below 6.5 mmol/l and for comparatively few with levels between 6.5 and 7.8 mmol/l. Many patients with cholesterol concentrations above 7.8 mmol/l will need medication, especially if there is associated hypertriglyceridaemia (*Lancet*, 1987), although this may not be the case in women or the elderly.

Lipid-lowering drugs are an important adjunct to dietary and life-style measures in high-risk patients with dyslipidaemia. Target levels for serum lipid concentrations suggested by the European Atherosclerosis Society (1992) are shown in Table 13.2. Adopting these targets would probably lead to 2–3% of all patients in the UK being treated with drugs. This would currently represent a 25 times increase, since we are one of the most conservative prescribers of lipid-lowering therapy (Reckless, 1990).

Table 13.2   Target levels for plasma cholesterol and LDL cholesterol

Global risk	Target level	
	Reduce plasma cholesterol to (mmol/l)	Reduce LDL cholesterol to (mmol/l)

Risk mildly increased
e.g. pretreatment cholesterol 5.2–7.8 mmol/l
    NO non-lipid risk factors
    Plasma cholesterol: HDL cholesterol ratio 4.5–5.0
	5–6	4–4.5

Risk moderately increased
e.g. pretreatment cholesterol 5.2–7.8 mmol/l
    PLUS one non-lipid risk factor
    or
    PLUS HDL cholesterol < 1 mmol/l
	5	3.5–4

High risk
e.g. presence of coronary or peripheral vascular disease
    or
    presence of familial hypercholesterolaemia
       or plasma cholesterol > 7.8 mmol/l
    or
    plasma cholesterol 5.2–7.8 mmol/l
       PLUS two non-lipid risk factors
    or
    plasma cholesterol 5.2–7.8 mmol/l
       PLUS one severe non-lipid risk factor
	4.5–5	3–3.5

Note: Triglyceride target level not yet determined: suggested value < 2.3 mmol/l

Initial drug therapy for those with hypercholesterolaemia is with bile acid sequestrant resins, such as cholestyramine or colestipol. The HMG-CoA reductase inhibitors (the 'statins') are being increasingly used and are extremely effective, particularly when used with low-dose cholestyramine.

Those with mixed hyperlipidaemias are usually treated with fibric acid derivatives (e.g. bezafibrate, ciprofibrate and gemfibrozil), especially if the triglyceride levels are markedly elevated.

Treatment of isolated hypertriglyceridaemia remains controversial. Mild elevations (3–6 mmol/l) are usually due to obesity or excess alcohol intake, but if fasting concentrations persist above 3 mmol/l, and are associated with depression of HDL-cholesterol levels (to less than 1.0 mmol/l), treatment should be considered. Nicotinic acid is sometimes very effective and is very popular in the USA, where it has been shown to be safe in long-term usage. Unfortunately, cutaneous flushing often limits its use. Acipimox is an analogue that may be more acceptable. Fish oils may be of benefit in reducing triglyceride levels as part of the basic diet but have not proved useful pharmacologically.

The benefits of lipid-lowering drug therapy

There have been several randomised trials, using angiography, looking at the regression of atheroma. These have shown that coronary atherosclerosis can be arrested or reversed by drug therapy and is associated with a significant reduction in clinical events (Thompson, 1992). Whilst it has been thought that a treatment effect may not be seen for over 2 years, as seen in the Helsinki Heart Study (1987a, 1987b) and Lipid Research Clinics Primary Prevention Trial (Lipid Research Clinics Program, 1984), a marked reduction in serious adverse cardiac events may be seen within 6 months (Pravastatin Multi-National Study Group, 1993).

Other studies have shown the value of combined therapy with drugs and diet in the secondary prevention of coronary heart disease (Nikkila et al, 1984; Blankenhorn et al, 1987), and special consideration should, therefore, be given to patients with coronary heart disease, especially if they have undergone coronary artery bypass surgery or coronary angioplasty (Pearson and Marx, 1993). In the list of treatment group priorities suggested by the British Hyperlipidaemia Association (Betteridge et al, 1993), these types of patient are given first priority (Table 13.3). Target cholesterol levels are lower than those for primary prevention.

Such guidelines need to be used flexibly, and the threshold for treatment needs consideration in the presence of other factors. For example, premenopausal women are at a lower risk of coronary heart disease, so cholesterol intervention levels could be increased by 1 mmol/l. In postmenopausal women, the risk of coronary heart disease rises steeply, possibly related to rising LDL levels. These changes may be ameliorated by hormone replacement therapy (Khaw, 1992).

The relationship between plasma cholesterol and coronary heart disease rises less steeply in the elderly (over 65 years of age). Whilst the benefits of cholesterol lowering would seem to be greater (since vascular events are more common) in this age group, it is not known whether intervention at this late stage will produce any effect. Trial results from the USA are awaited, and, in the meantime, it might be reasonable to raise intervention levels raised by 1 mmol/l.

Table 13.3 Priorities and action limits for lipid-lowering drug therapy in diet-resistant subjects

Priority	Subject category	Total cholesterol (mmol/l)	LDL cholesterol (mmol/l)
First	Patients with existing CHD, or post-CABG, angioplasty or cardiac transplant	> 5.2	> 3.4
Second	Patients with multiple risk factors or genetically determined hyperlipidaemia, e.g. FH	> 6.5	> 5.0
Third	Males with asymptomatic hypercholesterolaemia	> 7.8	> 6.0
Fourth	Postmenopausal females with asymptomatic hypercholesterolaemia	> 7.8	> 6.0

SMOKING

The habit of smoking is a complex addiction, with a high level of dependence. It appears to serve multiple functions and exerts its addictive influence by satisfying a physical need, providing stimulation and pleasure and relieving anxiety and tension.

Smoking is the most important risk factor for first and subsequent heart attacks. The risk of the first heart attack is halved within 5 years of stopping smoking (Doll and Peto, 1976). Stopping smoking after myocardial infarction is associated with a substantial reduction in the risk of non-fatal recurrence and death, in both the long and short term (Mulcahy, 1983; Cook et al, 1986), and the onset of angina may also be delayed (Daly et al, 1985). Additionally, stopping smoking reduces the excess risk of chronic bronchitis and cancer.

It has been estimated that a 20% reduction in cigarette smoking could result in 8000 fewer deaths in the UK every year. Non-smoking policies are widespread in hospitals these days, and cigarette sales from ward trolleys and hospital shops should become obsolete. Advice on smoking should start on the coronary care unit, and a nurse who is a non-smoker will be a more credible role model. Like all rehabilitation advice, its value depends heavily upon the attending medical and nursing staff adopting an informed, committed and uniform approach. Similar education of the patient's family is equally important, and giving such information at the bedside when the patient is suffering from obvious smoking-related symptoms often reinforces the importance of such advice.

A realistic plan can be drawn up, with the aim of complete cessation of smoking. Cutting down is not the answer, nor is switching to a low-tar cigarette. This is because the smoking pattern will change to extract the same amount of nicotine from weaker or fewer cigarettes. Smokers will automatically puff harder to titrate up the amount of nicotine (Woodward and Tunstall-Pedoe, 1993), and, of course, with this comes the other harmful constituents of tobacco smoke – carbon monoxide, thiocyanates and tar. Although it is widely held that switching to cigars or a pipe will reduce the cardiovascular risk, this is not the case (Kaufman et al, 1987). Anyone who has tried a pipe (without inhaling) will already realise this from the immediate symptoms of tachycardia and tremor.

The benefits, including improved health and finances, improvement of the senses of taste and smell and a greater physical attraction when freed from the smell of smoke, should be stressed. Many smokers advance the excuse that they will put on weight if they stop smoking. This is not an inevitable consequence; anyway, they would need to put on 2 stone in weight to nullify the benefits of stopping smoking.

During the initial period of withdrawal, the patients (and their relatives) should be warned that they may become irritable and unable to concentrate. There may be mood swings, gastrointestinal upsets or even an initial worsening of their 'smokers' cough. Reassurance that these effects are temporary is required. It is important to ensure that the patient does not succumb to the common temptation of 'just one more'. Distraction is useful when craving is present. Nicotine replacement therapy can help smokers to stop smoking but only if they are sufficiently motivated. Nicotine chewing gum may help by maintaining blood nicotine levels and easing withdrawal symptoms in the early stages. This has mainly been superseded by transdermal nicotine patches, which may assist phased withdrawal from smoking. Caution is advised in those with established cardiac disease, because of cardiostimulation.

Although the hospital setting is ideal for smoking cessation, it is necessary for periodic checks to be made after discharge on compliance with advice. General practitioners can influence their patients very effectively by advice, coercion and support: a patient's most common reason for stopping smoking is because his doctor told him to (Russell et al, 1979)!

Patients may often try to deceive their doctors about continued smoking, and objective markers such as blood carboxyhaemoglobin concentrations or plasma cotinine concentrations can clarify the situation. Such deception may increase unless the current controversy of not performing cardiac surgery on smokers is resolved (Underwood et al, 1993). Nearly all patients requiring bypass surgery have smoked for long periods, and many will not have given up prior to surgery, despite advise. The operative risks and chances of bypass failure are very high in current smokers, and whilst no smoker should be denied urgent surgery, elective surgery should perhaps only be offered to those who stop smoking. After 2–3 months of doing so, symptoms often improve, but even if they do not, surgery then carries a lower operative morbidity, fewer postoperative chest problems and improved graft patency (Powell and Greenhalgh, 1994).

HYPERTENSION

It is widely accepted that control of hypertension will reduce the incidence of cerebrovascular disease and renal failure, but the benefits for coronary heart disease, although likely, are still uncertain. Nevertheless, the most common cause of death in patients with hypertension is myocardial infarction, which occurs two to three times more commonly than stroke. Although there is currently no convincing evidence that secondary intervention improves outcome, hypertension should be treated, since the risk of heart failure, angina and stroke will be reduced (Sleight, 1993). Uncomplicated hypertension causes no symptoms and should be detected by routine screening every 5 years (Severs et al, 1993).

Clinical application of ambulatory blood pressure monitoring and self-measurement of blood pressure in the management of hypertension are still limited but are undergoing evaluation (Appel and Stason, 1993).

Non-pharmacological treatment should be employed in all patients, regardless of their need for medication (World Health Organization/International Society of Hypertension, 1993). This should include advice on exercise, weight reduction and dietary restriction of salt and alcohol. It is probably more important to stop smoking than to treat mildly raised blood pressure.

If drug therapy is required, it must be made clear that it is usually permanent, and patients should not just complete the 'course' of tablets. Special attention must be paid to the related contraindications of any antihypertensive agent employed. For example, beta-blockers are usually not advisable in patients with cardiac conduction defects or heart failure, and diuretics may adversely affect plasma lipid, urate and potassium levels.

Rapid reduction of blood pressure is seldom required but should be considered urgent in two groups of patients seen on coronary care:

1. *Those with hypertensive heart failure.* Pulmonary oedema and hypertension often coexist, and one may precipitate the other. Often the blood pressure falls with effective treatment of left ventricular failure. If not, vasodilator therapy (e.g. sodium nitroprusside) should be instituted.

2. *Those with hypertension complicating myocardial infarction.* Many patients with acute myocardial infarction will be hypertensive on admission to hospital. Hypertension will often respond to pain relief and sedation, but those whose systolic blood pressure remains over 160 mmHg should be treated. This reduces the risk of several cardiac complications, including cardiac rupture.

The first ISIS study (ISIS-1 Collaborative Group, 1988) showed that acute administration of intravenous atenolol reduced mortality, although caution is needed in those at risk of heart failure (as tachycardia and hypertension may be a compensatory mechanism in response to left ventricular dysfunction). This is usually not the case if there is a loud first heart sound, wide pulse pressure and no dyspnoea.

The aim of treatment in hypertension is to lower the blood pressure as safely as possible, rather than as quickly as possible. In patients with chronic hypertension, sudden reduction of the blood pressure may cause a stroke. This is because cerebral autoregulation is set to higher levels (Figure 13.2) and 'normal' blood pressures will be insufficient to perfuse the brain, resulting in cerebral ischaemia and infarction.

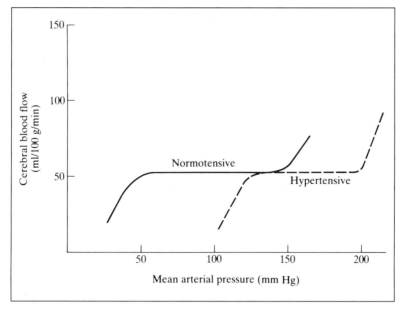

Fig. 13.2 Cerebral autoregulation of blood flow. Note that the control mechanism is set at a higher level in patients with hypertension

STRESS

A marked reduction in the intensity of Type A behaviour has been seen in patients undergoing regular counselling (Gill et al, 1985), suggesting that it can be modified, at least in the short term. Intervention by counselling after acute myocardial infarction may lead to a dramatic and sustained fall in cardiovascular mortality (Friedman et al, 1986), and some would suggest that counselling should be a routine component of post-infarction management (Lloyd, 1991). Methods of relaxation are numerous and varied, and one that is suitable to the individual, e.g. progressive relaxation, meditation, biofeedback, yoga, self-hypnosis, group therapy or listening to music, should be chosen. Biofeedback relaxation therapy may lower blood pressure for up to 6 months following therapy.

Polyphasic activities during everyday life (e.g. watching television, eating and reading simultaneously) must be avoided. The role of frequent, moderate exercise is often underplayed. Jogging, for example, is ideal for reducing muscular tension and giving the patient an opportunity for privacy and self-appraisal whilst running.

The risk of developing persistent psychological disturbance is greater for those patients who were psychiatrically ill before their myocardial infarction, and they will need to be supported during convalescence. Drug therapy needs careful consideration in view of the frequent cardiovascular side effects of antidepressant medication. The new serotonin uptake inhibitors are better than traditional tricyclic drugs.

EXERCISE

Exercise training programmes have been recommended to aid recovery from myocardial infarction (see Chapter 12), although these need not be of very high intensity (Worcester et al, 1993). Approximately 30 minutes of moderate aerobic exercise on alternate days, or 20 minutes daily, is the usual advice, although this should be related to individual capacity.

Physical fitness is psychologically beneficial, and exercise favourably influences lipid levels (raising HDL concentrations), glucose tolerance, fibrinolytic activity and blood pressure, as well as helping to combat obesity (Royal College of Physicians, 1991). Unfortunately, exercise probably does not influence prognosis following acute myocardial infarction. There is no evidence that it prevents progression of the disease, promotes coronary collateral circulation or reduces the risk of further heart attacks. Care is required in previously sedentary subjects, particularly if overweight. Those with advanced coronary heart disease should initially be supervised.

DRUG THERAPY

Aspirin

Administration of aspirin acutely and long term greatly reduces the risk of subsequent vascular events, including reinfarction (Anti-platelet Trialists' Collaboration, 1994). The beneficial dose is unknown, but is probably in the range of 75–300 mg daily.

Beta-blockers

The use of certain beta-blockers (timolol, metoprolol or propranolol) following myocardial infarction reduces the risk of death and non-fatal reinfarction by about one fifth (Yusuf et al, 1985). This benefit cannot be assumed for other beta-blockers, and, indeed, those with intrinsic sympathomimetic activity (e.g. pindolol and oxprenolol) may increase mortality. The evidence for continuation of beta-blockers beyond 2 years after myocardial infarction is not yet established, but most physicians would continue the drug indefinitely unless there were problems.

Calcium antagonists

These have no benefit following complicated myocardial infarction, but diltiazem may be of value in preventing reinfarction, particularly following non-transmural myocardial infarction (Gibson et al, 1986).

ACE-inhibitors

The routine use of ACE-inhibitors in unselected patients following acute myocardial infarction has been addressed in the ISIS-4 (1995) and GISSI-3 (1994) studies, which seem to show a small benefit with early administration. In addition, the SAVE (Pfeffer et al, 1992) and AIRE (Acute Infarction Ramipril Efficacy) (1993) studies have shown that ACE-inhibitors commenced within 1 week of myocardial infarction reduce the incidence of mortality and serious cardiovascular events. Whilst the SAVE (Survival and Ventricular Enlargement) and SOLVD (Studies of Left Ventricular Dysfunction) prevention studies provided good evidence of improved prognosis in patients with asymptomatic left ventricular dysfunction (Vannan et al, 1993), the use of ACE-inhibitors following acute myocardial infarction probably only needs consideration in those patients with overt cardiac failure or ejection fractions under 40%, secondary to significant left ventricular damage (St John Sutton, 1994).

SURGICAL THERAPY

The role of surgery following myocardial infarction is discussed in Chapter 14. Coronary bypass surgery is now established as an adjunct for prolonging survival following myocardial infarction. It is likely that coronary angioplasty will be shown to do the same, and both surgical interventions can improve symptoms.

ASSESSING PROGNOSIS FOLLOWING MYOCARDIAL INFARCTION

Patients who survive a myocardial infarction are at increased risk of death and reinfarction. Prognostic assessment of patients following acute myocardial infarction is important, so that therapy may be optimised and new treatments evaluated. Stratification of patients according to risk is a continuous process and should not be based upon a single assessment; prognosis may change because of medical intervention (Krone, 1992).

Most of the patients who die from heart attacks do so within the first few weeks, the majority of these from ventricular fibrillation before reaching hospital. In-hospital deaths are usually due to heart failure or reinfarction and relate strongly to the age of the patient. Of those patients receiving thrombolytic therapy, the mortality rate lies between 4% (for patients under 55 years of age) and 25% (for those over 75 years of age). The overall mortality at 1 year is 10–15%, and there is some concern that although patients treated by thrombolysis have a relatively good short-term prognosis, long-term mortality and recurrent non-fatal ischaemic events are very common (Stevenson et al, 1993). This may relate to early reocclusion of the infarct-related artery. For those who survive 1 year, the annual mortality is believed to be less than 5%. The net reduction in mortality for patients thrombolysed within 24 hours of acute myocardial infarction is about 20% (Fibrinolytic Therapy Trialists' Collaborative Group, 1994).

A number of strategies have been devised for long-term risk stratification in post-infarction patients, attempting to predict future cardiac events, particularly sudden death and reinfarction (Glover and Littler, 1987; Campbell et al, 1988). It is often possible to recognise many patients at high risk (Table 13.4); most will have shown problems within the early weeks following acute myocardial infarction. However, effective strategies for identifying and treating all high-risk patients have not yet been developed. The most important determinants seem to be:

● The extent of myocardial damage
● The extent of coronary arterial disease

The extent of myocardial damage

The size of the myocardial infarct influences outcome, and loss of more than 40% of the left ventricular myocardium is usually associated with cardiogenic shock and death. The degree of damage may be assessed clinically, electrocardiographically or by imaging techniques, often aided by monitoring enzyme concentrations in the blood. For example, there is a strong correlation between the peak creatine kinase (CK) level and 4-year mortality (Thompson et al, 1979). This and other enzymatic markers of myocardial infarction are linked closely to other prognostic indices, including the site and thickness of the infarct, the degree of left ventricular dysfunction and the frequency of ventricular dysrhythmias. The prognosis is best in patients with left ventricular ejection fractions of 50% or more at rest; those with an ejection fraction of less than 35% are at greatest risk. Assessment may be made by biplane ventriculography at the time of coronary angiography or, non-invasively, by echocardiography or radionuclide scanning.

The location of the infarct is prognostically important: mortality is lower with inferior, as opposed to anterior, infarction, even when estimates of infarct size are identical. Infarct extension, mural thrombus, left ventricular aneurysm and cardiac

Table 13.4 Factors associated with a poor prognosis following acute myocardial infarction

Age > 60 years
Male sex
Poor left ventricular function (heart failure, hypotension)
Post-infarction angina
Cardiomegaly on the chest X-ray
Previous evidence of coronary heart disease
ECG:
● Persistent ST/T wave changes
● Ventricular ectopic activity
● Atrial fibrillation
● Conduction defects
● Left ventricular hypertrophy
Other coexisting diseases:
● Hypertension
● Diabetes

rupture are also much more common with anterior myocardial infarction (Bulkley, 1981). As might be expected, short-term prognosis is better with non-transmural, as opposed to full-thickness, infarcts. However, even non-transmural infarcts do not seem to have a good long-term prognosis, probably because coronary heart disease continues to progress, leading to further cardiac events in later years (De Wood et al, 1986). This justifies a rigorous search for inducible ischaemia in the recovery period, with early referral for coronary angiography and revascularisation.

The extent of coexisting coronary arterial disease

Most patients who present with acute myocardial infarction have two or more diseased coronary vessels. If there is poor perfusion of the surviving myocardium following the infarct, not only will left ventricular function be impaired, but the surviving myocardium will also be placed in jeopardy from further coronary events. Poor angiographic findings carry a poor prognosis, unless revascularisation is possible (CASS, 1983). Early clues to extensive coronary arterial disease may be reciprocal ST segment depression on the presenting ECG and persistent or recurrent ischaemic pain. Later, ST segment monitoring using Holter systems, or exercise stress tests, may be useful in selecting these high-risk patients for surgical intervention (Bosch et al, 1987). Limited exercise stress testing prior to discharge from hospital is safe, provided there is no heart failure, hypotension, ventricular dysrhythmia or post-infarct angina (Crean and Fox, 1987). The 'Naughton' protocol is a suitable low-intensity test. Alternative approaches to the standard treadmill assessment include the use of a bicycle or the use of pharmacological stress with dipyridamole or dobutamine (Bach and Armstrong, 1992). Patients identified as being at risk on the basis of stress testing should undergo coronary angiography.

The number and distribution of coronary vessels stenosed affects prognosis (Table 13.5). A significant stenosis may be defined as one that occludes 70% or more of the internal diameter of the coronary vessel (50% for the left main stem artery). Involvement of the right coronary artery is generally less serious than involvement of the left coronary artery. A severe stenosis in the left anterior descending artery proximal to the first septal branch is very serious and carries the same prognosis as three-vessel disease.

Table 13.5 Survival and coronary artery stenosis (CASS, 1983)

Number of vessels	Survival (%)	
> 70% stenosed	1 year	5 years
One	98	89
Two	96	88
Three	89	67
Left main stem (> 50% stenosis)	71	57

Dysrhythmias and prognosis

Dysrhythmias following acute myocardial infarction are either manifest or latent.

Manifest dysrhythmias

Early dysrhythmias following acute myocardial infarction reflect short-lived electrical instability and are usually self-limiting, without any prognostic significance. Atrial fibrillation, however, developing in the first 72 hours following infarction is associated with a higher mortality, often reflecting post-infarction complications, such as heart failure. Ventricular dysrhythmias are very common in the first 48 hours and are usually transient. Asymptomatic, but frequent, ventricular ectopic beats indicate an adverse prognosis, but treatment may not influence outcome. After 48 hours, the presence of ventricular dysrhythmias is a poor prognostic factor, often indicating poor cardiac function. Many of these patients die in hospital.

Latent dysrhythmias

There are a number of methods of assessing patients with myocardial irritability, and many studies have shown that this condition strongly is associated with sudden cardiovascular death in the first year following myocardial infarction (Mattioni, 1992). Ventricular irritability might be determined by predischarge Holter monitoring or exercise stress testing (Pratt et al 1984), when the finding of complex ventricular dysrhythmias (ventricular tachycardia, multifocal ectopics, etc.) may be an indication for early angiography. Measuring 'late potentials' is an alternative method of stratifying post-infarction dysrhythmia risk (Lander et al, 1993). There is a higher incidence of dysrhythmic events or sudden death in patients with late potentials, in comparison to those with a normal signal averaged ECG. Finally, programmed ventricular stimulation, an invasive electrophysiological test, can be used to induce ventricular dysrhythmias. Whilst this is not a routine investigation, it has been used to highlight a small group with high mortality, and this prognostic indicator may be superior to any other (Cripps et al, 1988).

Whilst it was previously thought that beta-adrenergic blocking agents may have contributed towards an improved post-infarction prognosis by the suppression of dysrhythmias, analysis of the Beta-blockers in Heart Attack Trial (BHAT, 1982) suggests that the beneficial effect of beta-blockers is not mediated through the reduction of ectopic frequency. However, where beta-blockers have been contra-indicated or replaced by other antidysrhythmic agents, prognosis has not been so good, which suggests that the replacement drug has failed to control ventricular dysrhythmias or has even induced a proarrhythmic effect. This was the conclusion in the Cardiac Arrhythmia Suppression Trial (CAST), where flecainide and encainide were used following acute myocardial infarction (Echt et al, 1991).

The current conclusion from the antidysrhythmic trials must be that whilst treating symptomatic dysrhythmias is justified, asymptomatic dysrhythmias should probably be left untreated. The use of amiodarone for the treatment of asymptomatic ventricular dysrhythmias may be an exception to this (Burkart et al, 1990).

References

AIRE (Acute Infarction Ramipril Efficacy) Investigators (1993) Effect of Ramipril on mortality and morbidity of survivors of acute myocardial infarction with clinical evidence of heart failure. *Lancet*, **342:** 821–828.

Anti-platelet Trialists' Collaboration (1994) Overview I. Prevention of death, myocardial infarction and stroke by prolonged anti-platelet therapy in various categories of patients. *British Medical Journal*, **308:** 81–106.

Appel L J and Stason W B (1993) Ambulatory blood pressure monitoring and blood pressure self-measurement in the diagnosis and management of hypertension. *Annals of Internal Medicine*, **118:** 867–882.

Bach D S and Armstrong W F (1992) Dobuatamine stress echocardiography. *American Journal of Cardiology*, **69:** 90H–96H.

Betteridge D J, Dodson P M, Durrington P N, Hughes E A, Laker M F, Nicholls D P, Rees J A E, Seymour C A, Thompson G R, Winder A F, Wincour P H and Wray R (1993) Management of hyperlipidaemia: guidelines of the British Hyperlipidaemia Association. *Postgraduate Medical Journal*, **69:** 359–369.

BHAT: the Beta-blocker Heart Attack Trial Research Group (1982) A randomised trial of propranolol in patients with acute myocardial infarction. 1. Mortality results. *Journal of the American Medical Association*, **247:** 1707-1714.

Bingham S (1991) Dietary aspects of a health strategy for England. *British Medical Journal*, **303:** 353–355.

Blankenhorn D M, Nessim S A, Johnson R L, Sanmarco M E, Azen S P and Cashin-Hemphill L (1987) Beneficial effects of combined colestipol-niacin therapy on coronary atherosclerosis and coronary venous bypass grafts. *Journal of the American Medical Association*, **257:** 3233–3240.

Bosch X, Theroux P, Waters D D, Pelletier G B and Roy D (1987) Early post-infarction ischaemia: clinical, angiographic and prognostic significance. *Circulation*, **75:** 988–995.

British Hyperlipidaemia Association (1993) Guidelines on the management of hyperlipidaemia. *Postgraduate Medical Journal*, **69:** 359–369.

Bulkley B H (1981) Size and sequelae of myocardial infarction. *New England Journal of Medicine*, **305:** 337–338.

Burkart F F, Pfisterer M, Kiowski W et al (1990) Effect of anti-arrhythmic therapy on mortality in survivors of myocardial infarction with asymptomatic complex ventricular arrhythmias: Basel Antiarrhythmic Study of Infarct Survival (BASIS). *Journal of the American College of Cardiology*, **16:** 1711–1718.

Campbell S, A'Hern R, Quigley P et al (1988) Identification of patients who are at low risk of dying after acute myocardial infarction by simple clinical and sub-maximal exercise test criteria. *European Heart Journal*, **9:** 938–947.

CASS – The Coronary Artery Surgery Study (1983) A randomised trial of coronary artery bypass surgery: survival data. *Circulation*, **68:** 939–950.

Cook D G, Shaper A G, Pocock S J and Kussick S J (1986) Giving up smoking and the risk of heart attacks: a report from the British Regional Heart Study. *Lancet*, **ii:** 1376–1379.

Crean P A and Fox K M (1987) Exercise electrocardiography in coronary artery disease. *Quarterly Journal of Medicine*, **62:** 7–13.

Cripps T C, Bennett D and Camm A J (1988) Prospective evaluation of clinical assessment, exercise testing and signal-averaged electrocardiogram in predicting outcome after myocardial infarction. *American Journal of Cardiology*, **62:** 995–999.

Daly L E, Graham I M, Hickey N and Mulcahy R (1985) Does stopping smoking delay onset of angina after infarction? *British Medical Journal*, **291:** 935–937.

De Wood M, Stifter W F, Simpson C S et al (1986) Coronary angiographic findings soon after non-Q-wave myocardial infarction. *New England Journal of Medicine*, **315:** 412–422.

Doll R and Peto R (1976) Mortality in relation to smoking: 20 years' observations on male British doctors. *British Medical Journal*, **ii:** 1525–1536.

Echt D S, Liebson P R, Mitchell L B et al (1991) Mortality and morbidity in patients receiving encainide, flecainide or placebo: the Cardiac Arrhythmia Suppression Trial (CAST). *New England Journal of Medicine*, **324:** 781–788.

European Atherosclerosis Society (1992) Prevention of coronary heart disease: scientific background and new clinical guidelines. *Nutrition, Metabolism and Cardiovascular Diseases*, **2:** 113–156.

Fibrinolytic Therapy Trialists' Collaborative Group (1994) Indications for fibrinolytic therapy in suspected acute myocardial infarction: collaborative overview of early and major mortality from all randomised trials of more than 1000 patients. *Lancet*, **343:** 311–322.

Friedman M, Thorensen C E and Gill J J (1986) Alteration of Type A behaviour and its effect on cardiac recurrences in post-myocardial infarct patients: summary results in the Recurrent Coronary Prevention Project. *American Heart Journal*, **112:** 653–665.

Garrow J S (1981) *Treating Obesity Seriously*. Edinburgh: Churchill Livingstone.

Gibson R S, Boden W E, Theroux P, Strauss H D and Pratt C M (1986) Diltiazem and re-infarction in patients with non-Q-wave myocardial infarction. *New England Journal of Medicine*, **315:** 423–429.

Gill J J, Price V A, Friedman M, Thorensen C E, Powell L H, Ulmer D, Brown B and Drews F R (1985) Reduction in type A behaviour in healthy middle aged American military officers, *American Heart Journal*, **110:** 503–514.

GISSI-3 (Gruppo Italiano per lo Studio della Sopravvivenza nell'Infarto Miocardico) (1994) Effects of Lisinopril and transdermal glyceryl trinitrate singly and together on 6-week mortality and ventricular function after acute myocardial infarction. *Lancet*, **343:** 1115–1122.

Glover D R and Littler WA (1987) Factors influencing the survival and mode of death in severe ischaemic heart disease. *British Heart Journal*, **57:** 125–132.

Helsinki Heart Study (1987a) Primary prevention trial with gemfibrozil in middle-aged men with dyslipidaemia. Safety of treatment, changes in risk factors and incidence of coronary heart disease. *New England Journal of Medicine*, **317:** 1237–1245.

Helsinki Heart Study (1987b) Lipid alterations and decline in the incidence of coronary heart disease. *Journal of the American Medical Association*, **260:** 641–651.

ISIS-1 Collaborative Group (1988) mechanisms for the early mortality reduction produced by beta-blockade started early in acute myocardial infarction. *Lancet*, **i:** 921–923.

ISIS-4 Collaborative Group (1995) A randomised factorial trial assessing early oral Captopril, oral mononitrate, and intravenous magnesium sulphate in 58,050 patients with suspected acute myocardial infarction. *Lancet*, **345:** 669–685.

Jowett N I and Galton D J (1987) The management of the hyperlipidaemias. In *Drugs for Heart Disease*, 2nd edn (ed.) Hamer J. London: Chapman & Hall.

Kaufman D W, Palmer J R, Rosenberg L and Shapiro S (1987) Cigar and pipe smoking and myocardial infarction in young men. *British Medical Journal*, **294:** 1315–1316.

Keys A (1980) *Seven Countries*. London: Harvard University Press.

Khaw K T (1992) Hormone replacement therapy. *British Medical Bulletin*, **48:** 249–476.

Krone R J (1992) The role of risk stratification in the early management of a myocardial infarction. *Annals of Internal Medicine*, **116:** 223–237.

Lancet (1987) Prevention of coronary heart disease. *Lancet*, **i:** 601–602.

Lander P, Berbari E J, Rajagopalan C V, Vatterott P and Lazzara R (1993) Critical analysis of the signal-averaged electrocardiogram. *Circulation*, **87:** 105–117.

Law M R, Wald N J and Thompson S G (1994) By how much and how quickly does reduction in serum cholesterol concentration lower risk of ischaemic heart disease? *British Medical Journal*, **308:** 367–373.

Lipid Research Clinics Program (1984) The Lipid Research Clinics Primary Prevention Trial Results. 1. Reduction in incidence of coronary heart disease. *Journal of the American Medical Association*, **251:** 351–364.

Lloyd G G (1991) Myocardial infarction and the mind. *Hospital Update*, **December:** 943–944.

Mattioni T A (1992) Long-term prognosis after myocardial infarction. Who is at risk for sudden death? *Postgraduate Medicine*, **92:** 107–108, 111–114.

Mulcahy R (1983) Influence of cigarette smoking on morbidity and mortality after smoking. *British Heart Journal*, **49:** 410–415.

Neaton J D and Wentworth D (1992) Serum cholesterol, blood pressure, cigarette smoking and death from coronary heart disease. Overall findings and differences by age for

316,099 white men. Multiple Risk Factor Intervention Trial (MRFIT) Research Group. *Archives of Internal Medicine*, **152:** 56–64.

Neaton J D, Blackburn H, Jacobs D, Kuller L, Lee D J, Sherwin R, Shih J, Stamler J and Wentworth D (1992) Serum cholesterol level and mortality findings for men screened in the Multiple Risk Factor Intervention Trial. *Archives of Internal Medicine*, **152:** 1490–1500.

Nikkila E A, Viikiukoski P, Valle M and Frick M H (1984) Prevention of progression of coronary atherosclerosis by treatment of hyperlipidaemia: a seven year prospective angiographic study. *British Medical Journal*, **289:** 220–223.

Oliver M F (1986) Prevention of coronary heart disease; propaganda, promises, problems and prospects. *Circulation*, **73:** 1–9.

Pearson T A and Marx H J (1993) The rapid reduction in cardiac events with lipid lowering therapy: mechanisms and implications. *American Journal of Cardiology*, **72:** 1072–1073.

Pfeffer M A, Braunwald E, Moyle L A, Basta L, Brown E J and Cuddy T E (1992) Effect of Captopril on mortality and morbidity in patients with left ventricular dysfunction after myocardial infarction: results of the survival and ventricular enlargement trial (SAVE). *New England Journal of Medicine*, **327:** 669–677.

Powell J T and Greenhalgh R M (1994) Arterial bypass surgery and smokers. *British Medical Journal*, **308:** 607–608.

Pratt C M, Seals A A and Luck J C (1984) The clinical significance of ventricular arrhythmias after myocardial infarction, *Cardiology Clinics*, **2:** 3–11.

Pravastatin Multi-National Study Group (1993) Effects of pravastatin in patients with serum total cholesterol levels from 5.2 to 7.8 mmol/l plus two additional atherosclerotic risk factors. *American Journal of Cardiology*, **72:** 1031–1037.

Reckless J P D (1990) The economics of cholesterol lowering. *Clinical Endocrinology and Metabolism*, **4:** 947–972.

Royal College of Physicians (1991) Medical aspects of exercise; benefits and risks. *Journal of the Royal College of Physicians of London*, **25:** 193–196.

Russell M A, Wilson C, Taylor C and Baker C D (1979) Effect of general practitioners' advice against smoking. *British Medical Journal*, **ii:** 231–235.

Severs P, Beevers G, Bulpitt C, Lever A, Ramsay L, Reid J and Swales J (1993) Management guidelines in essential hypertension: report of the second working party of the British Hypertension Society. *British Medical Journal*, **306:** 983–987.

Sleight P (1993) Is cardioprotection important in the treatment of hypertension? Consideration for the ideal agent. *Journal of Hypertension*, **11**(supplement): S49–S53.

Stevenson R, Ranjadayalan K, Wilkinson P, Roberts R and Timmis A D (1993) Short and long term prognosis of acute myocardial infarction since introduction of thrombolysis. *British Medical Journal*, **307:** 349–353.

St John Sutton M (1994) Should ACE inhibitors be used routinely after infarction? Perspectives from the SAVE trial. *British Heart Journal*, **71:** 115–118.

Thompson D R (1983) Dietary advice and heart disease: a nursing dilemma? *International Journal of Nursing Studies*, **20:** 245–253.

Thompson G R (1992) Progression and regression of coronary artery disease. *Current Opinions in Lipidology*, **3:** 263–267.

Thompson P L, Fletcher E E and Katavatis V (1979) Enzymatic indices of myocardial necrosis: influence on short and long term prognosis after myocardial infarction. *Circulation*, **59:** 113.

Tunstall-Pedoe H (1991) The Dundee coronary risk-disk for management of change in risk factors. *British Medical Journal*, **303:** 744–747.

Ulbricht T L V and Southgate D A T (1991) Coronary heart disease: seven dietary factors. *Lancet*, **338:** 985–992.

Underwood M J, Bailey J S, Shiu M and Higgs R (1993) Should smokers be offered coronary bypass surgery? *British Medical Journal*, **306:** 1047–1050.

Vannan M A, Taylor D J E, Webb-Peploe M W and Konstam M A (1993) ACE inhibitors after myocardial infarction. *British Medical Journal*, **306:** 531–532.

Watts G F, Lewis B, Boult J N H et al (1992) Effects on coronary artery disease of lipid-lowering diet or diet plus cholestyramine in the STARS study. *Lancet*, **i:** 563–569.

Woodward M and Tunstall-Pedoe H (1993) Self-titration of nicotine: evidence from the Scottish Heart Health Study. *Addiction,* **88:** 821–830.

Worcester M C, Hare D L, Oliver R G, Reid M A and Goble A J (1993) Early programmes of high and low intensity exercise and quality of life after acute myocardial infarction. *British Medical Journal,* **307:** 1244–1247.

World Health Organization (1990) *Diet, Nutrition and the Prevention of Chronic Disease.* Report of a WHO study group. WHO Technical Report Series No. 797. Geneva: WHO.

World Health Organization/International Society of Hypertension (1993) Guidelines for the management of mild hypertension. *Bulletin of the World Health Organization,* **71:** 503–517.

Yusuf S, Peto R, Lewis J, Collins R and Sleight P (1985). Beta-blockade during and after myocardial infarction: an overview of randomised trials. *Progress in Cardiovascular Diseases,* **27:** 335–371.

14

Role of Surgery in Coronary Heart Disease

The main role of surgery in coronary heart disease is to improve the blood supply to the ischaemic myocardium. Operations may also be required for mechanical defects that have arisen as a consequence of a myocardial infarction (e.g. mitral incompetence or ruptured interventricular septum). Surgery is most often and most safely performed electively but is sometimes required urgently when these complications occur suddenly (Table 14.1).

Although many operations have been described in the past for improving myocardial blood supply, coronary artery surgery is really a recent innovation, having only been practised since the late 1960s (Favaloro, 1969). Since that time, the number of operations performed has increased exponentially, placing an ever-increasing demand on the existing limited facilities of the NHS (English, 1984).

The most frequently performed operation for coronary heart disease is coronary artery bypass grafting (CABG). This has become an important adjunct to current medical therapy and is highly effective in the treatment of angina. As experience of this operation has improved, there has been a major fall in operative mortality and morbidity, which is attributed to better patient selection and preoperative assessment.

In the early 1980s, cardiac surgeons attempted to attain a greater degree of revascularisation by bypassing more of the diseased vessels. The original 'triple bypass' then became a much longer affair, often involving five or six separate bypass vein grafts. These days, the approach is more realistic, given that these costly and time-consuming operations are palliative and do not arrest the progres-

Table 14.1 Some indications for surgery in coronary heart disease

Elective surgery
Poorly controlled stable angina
Occlusion of the left main stem coronary artery
Three-vessel coronary arterial disease
Left ventricular aneurysm producing symptoms
Malignant dysrhythmias uncontrolled by medical therapy

Emergency surgery
Crescendo angina uncontrolled by medical therapy
Mechanical defects – mitral incompetence
                – ventriculoseptal defect
Cardiogenic shock
Following unsuccessful coronary angioplasty

sion of the underlying atherosclerotic process. Whilst incomplete revascularisation can lead to premature death or recurrence of angina, grafting is more often restricted to tight stenoses with adequate run-off; without adequate run-off, grafts will usually occlude. The typical operation involves between two and four grafts.

CORONARY ARTERY BYPASS SURGERY

Indications

Britain's first consensus development conference for coronary artery bypass grafting met in November 1984 and considered the indications for coronary bypass surgery in the UK (Consensus Development Conference, 1984). These indications are similar to those of the American College of Cardiology and the American Heart Association (ACC/AHA, 1991). The general approach for patients with stable angina and for asymptomatic patients following myocardial infarction is shown in Figures 14.1 and 14.2.

The main indication for coronary bypass surgery is relief of symptoms, although it is now known that coronary artery surgery can improve prognosis. The European Coronary Surgery Study Group (1980) showed that the 5-year survival rate for three-vessel and left main stem disease was greater in those treated surgically than medically (Table 14.2). Disease of the left main stem artery is associated with serious coronary events, including myocardial infarction and sudden death (Mock et al, 1982). Although disease of this artery is usually symptomatic, it may only be revealed at coronary angiography. Some centres consider 50% occlusion of the left main stem sufficient for urgent surgery, regardless of symptoms.

The prognosis of patients with severe symptoms or strongly positive stress tests will improve with surgery, especially if there is impaired left ventricular function. Those with moderate angina or single or double artery disease (excluding the left main stem) are probably better managed by medical therapy or coronary angioplasty if the lesions are accessible.

Patient selection

Patients vary markedly in their reaction to anginal symptoms. The decision to proceed to coronary artery bypass surgery needs careful consideration. Surgery for degenerative disease never cures, and bypass surgery should be postponed in those

Table 14.2   Results of the European Coronary Surgery Study Group (1980)

Group	5-year survival (%)	
	Medical	Surgical
Left main stem	62	93
Three vessels	85	95
Two vessels	88	92

with mild to moderate coronary heart disease and good left ventricular function. Operative risk is also greater in the elderly and for female patients, presumably because the smaller vessels and compact anatomy compromise surgical techniques and graft patency. Young men are often referred as urgent candidates for bypass surgery, but buying time with angioplasty is preferable, since most will develop

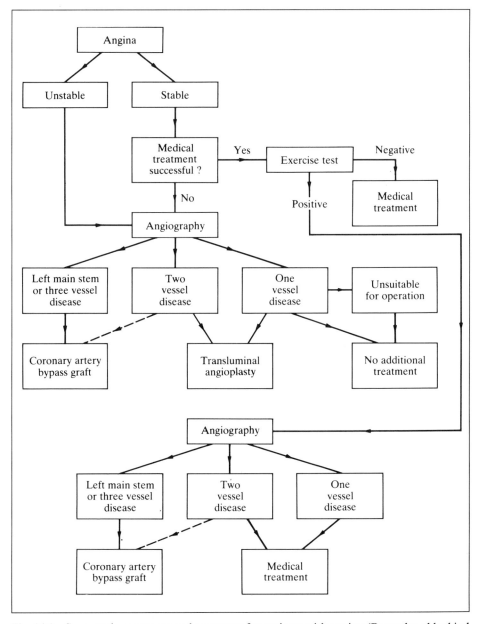

Fig. 14.1   Suggested assessment and treatment for patients with angina (Reproduced by kind permission of the *British Medical Journal*)

clinically-important graft atheroma within 5 years of coronary bypass. Diabetes and hypertension also increase perioperative risk. In addition, many surgeons will not consider operating on patients who have not stopped smoking or reduced their body weight to acceptable levels, because of the associated higher perioperative risk and outcome. Long-term follow-up of patients in the Coronary Artery Surgical Study (CASS) has reported on the effects of smoking. Ten-year survival in patients following coronary artery bypass surgery was 84% in those who stopped smoking and 68% in those who continued to smoke (Cavender et al, 1992). Smokers had more hospital admissions, were more likely to have developed angina and were more likely to be unemployed.

Poor operative risk factors need to be balanced against poor prognostic features of the disease itself, including low exercise tolerance and stenoses at dangerous sites (left main stem, proximal left anterior descending artery) or three-vessel disease. Poor left ventricular function, as may be assessed by ventriculography, echocardiography or MUGA scanning, is associated with a poor operative risk, but the worse this is, the worse the prognosis without intervention. Survival following surgery is superior compared to that after medical therapy, and it may be justified to take the risk. Occasionally, a severely-reduced ejection fraction is

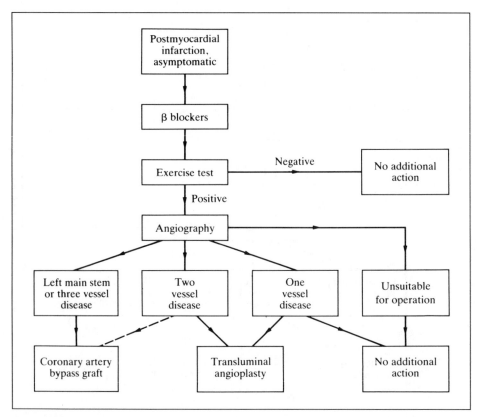

Fig. 14.2 Suggested assessment and treatment for asymptomatic patients who survive myocardial infarction (Reproduced by kind permission of the *British Medical Journal*)

related to myocardial ischaemia, rather than myocardial scarring. Thallium-201 scintigraphy may help to distinguish between poorly-functioning ischaemic myocardium and non-functioning scar tissue.

The availability and suitability of the saphenous vein needs to be assessed. Varicosities and previous saphenous vein surgery do not preclude bypass grafting. The short saphenous vein may be used instead (although this is more difficult), but arm veins are unsatisfactory. Synthetic grafts do not seem to be helpful either; patency is less than 50% at 1 year.

Operative procedure

The heart is exposed through a median sternotomy. Limited grafting procedures may be carried out on the beating heart, but most cases require cardioplegia with extracorporeal cardiopulmonary bypass. This is established via cannulae in the right atrium and ascending aorta, blood passing outside the body for oxygenation. The body temperature is reduced to about 26°C and cardiac arrest induced with a cardioplegic solution. The heart can be stopped for up to 2 hours to allow anastomoses. Whilst this is going on, a second group of surgeons is stripping the long saphenous vein from the leg. It is then flushed with heparinised blood and checked for leaks. Endarterectomy of the major coronary arteries is sometimes carried out first, if there is diffuse disease or complete stenosis. The distal ends of the bypass vein grafts are sutured to as many vessels as require it. The aorta is then unclamped, the patient rewarmed and normal cardiac rhythm established by defibrillation. Using special side-biting clamps, the proximal ends of the grafts are sutured to the ascending aorta, cardiopulmonary bypass is stopped, the cannulae removed and the chest closed.

Postoperative management

Patients are normally ventilated until haemodynamically stable. Arterial lines and Swan–Ganz catheters are used to monitor intracardiac pressures for the first 24 hours, after which time the majority of patients can leave the intensive care unit. Patients are mobilised quickly and are often fit for discharge from hospital within 7 days. The majority of patients are able to return to work between 2 and 6 months after the operation. Aspirin (with or without dipyridamole) should be started within 6 hours of surgery and continued for at least 12 months (Anti-platelet Trialists' Collaboration 1994). This considerably reduces the risk of graft occlusion and will, additionally, help to prevent other major clinical vascular events, such as myocardial infarction or stroke.

Problems following surgery

Early effects

The morbidity and mortality rates following coronary artery surgery have fallen with increasing surgical expertise; in most centres the overall mortality is less than 3% (Treasure, 1983). Although the main determinant of operative risk is left ventricular function, several other factors have been implicated, including emergency surgery, previous myocardial infarction (especially if very recent), left main stem or multivessel disease, mitral regurgitation and hypertension.

The most common problem is dysrhythmia, affecting up to one third of all patients in the first 5 days. Most are benign supraventricular dysrhythmias. Temporary heart block occurs in 5–10% of patients.

Perioperative myocardial infarction is not uncommon, but the majority of these do not have significant sequelae. Optimising antianginal therapy helps, and careful attention to perioperative ischaemia is important, particularly during induction of anaesthesia and during extracorporeal bypass. Perioperative myocardial infarction is a risk factor for premature death, and the current frequency is down to about 2.5%. Global left ventricular damage is more difficult to diagnose but is probably frequent. A low-output period may follow, particularly if the left ventricular function was poor to start with. Some patients need to be supported by extracorporeal bypass whilst the ventricular myocardium recovers. Pain from the sternotomy and cracked ribs can cause discomfort for a few weeks, as can pain around the long incision made for removing the saphenous vein. Cerebral embolisation is rare, since the operation is essentially closed apart from the cardiopulmonary bypass cannulae. A small number of patients have a temporary impairment of concentration or memory attributable to small atheromatous emboli being ejected from the aorta at the time of the operation (Smith et al, 1986). Whilst embolic events have been considered to be the major cause of stroke during heart surgery, hypoperfusion of the brain may be contributory. Current evidence seems to suggest that these complications are due to cardiopulmonary bypass rather than the operation itself (Allen, 1986). Perioperative stroke is a sufficiently common complication (about 2% risk), particularly in the elderly, that it should be discussed preoperatively.

Immediate and complete relief from angina is reported in about 80% of patients, and most of the remainder have marked improvement in their symptoms. Between 60 and 80% of patients are free from angina at 1 year, and the various trial reports indicate that results are improving as the skill of the surgeons increases (Hampton, 1984).

Left ventricular function may improve postoperatively if poor function has been due to myocardial ischaemia rather than infarction. What may have appeared to be dead muscle preoperatively may sometimes be revived following reperfusion. These areas of reversibly-impaired contractility are termed 'stunned' or 'hibernating' myocardium. Preoperative scanning may be of benefit in identifying areas that may be salvageable and may be used to predict an improved operative success. PET scanning can detect stunned myocardium, and MUGA scanning can detect aneurysmal sections.

The only operative treatment for irreversible and severely-impaired left ventricular dysfunction following myocardial infarction is cardiac transplantation, although there are promising reports of a new surgical technique called *cardiomyoplasty*. Skeletal muscle from the leg is applied around the left ventricular wall and is electrically stimulated to assist contractile function. Clearly, this advance is of importance, since the number of potential recipients of transplanted hearts greatly outnumbers that of organ donors.

Long-term effects

The long-term effects of coronary artery bypass surgery are determined by changes in left ventricular function, patency of the grafts and progression of generalised atherosclerosis. The 1-year survival is 95%, and 5-year survival 88%. An early return of angina is due to either incomplete revascularisation or graft occlusion. Many grafts (8–18%) become occluded in the first month, especially if endarterectomy has been required. Operative technique, including the meticulous preparation of the saphenous vein graft before anastomosis, is obviously important, to minimise the risk of thrombosis. At 1 year, a further 10–15% of the grafts have become occluded, after which the rate falls to about 2%- per year (Angelini & Bryan, 1992). Early occlusion is usually due to thrombosis, and anticoagulants or antiplatelet agents are usually prescribed for the first year to minimise this complication. Later on, occlusion may be due to atheroma or fibrointimal hyperplasia. Myointimal hyperplasia may possibly be slowed by antiplatelet drugs. Preventing, retarding or reversing graft atheroma requires attention to classical risk factors, including hypertension, smoking and hypercholesterolaemia. Aggressive treatment of hyperlipidaemia, often with lipid-lowering agents, is usually needed to reduce the cholesterol level to below a target of 5 mmol/l. Failure to control lipid levels results in an increased rate of graft occlusion, as well as progress of atheroma in native vessels.

The return of angina typically occurs suddenly, at rest, 7 years after the operation. Overall, one third of patients experience recurrent angina after 10 years, although it will not necessarily be so severe. The diagnosis may be confirmed by exercise stress testing, and drug therapy should be restarted. Angiography should not be performed until the symptoms are limiting. Reoperation will produce nearly as good results (60% angina-free at 1 year), although operative mortality is higher, probably because of technical difficulties, which may need preoperative consideration. Up to 7% of patients require a second procedure in the first 10 years; most of these are young patients.

Coronary bypass using the internal mammary artery

Most patients undergoing coronary arterial surgery receive saphenous vein grafts, but around 40% now have bypasses using the internal mammary artery. Although technically more difficult, arterial grafts will fare much better than traditional saphenous vein grafts, because the graft has its own blood supply left intact and thus forms a 'living' graft with the potential for growth (*Lancet*, 1984). The left internal mammary artery (LIMA) is usually selected for bypass grafting, mostly for cases of proximal occlusion of the left coronary artery. The internal mammary artery is mobilised from its origin at the subclavian artery and its branches tied. It is then anastomosed directly onto the left coronary artery, distal to the occlusion.

This operation has been playing an increasing role in coronary bypass surgery, and an arterial graft is the conduit of choice in surgery involving the anterior descending coronary artery. It is particularly suited to the younger patient, in whom a longer surviving graft is required. At 10 years, when on average 50% of saphenous vein grafts will have stenosed, about 90% of LIMA grafts are still functioning. Improved survival has also been confirmed in patients with LIMA grafts, when used either alone or in association with saphenous vein grafts.

The right internal mammary can also be used for this procedure, and both the left and the right internal mammary arteries have been used as free grafts from the ascending aorta to the left anterior descending artery, with as good results (Loop et al, 1986).

Recently, the gastro-epiploic artery has been used as an alternative conduit. Using this in association with double internal mammary grafts, it is possible completely to revascularise the heart arterially (Suma et al, 1989).

Bypass surgery following acute myocardial infarction

Traditionally, coronary arterial surgery is delayed for several weeks following myocardial infarction, because of the increased operative risks. However, it is becoming clear that it is not the time interval that is critical but rather the clinical state of the patient. In patients under the age of 70 years, with an ejection fraction greater than 30%, the risks do not appear to be excessive (Applebaum et al, 1991). The place of peri-infarction bypass surgery will have to await studies to compare results with thrombolysis and coronary angioplasty.

OPERATIONS FOR THE COMPLICATIONS OF MYOCARDIAL INFARCTION

There are three commonly performed operations in patients who have developed mechanical post-infarction complications. These are resection of left ventricular aneurysms, replacement of the mitral valve and repair of the interventricular septum.

Resection of left ventricular aneurysms

After myocardial infarction, parts of the damaged left ventricle may be akinetic (i.e. do not move) or dyskinetic (i.e. move paradoxically). The latter areas, if sufficiently large, will act as a chamber that fills during diastole but does not contribute to ejection of blood during systole, since the area bulges outwards. This situation will usually improve as the infarct heals. Left ventricular aneurysms usually produce problems several weeks or even months after acute myocardial infarction and present with angina, heart failure, dysrhythmias or thrombo-embolic events. Surgery will usually help overall left ventricular function, but the prognosis is dependent upon how well the left ventricle performs postoperatively, as well as on the overall perfusion of the remaining myocardium. Hence, coronary artery bypass grafting is often performed at the same time as resection of the aneurysm.

Mitral valve replacement

This may be required if there has been acquired mitral regurgitation due to papillary muscle rupture or dysfunction. The degree of valvular incompetence can vary from slight to massive. Whilst mild degrees of mitral regurgitation may be treated with diuretics and vasodilatory drugs, uncontrolled heart failure requires valve repair or replacement. Acute rupture is usually fatal within 1–2 days, and although operation carries a high mortality, normal valve function may be restored by replacement with a prosthetic valve.

Repair of a ruptured interventricular septum

Rupture of the interventricular septum occurs in about 1–3% of all myocardial infarcts (mostly anterior) and, if untreated, will be lethal in nearly all patients, usually within a few days. The clinical picture varies considerably, but patients usually present within the first 4 days following myocardial infarction with severe heart failure, with the presence of a loud pansystolic murmur at the left sternal edge. Initial therapy is with diuretics and vasodilators, such as sodium nitroprusside. Insertion of an intra-aortic balloon pump may augment coronary, cerebral and renal blood flow. Early surgical repair is the best option, although operative mortality may be as high as 30%. However, those who survive do well, with as many as 70% surviving 5 years or more.

SURGERY FOR TACHYDYSRHYTHMIAS

Surgery has been shown to be effective in the treatment of tachydysrhythmias in patients with or without accessory atrioventricular connections. Electrophysiological investigation is normally carried out to determine the site and mechanism of the dysrhythmia. Operative therapy is then carried out to destroy or remove the abnormal focus or to interrupt the accessory pathway.

1. Areas of irritable myocardium can be surgically excised or destroyed by catheter ablation. An electrical direct current shock is delivered via a pacemaker catheter to the focus, which destroys its ability to conduct or generate impulses. Radiofrequency ablation and cryodestruction may also be used.

2. Destruction or surgical incision of the AV node or other atrioventricular pathways will prevent transmission of supraventricular tachycardias. A permanent ventricular pacemaker may then need to be inserted, unless the 'slow pathway' has been selectively destroyed (Jackman et al, 1992).

3. Implantable cardioverter defibrillators (ICDs) with an output of 1–30 J have been used to sense serious dysrhythmias and deliver a direct current shock to restore sinus rhythm (Mirowski et al, 1980). If the initial discharge is ineffective, they are able to recycle and deliver further shocks of increasing strength. Progress over the last 15 years has reduced these devices to a weight of 125 g and a cost of about £15 000 to implant. About 25 000 of these devices have been used worldwide, and they now have multiprogrammable functions, including antitachycardia pacing, low-energy cardioversion and defibrillation. Most have been implanted to recognise and treat ventricular tachycardia and fibrillation. The new unipolar, transvenous defibrillation systems are easier to insert (rather like a pacemaker) and should substantially reduce morbidity, time and costs of defibrillator implantation (Bardy et al, 1993).

PERCUTANEOUS TRANSLUMINAL CORONARY ANGIOPLASTY (PTCA)

A procedure for dilatation of the coronary arteries was first described by Gruntzig in September 1977. It has since become an established and effective way of treating many serious arterial stenoses (Gruntzig, 1984; Landau et al, 1994). In the UK, about 170 procedures per million of the population are carried out annually, whilst in the USA, this figure is 1000 procedures per million population per year. Angioplasty has obvious clinical and financial advantages over bypass surgery, since it is performed under local anaesthetic and patients are fully mobile 24 hours after the procedure, allowing early discharge from hospital. Initially, the main limitation of the procedure was the low number of patients thought to be treatable by this technique (Cumberland, 1985), but as equipment and expertise have improved, many more angioplasties are able to be carried out. In 1984, it was estimated that 40 000 coronary angioplasties had been carried out in the USA, which by 1990, had risen to over 300 000 procedures. Typical coronary lesions suitable for angioplasty are listed in Table 14.3.

The procedure involves introducing a thin, double-lumen balloon catheter through a guiding catheter into the affected coronary artery. Steerable wire guiding systems help with access to more difficult arteries, such as the circumflex artery. The balloon is advanced to lie within the stenosis and then inflated to a pressure of 3–8 atmospheres for 60–120 seconds. This may be repeated several times, until there is angiographic evidence of improved patency. This can be confirmed by measuring the pressure gradient across the stenosis. On average, a 50% improvement in patency is obtained, which is thought to be produced by a combination of atheroma splitting, atheroma compression, stretching of the arterial media and endothelial desquamation. Chest pain is often experienced during dilatation, so the procedure is usually covered with drugs that reduce coronary arterial spasm. Nifedipine (10 mg sublingually) may be given at the start of the procedure, and intracoronary nifedipine or nitrates can be given if there is observed spasm at the time of angioplasty. Heparin is given until the patient leaves hospital, and nifedipine and nitrates may be given longer term. Antiplatelet therapy substantially reduces the risk of reocclusion (Anti-platelet

Table 14.3   Selection criteria for PTCA

Ideal criteria
Single, short, non-calcified lesions
Proximal lesions
Stable angina

Possible criteria
Multiple lesions in one vessel
Multiple lesions in two or more vessels
Distal lesions
Unstable angina
Acute myocardial infarction
Occluded saphenous vein grafts

Trialists' Collaboration, 1994). About 3–5% of patients sustain a myocardial infarction during the procedure, and a further 3–7% need emergency coronary artery bypass surgery. Overall, the mortality is less than 2%.

Although the patency of coronary arteries improves in the early weeks following PTCA, due to healing and remodelling, restenosis occurs in about one third of patients within 3 months, but seldom before 4 weeks or after 6 months (Gruntzig, 1984). Second angioplasties are often easier to perform, with less risk and a higher degree of patency being obtained. Expandable wire mesh stents can reduce the risk of restenosis, particularly at high-risk sites, such as the proximal left anterior descending coronary artery (Kimura et al, 1993). The potentially-thrombogenic surface of the stents means that aggressive anticoagulation with heparin and anti-platelet therapy are needed acutely. One year after angioplasty, 95% of patients are symptomatically improved, and 80% have normal exercise stress tests.

PTCA may also be used to recanalise saphenous vein grafts used for bypass surgery, since the perioperative mortality for second bypass operations is higher. However, complications and restenosis are much more common; stent insertion may be very helpful here.

Laser-assisted angioplasty and atherectomy

Newer techniques, including atherectomy using a side-cutting, directional atherectomy catheter, have been introduced, as have several laser systems. The potential for a laser to clear the lumen during angioplasty was first described during coronary artery bypass surgery in 1982, but development has been held back because of vessel perforation. However, reports are emerging of successful utilisation of this technique (Cumberland et al, 1986), which may prove very useful in completely-occluded vessels that cannot be treated by traditional PTCA. The laser can be used to clear a path for passage of the dilatation balloon catheter.

Coronary atherectomy is often used to treat non-calcified coronary stenoses and involves a catheter with a windowed cylinder being pressed against the atheromatous stenosis, by blowing up an angioplasty balloon within the coronary vessel. A rotating blade then shaves plaque from the vessel wall. At present, no major advantage has been shown over normal PTCA (Adelman et al, 1993; Topol et al, 1993).

Angioplasty or bypass surgery?

Several trials are taking place to compare PTCA with bypass surgery, including the Coronary Artery Bypass Revascularisation Investigation (CABRI), the German Angioplasty Bypass Investigation (GABI) and the American Bypass Angioplasty Revascularisation Investigation (BARI).

Interim results of the UK Randomised Intervention Treatment of Angina (RITA) trial found that bypass grafting involved longer initial hospitalisation and convalescence than PTCA, but during the 2.5 years follow-up, CABG provided greater relief of angina and a lower risk of further intervention (RITA Trial Participants, 1993). Hence, CABG is probably the best solution to treat patients who have repeated hospital admissions for angina. However, for those who cannot face the thought of CABG, or those at anaesthetic risk due to concomitant disease (e.g. chronic bronchitis), PTCA may be more suitable, although further intervention and CABG may well be needed later (Goldhaber, 1993). Another trial comparing medical treatment with PTCA in patients with stable angina due to single-vessel disease found greater improvement of symptoms with PTCA, but only marginally (Parisi et al, 1992).

The benefits of PTCA must be weighed against the drawbacks; many patients treated by angioplasty required further attempts or CABG. Elderly patients should perhaps be treated by angioplasty rather than bypass surgery, in view of the poor tolerance of open-heart surgery. Angioplasty is usually well tolerated, and long-term follow up gives results identical to those of CABG (Bonnier et al, 1993).

PTCA following acute myocardial infarction

Early coronary artery recanalisation reduces infarct size and improves survival, and the sooner patients are treated, the better the result. PTCA is being investigated as an alternative or adjunct to coronary thrombolysis.

Primary PTCA for acute myocardial infarction was first carried out in 1983, using balloon dilatation to disrupt the thrombus, as well as the underlying stenosis (Hartzler et al, 1983). The advantages and disadvantages of this are shown in Table 14.4. It has been shown to be a safe procedure, and patency rates in excess of 90% are usually obtained, with rapid restoration of blood flow and reperfusion of the left ventricular myocardium (Kahn et al, 1990). Patients are less likely to experience post-infarction angina and have better left ventricular function,

Table 14.4 Comparative advantages of primary PTCA and thrombolysis

---

Primary PTCA
Advantages
    Coronary anatomy defined; prognosis may be established
    Up to 98% of vessels recanalised immediately
    Residual stenosis cleared
    Left ventricular function improves
    Intraplaque haemorrhage minimised
    Less post-infarction angina and reinfarction

Disadvantages
    Expensive (over £1000)
    Specialised (requires catheter laboratory and expertise)
    Slower to institute

Thrombolysis
Advantages
    Cheap (mostly under £100)
    Quick and simple to administer
    Avoids risks of invasive study
    Infarct-related artery opened in over half of cases within 2 hours

Disadvantages
    Systemic and plaque haemorrhage may occur
    Slow and unpredictable restoration of coronary blood flow
    Residual stenoses remain; post-infarction ischaemia likely
    Coronary anatomy unknown; angiography may be required later

---

compared to those treated with thrombolytic therapy. The most impressive results so far have been seen in patients with single-vessel disease (Stone et al, 1990) and in those with hypotension or cardiogenic shock, who have shown improved survival, providing angioplasty is not delayed more than 6 hours. Unfortunately, logistics and facilities mean that this approach to acute myocardial infarction is limited, and it is often reserved for those patients in whom thrombolytic therapy is contraindicated (Lange and Hillis, 1993).

Emergency angioplasty following thrombolysis does not currently seem to confer additional benefits (TIMI Study Group, 1989).

HEART TRANSPLANTATION SURGERY

The first human heart transplant was carried out in December 1967, and cardiac transplantation is now sufficiently commonplace not to attract public attention. Up to January 1990, 12 631 heart transplants had been performed worldwide. Cardiac transplantation is usually carried out in patients with cardiomyopathy, mostly the result of advanced ischaemic left ventricular damage. Those with primary cardiomyopathies are probably better recipients, since they are less likely to be affected by those factors that lead to myocardial damage in ischaemic cardiomyopathy. Less commonly, transplantation has been performed for certain forms of congenital heart disease or following difficult and unsuccessful valve replacement (Schofield, 1991).

One of the greatest advances in transplant surgery has been the development of drugs to suppress rejection, in particular cyclosporin A (Sandimmun). Its introduction has allowed a reduction in the high-dose steroid therapy previously used, which permits better surgical healing.

It has been estimated that, at any time, up to 900 potential recipients exist in the UK. Of those patients selected for heart transplantation, only 5% will live for 6 months unless a donor heart is found. Following transplantation, cumulative survival is now in the order of 90% at 1 year and 78% at 5 years. There seems to be little doubt about the value of cardiac transplantation in prolonging the quantity and quality of patients' lives. Cost–benefit studies (Buxton et al, 1985) show significant improvement in key aspects of life-style, and 91% of patients are able to resume normal lives. Medical research and progress needs transplant programmes to continue, despite the financial implications.

References

ACC/AHA (1991) Guidelines and indications for coronary artery bypass graft surgery. *Circulation,* **83:** 1125–1173.

Adelman A G, Cohen E A and Kimball B P (1993) A comparison of directional atherectomy with ballon angioplasty for lesions of the left anterior descending coronary artery. *New England Journal of Medicine,* **329:** 228–233.

Allen C M C (1986) Cabbages and CABG. *British Medical Journal,* **297:** 1485–1486.

Angelini G D and Bryan A J (1992) Extending the use of autologous arterial conduits in myocardial revascularisation. *British Heart Journal,* **68:** 161–162.

Anti-platelet Trialists' Collaboration (1994) Overview II. Maintenance of vascular graft or arterial patency by anti-platelet therapy. *British Medical Journal*, **308:** 159–168.

Applebaum R, House R and Rademaker A (1991) Coronary artery bypass grafting within 30 days of acute myocardial infarction. Early and late results in 406 patients. *Journal of Thoracic and Cardiovascular Surgery*, **102:** 745–752.

Bardy G H, Johnson G and Poole J E (1993) A simplified, single lead unipolar transvenous cardioversion-defibrillating system. *Circulation*, **88:** 543–547.

Bonnier H, de Vries C, Michels R and El Gamal M (1993) Initial and long term results of coronary angioplasty and coronary bypass surgery in patients older than 75 years. *British Heart Journal*, **70:** 122–125.

British Medical Journal (1984) Consensus development conference: Coronary artery bypass grafting. *British Medical Journal*, **289:** 1527.

Buxton M, Acheson R, Caine N, Gibson S and O'Brien V (1985) *Costs and Benefits of the Heart Transplantation Programmes at Harefield and Papworth Hospitals: Final Report*. London: HMSO.

Cavender J B, Rodgers W J and Fisher L D (1992) Effects of smoking on survival and morbidity in patients randomised to medical or surgical therapy in the Coronary Artery Surgery Study (CASS). *Journal of the American College of Cardiology*, **20:** 287–294.

Consensus Development Conference (1984) Coronary artery bypass grafting. *British Medical Journal*, **289:** 1527–1529.

Cumberland D C (1985) The current status of percutaneous coronary angioplasty. *Acta Radiologica*, **26:** 497–505.

Cumberland D C, Starkey I R, Oakley G D, Fleming J S, Smith G H, Goiti J J, Tayler D I and Davis J (1986) Percutaneous laser-assisted coronary angioplasty. *Lancet*, **ii:** 214–215.

English T A H (1984) The UK cardiac surgical register (1977–1982). *British Medical Journal*, **289:** 1205–1208.

European Coronary Surgery Study Group (1980). Second interim report. *Lancet*, **ii:** 491–495.

Favaloro R G (1969) Saphenous vein grafts in the surgical treatment of coronary artery disease. *Journal of Thoracic and Cardiovascular Surgery*, **58:** 178–185.

Goldhaber S Z (1993) Coronary disease. Angioplasty or coronary bypass graft? *Lancet*, **341:** 599–600.

Gruntzig A R (1984) Percutaneous transluminal angioplasty: six years' experience. *American Heart Journal*, **107:** 818–819.

Hampton J R (1984) Coronary artery bypass grafting for the reduction of mortality: analysis of the trials. *British Medical Journal*, **289:** 1166–1170.

Hartzler G O, Rutherford B D and McConahay D R (1983) PTCA with and without thrombolytic therapy for treatment of acute myocardial infarction. *American Heart Journal*, **106:** 965–973.

Jackman W M, Beckman K J and McClelland J H (1992) Treatment of supraventricular tachycardia due to atrioventricular nodal reentry by radiofrequency catheter ablation of slow pathway conduction. *New England Journal of Medicine*, **327:** 313–318.

Kahn J K, Rutherford B D and McConahay D R (1990) Results of primary angioplasty for acute myocardial infarction with multivessel disease. *Journal of the American College of Cardiology*, **16:** 1089–1096.

Kimura T, Nosaka H, Yokoi H, Iwabuchi M and Nobuyoshi M (1993) Serial angiographic follow-up after Palmaz–Schatz stent implantation: comparison with conventional balloon angioplasty. *Journal of the American College of Cardiology*, **21:** 1557–1563.

Lancet (1984) Coronary bypass with the internal mammary. *Lancet*, **ii:** 1253–1254.

Landau C, Lange R A and Hillis L D (1994) Percutaneous transluminal coronary angioplasty. *New England Journal of Medicine*, **330:** 981–993.

Lange R A and Hillis L D (1993) Immediate angioplasty for acute myocardial infarction. *New England Journal of Medicine*, **328:** 726–728.

Loop F D, Lyle B W, Cosgrove D M, Golding L A R, Taylor P C and Stewart R W (1986) Free (aorta-coronary) internal mammary artery grafts: late results. *Journal of Thoracic and Cardiovascular Surgery*, **92:** 827–831.

Mirowski M, Reid P R, Mower M M, Watkins L, Gott V L, Schayble J F, Langer A, Heilman M S, Kolenik S A, Fischell R E and Weisfeldt M L (1980) Termination of malignant ventricular arrhythmias with an implanted automatic defibrillator in human beings. *New England Journal of Medicine*, **303:** 322–324.

Mock, M, Ringqvist I, Fisher L, Davis K, Chaitman B R, Kouchoukos N, Kaiser G, Alderman E, Ryan T, Russell R, Mullen S, Fray D and Killip T (1982) The survival of medically treated patients in the Coronary Artery Surgery Study (CASS) registry. *Circulation*, **66:** 562–568.

Parisi A F, Folland E H, Hartigan P for the Veterans Affairs ACME Investigators (1992) A comparison of angioplasty with medical therapy in the treatment of single vessel coronary artery disease. *New England Journal of Medicine*, **326:** 10–16.

RITA Trial Participants (1993) First report of a randomised trial of coronary angioplasty versus coronary artery surgery. *Lancet*, **341:** 573–580.

Schofield P M (1991) Indications for cardiac transplantation. *British Heart Journal*, **65:** 55–56.

Smith P L, Treasure T, Newman S P, Joseph P, Ell P J, Schneidau A and Harrison M J (1986) Cerebral consequences of cardiopulmonary bypass. *Lancet*, **i:** 823–825.

Stone G W, Rutherford B D and McConahay D R (1990) Direct coronary angioplasty in acute myocardial infarction in patients with single vessel disease. *Journal of the American College of Cardiology*, **15:** 534–543.

Suma H, Takeuchi A and Hirota Y (1989) Myocardial re-vascularisation combined arterial grafts utilising the internal mammary and the gastroepiploic arteries. *Annals of Thoracic Surgery*, **47:** 712–715.

TIMI Study Group (1989) Comparison of invasive and conservative strategies after treatment with intravenous TPA in acute myocardial infarction: results of the thrombolysis in myocardial infarction (TIMI) phase II trial. *New England Journal of Medicine*, **320:** 618–627.

Topol E J, Leya F and Pinkerton C A (1993) A comparison of directional atherectomy with coronary angioplasty in patients with coronary artery disease. *New England Journal of Medicine*, **329:** 221–227.

Treasure T (1983) Coronary artery bypass surgery. *British Journal of Hospital Medicine*, **30:** 259–263.

15

Therapeutics

The following is a list of some of the drugs frequently used on the coronary care unit, with doses and common side-effects. Trade names are shown in brackets. It is not fully comprehensive or complete and serves only as a guide. Further information should always be sought from the hospital pharmacy department, manufacturers' data sheets, the *Monthly Index of Medical Specialities* (MIMS) or the *British National Formulary* (BNF), particularly if the drug is unfamiliar. The BNF is published jointly by the British Medical Association and the Pharmaceutical Society of Great Britain and, additionally, contains useful sections on drug interactions, intravenous additives and advisory labelling.

ADENOSINE

Adenosine (Adenocor) is an endogenous nucleoside that will produce AV nodal block when injected intravenously. Because of its very brief half-life, it is very safe. It has become the treatment of choice for re-entry tachycardias and, additionally, may have a diagnostic role in regular broad-complex tachycardias and intra-atrial tachycardias (see Chapter 9).

Dose 3 mg by rapid intravenous injection. If ineffective, a second bolus of 6 mg should be given, followed by a third bolus of 12 mg.

Side-effects Transient chest pain and flushing. In asthmatics, it may cause bronchospasm.

ADRENALINE

Adrenaline is the first drug given for all types of cardiac arrest. Adrenaline has strong alpha- and beta-adrenergic agonist activity, which increases heart rate and contractility, as well as having a powerful vasoconstrictor action. Administration during cardiac arrest will result in peripheral vasoconstriction, which augments the effect of chest compression, leading to increased cerebral and coronary perfusion. The beta-agonist properties (positive chronotropic and inotropic effects) help myocardial function following attainment of sinus rhythm.

Dose 1 mg intravenously (10 ml of a 1:10 000 solution), which may be repeated every 2 minutes. In asystolic arrests, a single 5 mg dose of adrenaline should be considered if initial smaller doses have not helped. However, its value is unproven.

AMILORIDE

Amiloride (Midamor) is a potassium-conserving diuretic, which acts by direct action on the distal renal tubules. Diuresis occurs over 24 hours, but full activity may be delayed for 2–3 days. It should not be used in renal failure, potassium supplements or ACE-inhibitors unless serum potassium is closely monitored.

Dose 5–20 mg orally.

AMINOPHYLLINE

Aminophylline has been used in patients with acute left ventricular failure. It is a phosphodiesterase-inhibitor and works by relieving bronchospasm (cardiac asthma) and increasing the force of cardiac contraction, to augment cardiac output. In addition, patients with inferior myocardial infarction usually develop AV nodal dysfunction because of oedema rather than necrosis; this may be mediated by adenosine. Atropine is not always helpful here, and aminophylline may be tried (Shah et al, 1987). However, intravenous aminophylline may produce serious ventricular dysrhythmias, and its use requires very careful consideration following acute myocardial infarction.

Dose 250 mg (5 mg/kg) by very slow intravenous injection (over 20 minutes).

Side-effects Dysrhythmias and convulsions. Increased toxicity in smokers.

AMIODARONE

Amiodarone (Cordarone X) is really the only potent Class III antidysrhythmic agent. It prolongs the duration of the action potential and increases the effective refractory period of both the atria and the ventricles. Intravenously, it may also have quinidine-like effects and some beta-blocking properties. It is of value in many different atrial and ventricular dysrhythmias, including re-entry tachycardias.

Dose The dose is usually 150–300 mg intravenously (5 mg/kg over 20–120 minutes), followed by intravenous infusion of 1 g over 24 hours. It should be given by a centrally-placed cannula or thrombophlebitis may result. Oral therapy is usually started at the same time, since this will only be maximal after 4–6 days. This is because the half-life of the drug is very long (30–45 days). The dose is 200 mg three times daily for 1 week, 200 mg twice daily for 1 week and then 200 mg per day. Some patients require a faster loading rate and higher maintenance doses.

Side-effects   Chronic use is limited by side-effects (McGovern et al, 1983), which are virtually all extracardiac:

- Corneal deposits are universal but usually not a problem. Periodic slit lamp examination is recommended
- Photosensitivity is very common, as is a bluish discoloration of the skin
- Thyroid dysfunction occurs in 2–3% of patients, and there may also be problems with biochemical analysis of serum thyroid hormone levels. Thyroid function tests should be carried out before treatment and then every 6 months during therapy
- Interstitial pulmonary fibrosis or pulmonary alveolitis
- Abnormal liver function tests
- Peripheral neuropathy

ANALGESICS

Narcotic analgesics (opiates) are used to relieve moderate to severe pain. Drugs in the group all have similar effects and side-effects but differ in their duration of action. Although primarily analgesics, they are also sedative in high doses, particularly when used in combination with other centrally-acting drugs (e.g. tranquillisers). They suppress cough, cause euphoria, stimulate the vomiting centres in the brain and remove the sensation of pain. They are usually given with an anti-emetic drug.

Narcotic analgesics are usually given by slow intravenous injection or infusion following acute myocardial infarction, since intramuscular absorption may be unpredictable if there is peripheral hypoperfusion of the patient. Diamorphine is probably the best choice of analgesic, since it produces a smaller fall in blood pressure. It also produces vasodilatation, thereby reducing myocardial work and oxygen consumption. It is also much more soluble and allows injection of smaller volumes of fluid.

Dose

- Diamorphine (heroin): 2.5–10.0 mg iv, repeated as required
- Morphine and cyclomorphine: 5–10 mg iv, repeated as required
- Papaveretum (Omnopon) is a mixture of the alkaloids of opium (20 mg is roughly equivalent to 12.5 mg of morphine)

Side-effects   Nausea, vomiting, constipation, urinary retention, bradycardia and respiratory depression.

ANGIOTENSIN CONVERTING ENZYME (ACE-) INHIBITORS

In patients with cardiac failure, the renin–angiotensin system is extremely active, resulting in angiotensin-mediated vasoconstriction, with increased sodium and water retention secondary to increased aldosterone secretion (Figure 15.1). The

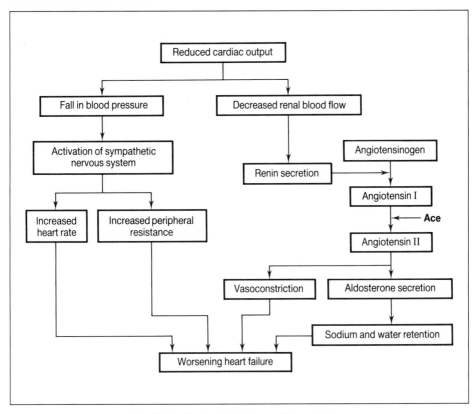

Fig. 15.1 Pathophysiology of heart failure

ACE-inhibitors inhibit the conversion of angiotensin-I to the potent vasoconstrictor angiotensin-II (allowing vasodilatation of arteries and veins) and reduce aldosterone secretion.

Captopril was introduced in 1981, and many more ACE-inhibitors have been developed since; currently, there are nine different ACE-inhibitors available in the UK, of which five (captopril, enalapril, lisinopril, perindopril and quinapril) are licensed for the treatment of heart failure. Despite claims of potential advantages of one compound over another, no clinically significant differences have yet been shown in the treatment of either hypertension or heart failure.

The benefits of these drugs for patients with congestive heart failure have been unequivocally demonstrated, resulting in symptomatic improvement and reduced mortality (Packer, 1992). For patients with acute myocardial infarction, the ISIS-4 study showed a small benefit with early routine use of ACE-inhibitors in unselected patients, but this is probably brought about by greater benefits in high-risk patients and no effect in others. Those patients with asymptomatic left ventricular dysfunction who are treated with ACE-inhibitors may not progress to overt heart failure, although this does not necessarily affect survival rates.

The situation for patients with overt cardiac failure or significant left ventricular damage, following recent myocardial infarction, is, however, clear. ACE-inhibition should be commenced within 1 week of myocardial infarction to reduce the risk of mortality and serious cardiovascular events (St John Sutton, 1994).

Dose

- Captopril (Capoten, Acepril): 6.25–150.0 mg daily in divided doses
- Enalapril (Innovace): 2.5–40.0 mg in divided doses
- Lisinopril (Zestril): 2.5–40.0 mg daily

Side-effects   Serious side-effects are less common now, since doses used are lower than in the past. Fear of first-dose hypotension is rarely a problem in mild to moderate heart failure, and hospital admission for initiation of therapy is seldom required. Rash and cough are common (particularly in women), and renal failure, hyperkalaemia and angio-oedema are important complications of therapy. Some side-effects occur with one ACE-inhibitor but not another.

ANTIDYSRHYTHMIC AGENTS

Suppression of serious dysrhythmias following acute myocardial infarction should be associated with a reduced mortality and morbidity, as well as relieving much of the anxiety in the patient with symptomatic dysrhythmias. Despite large advances in our understanding of the pathogenesis and pharmacological treatment of cardiac dysrhythmias, management is still largely unsatisfactory, many patients being treated empirically.

Antidysrhythmic drugs work essentially by one or more of the following mechanisms:

1. *Blocking the stimulus.* Certain exogenous factors are known to precipitate dysrhythmias in the sensitised heart. Increased levels of circulating catecholamines (from metabolic stress or anxiety), hypoxia, increased circulating free fatty acids and hyperglycaemia have all been implicated in provoking dysrhythmias. Therapy aimed at correcting these factors may reduce the incidence of dysrhythmias.

2. *Blocking impulse formation.* Many dysrhythmias are initiated or maintained by spontaneous ectopic activity (enhanced automaticity), and suppression of these abnormal impulses plays a major role in treatment.

3. *Inhibiting impulse transmission.* Impulse transmission can be blocked by interfering with different electrophysiological mechanisms and hence preventing impulse transmission.

Classification

There are many ways of classifying antidysrhythmic drugs. They may be classified by the type of rhythm disturbance they can be used to treat, the anatomical site of action or their electrophysiological action on isolated myocardium. This latter classification was devised by Vaughan Williams in 1969 and is still used today

(Vaughan Williams, 1984), but with our expanding knowledge of dysrhythmogenesis and drug actions, it is becoming incapable of supporting current clinical practice. It does, however, provide many theoretical and practical benefits for a rational approach in the treatment of dysrhythmias (see Chapter 10). Initial selection of a drug can often be simplified, and, should a second agent be required, selection from a different action group is frequently more successful than if an agent from the same group is employed. In addition, side-effects may be reduced.

There are four classes of drug in the Vaughan Williams classification, grouped on the basis of their *in vitro* effects on the action potentials of normal cardiac cells.

Class I: Membrane-stabilising agents

(Examples: lignocaine, flecainide, propafenone)
These agents depress membrane responsiveness and slow myocardial conduction by their membrane-stabilising activity. The fast sodium current is inhibited, and the phase 0 rise is thus reduced. These drugs also depress the rate of diastolic depolarisation (phase 4), which reduces spontaneous automaticity.

The group is subdivided into Classes Ia, Ib, and Ic, on the basis of the overall effect on the action potential: class Ia drugs (quinidine, disopyramide, procainamide) prolong it; class Ib drugs (lignocaine, mexiletine, moricizine) shorten it; and class Ic drugs (flecainide, encainide, propafenone) have no effect. Class Ia drugs are more cardiodepressant.

Class II: Beta-blockers

(Examples: propranolol, metoprolol, atenolol)
These drugs block catecholamine stimulation (which may induce cardiac dysrhythmias) of the myocardial cells. They also produce direct (membrane-stabilising) effects, similar to those of Class I drugs.

Class III: Drugs sustaining depolarisation

(Examples: amiodarone, sotalol)
The major action of these drugs is to prolong the duration of the action potential, with consequent lengthening of the effective refractory period. The membrane responsiveness, conduction velocity and rate of rise of the action potential in phase 0 are not affected. They impressively suppress ventricular ectopic activity and may be capable of chemical defibrillation (i.e. restoring sinus rhythm in patients with ventricular fibrillation).

Class IV: Calcium-channel blockers

(Examples: verapamil, diltiazem)
These agents inhibit the slow inward calcium current and depress phases 2 and 3 (plateau phase) of the action potential. These actions are of particular importance in the upper part of the AV node and will block circus movements during re-entry tachycardias.

This classification of antidysrhythmic drugs is based on presumed alterations in ionic conduction in normal myocardial fibres. However, these drugs probably have differing effects on the diseased myocardium, and many have properties of more than one class. Clinically, it is sometimes better to have a classification based on the action of the drugs on differing cardiac tissues (see Chapter 10). The Task Force of the Working Group on Arrhythmias of the European Society of Cardiology have suggested a new classification (the 'Sicilian Gambit'), based upon the mechanism of antidysrhythmic activity (Katritsis and Camm, 1994). The importance of this new proposal is that drug actions may be considered not only on the basis of antidysrhythmic activity, but also on what is now recognised to be of equal importance – their proarrhythmic properties.

Proarrhythmic effects of cardiac drugs

Most antidysrhythmic drugs have the potential actually to cause abnormalities of cardiac rhythm (Podrib et al, 1987). The CAST studies (1989, 1992) showed that post-infarction patients were more likely to die if treated with antidysrhythmic agents than with placebo, an effect attributed to the proarrhythmic effect of the agents used (e.g. flecainide). A different choice of drug may have provided us with a more optimistic view; empirical use of amiodarone in the CASCADE study (1993) was moderately successful in patients with poor left ventricular function following cardiac arrest.

ASPIRIN

Aspirin irreversibly blocks the enzyme cyclo-oxygenase and thus reduces the synthesis of various prostanoids. In platelets, the particular prostanoid involved is thromboxane A2, a potent vasoconstrictor and platelet aggregant. Administration of aspirin acutely and long term greatly reduces the risk of subsequent vascular events, including reinfarction (Anti-platelet Trialists' Collaboration, 1994), by prolonging the bleeding time and reducing thrombosis. The beneficial dose is unknown but is probably in the range of 75–300 mg daily.

The ISIS-2 study (1988) showed a 25% reduction in mortality when 160 mg aspirin was given within 4 hours of acute myocardial infarction, an effect that adds to the benefits of thrombolysis. In the first month after the heart attack, continuing treatment with aspirin reduces the risk of further myocardial infarction, vascular death and stroke by 25%. It also will greatly reduce the risk of vascular occlusion in those who have undergone coronary artery bypass grafting or angioplasty.

'Disprin CV' is an aspirin specifically designed for cardiovascular disease. The aspirin formulation (micro-encapsulated for sustained release) is not associated with as much gastrointestinal upset and reduces blood loss by a half in comparison to standard aspirin. It is, however, more expensive. The 100 mg formulation is recommended for prevention of coronary graft occlusion, whilst the 300 mg size is used for the other cardiovascular indications (transient ischaemic attack, post-myocardial infarction, unstable angina, etc.).

Dose 75–325 mg/day. For acute myocardial infarction, a dose of at least 150 mg should be chewed rather than swallowed to ensure absorption.

Side-effects Gastrointestinal discomfort or bleeding; bronchospasm.

ATROPINE

Atropine is an acetylcholine antagonist and gives rise to parasympathetic block-ade. It thus reduces vagal stimulation of the heart and is, therefore, useful for treating symptomatic bradycardia. A single dose of 3 mg is currently recommended in asystolic cardiac arrest to ensure complete vagal block, so that cholinergic over-activity on the conducting tissues is relieved. Repeat doses should be avoided, since they may reduce the electrical stability of the heart, making ventricular fibril-lation more likely.

Dose 0.3–0.6 mg intravenously for bradycardia, 3 mg intravenously during asysto-lic cardiac arrest.

Side-effects Dry mouth, confusion, tachycardia and urinary retention.

BETA-ADRENERGIC BLOCKING AGENTS

Since beta-adrenergic blocking agents first became clinically available in the early 1960s, they have been increasingly used in the treatment of coronary heart disease, dysrhythmias and hypertension (Vedin and Wilhelmsson, 1985).

Beta-blockers antagonise the effects of catecholamines, by occupying their recep-tors and competitively reducing occupancy. They will, therefore, reduce heart rate (particularly exercise-related tachycardias), myocardial contractility and systemic blood pressure. The overall effect is to reduce myocardial work and oxygen consumption. Unfortunately, the effects are sometimes offset by an increased oxygen requirement, due to an increase in left ventricular end diastolic pressure (LVEDP) and left ventricular ejection time. This may, to a certain extent, be balanced by the concomitant use of nitrates. Although there is only one type of adrenergic transmitter, there are two types of adrenergic receptor. These have been termed alpha and beta. Alpha-receptors seem to be associated with most of the usual adrenergic excitatory functions, such as vasoconstriction and dilatation of the pupils. Beta-functions, such as inhibition of vasoconstriction (resulting in vaso-dilatation) and inhibition of bronchial constriction (resulting in bronchial dilata-tion), are usually inhibitory. In tissues with both receptors, functions are balanced, but in tissues with only one type of receptor, adrenergic activity is either excitatory or inhibitory. The heart and the bronchi have only beta-receptors; stimulation is excitatory in the heart (causing positive inotropic and chronotropic effects) but inhibitory in the bronchi (causing bronchial relaxation). To explain these opposing actions, beta-receptors have been divided into two types, termed beta-1 (cardiac) and beta-2 (bronchial). Beta-blocking agents differ in their affinity for beta-1 and beta-2 receptors (see below).

The choice of agent is usually influenced by the following properties (see Table 15.1).

Half-life

Unlike the plasma half-life, the pharmacological half-life depends on the dose. Most beta-blockers can be prescribed twice daily, providing a big enough dose is given. Hydrophilic agents, however, are better suited to once-daily dosage, because they have longer plasma half-lives.

Cardioselectivity

Beta-blockers differ in their relative affinity for beta-1 or beta-2 sites. Timolol, propranolol and nadolol act on both sites and are termed 'non-specific'. However, atenolol and metoprolol act predominantly on the beta-1 cardiac sites and are, therefore, termed 'cardioselective'. These drugs (e.g. metoprolol and atenolol) may, therefore, be safer in patients with peripheral vascular disease or those prone to bronchospasm.

Cardioselectivity is relative and is lost at high doses. No beta-blocker is completely safe in the presence of bronchospasm.

Intrinsic sympathomimetic activity

Intrinsic sympathomimetic activity (ISA) is the property of coexistent partial agonist activity, i.e. the drug partially stimulates the beta sites. This property is believed to reduce the degree of cardiodepression. It is doubtful whether ISA confers any real advantages in the treatment of angina, but such drugs may have smaller effects on peripheral circulation, in congestive heart failure and in depression of the conducting tissue. These potentially-useful properties are not useful in those patients with angina at rest, although they are of value in patients with marked resting bradycardia. Patients with asthma or diabetes are less likely to develop problems with cardioselective agents, although beta-blockers are probably not first-line therapy in these cases. Catecholamines increase glycogenolysis and lipolysis and mobilise free fatty acids, to raise blood sugar levels. As a result, not only are catecholamine-induced symptoms of insulin-induced hypoglycaemia masked, but recovery from hypoglycaemia is also delayed.

Lipid solubility

The pharmacokinetics of beta-blockers varies widely, depending upon whether they are soluble in fat (lipophilic) or water (hydrophilic). Lipophilic agents (e.g. propranolol) are well absorbed orally and have a short half-life. They can cross the blood–brain barrier and may be responsible for central nervous system side-effects (e.g. nightmares) as a consequence. They are metabolised by the liver. Hydrophilic agents (e.g. atenolol), however, are poorly absorbed orally and are excreted unchanged by the kidneys. They have a long plasma half-life and do not easily cross the blood–brain barrier.

Table 15.1 Properties of beta-adrenoceptor blocking drugs

Generic name	Cardioselectivity	Intrinsic sympathomimetic activity	Membrane-stabilising activity	Potency (propranolol = 1)	Elimination half-life (hr)	Predominant route of elimination	Lipophilicity
Acebutolol	+	+	+	0.3	3–4	Renal	Low
Atenolol	+	0	0	1.0	6–9	Renal	Low
Labetalol	0	0	0	0.3	3–4	Hepatic	Low
Metoprolol	+	0	0	1.0	3–4	Hepatic	Moderate
Nadolol	0	0	0	1.0	14–24	Renal	Low
Oxprenolol	0	++	+	0.5–1.0	2–3	Hepatic	Moderate
Pindolol	0	+++	+	6.0	3–4	Renal (40%) Hepatic	Moderate
Propranolol	0	0	++	1.0	3–4	Hepatic	High
Sotalol	0	0	0	0.3	8–10	Renal	Low
Timolol	0	0	0	6.0–8.0	4–5	Renal (20%) Hepatic	Low

0   no effect
+   small effect
++   moderate effect
+++ strong effect

Variation in oral bioavailability is largely influenced by 'first-pass' metabolism of lipid-soluble compounds by the liver. A reduction of dose is, therefore, required in liver disease. Lipid-insoluble agents (atenolol, nadolol and sotolol) are excreted only by the kidneys.

Side-effects

Common side-effects include bradycardia, heart failure, bronchospasm, nightmares, insomnia, depression and peripheral coldness. There is no good evidence that beta-blockers induce coronary artery spasm (Sleight, 1986). A small number of patients will develop Raynaud's phenomenon, partly due to unopposed alpha-adrenergic action and partly due to a fall in cardiac output. Central nervous system side-effects are common with beta-blockers that cross the blood–brain barrier (lipid-soluble agents), especially propranolol. These may produce sedation, depression and nightmares.

Beta-blockers adversely affect serum lipid profiles (Jowett and Galton, 1987), although this may not be so severe with agents having strong ISA.

Sudden withdrawal of beta-blockade

Following sudden withdrawal of beta-blockade, there may be an increase in the number of beta-receptor sites. This manifests as an increased sensitivity to catecholamines, with an increase in myocardial work, heart rate and oxygen consumption. Angina, hypertension or even myocardial infarction may result. Patients should be warned of the dangers of suddenly stopping medication, and, if this is required, the dose should be tapered.

Therapeutic uses

There are major benefits on the oxygen supply/demand balance with the use of beta-blockers. Ninety per cent of patients with stable angina pectoris due to coronary atheroma demonstrate improved exercise tolerance and reduced chest pain with treatment (Frishman, 1981). With increased exercise capability, there is a secondary benefit in allowing patients to join training programmes. Beta-blockers also have Class II antidysrhythmic activity and are also of particular value in supraventricular dysrhythmias. Beta-blockers reduce catecholamine concentrations in ischaemic myocardium, decrease platelet stickiness and have been shown to modify type A behaviour (Sleight, 1986).

Beta-blockers and acute myocardial infarction

In an acute myocardial infarction, the amount of myocardial tissue that remains viable is the major determinant of patient survival. The extent of damage appears to depend upon the ratio between oxygen supply and demand. Increased demand is placed on the heart by increased sympathetic drive, producing increased chronotropic and inotropic effects. Since beta-blockers reduce myocardial work, their administration in the early phase of acute myocardial infarction might limit infarction size, as well as preventing oxygen-consuming tachydysrhythmias. Any benefits in the long term, however, would have to work by a different mechanism.

Over 65 trials (involving 50 000 patients) have so far been carried out to determine whether beta-blockers are of use in acute myocardial infarction (Yusuf et al, 1985). Despite the findings of such trials, there is still much confusion and conjecture over the use of beta-blockers in acute myocardial infarction. Certainly, there is no debate where the patient has heart failure, bronchospasm or heart block, where beta-blockade is clearly contraindicated. Patients with normal left ventricular function and no rhythm disturbances form a low-risk group, and treatment is probably not justified. Those forming a high-risk group have suffered larger infarcts, often resulting in poor left ventricular function and dysrhythmias. Treatment with beta-blockers will reduce the rate of reinfarction and sudden death if they can be tolerated. Those in the intermediate group will probably gain some benefit from beta-blockade.

The evidence that early commencement of beta-blockade improves outcome is difficult to interpret. It is necessary to treat 100–150 patients at average risk with an intravenous beta-blocker before one life is saved, so the benefit is not large (*Lancet*, 1986). This is probably not surprising since over 50% of myocardial damage takes place in the first 6 hours, and institution of any therapy often takes longer. However, acute intravenous beta-blockers may have a role in infarct limitation, so for selected patients, therapy is often desirable and safe. Intravenous beta-blockade reduces pain, recurrent ischaemia and mortality in patients with acute myocardial infarction. The TIMI II-B study has confirmed the additional benefits of beta-blockade when given in conjunction with thrombolysis, in part by reducing the incidence of cardiac rupture. Despite these benefits, intravenous beta-blockade is not often given acutely in the UK, and it is not clear why. Metoprolol and atenolol are safe to use provided there is no bradycardia, hypotension or heart failure. Doses for intravenous use are

- Metoprolol: 5 mg over 2 minutes, repeated up to a total of 15 mg
- Atenolol: 5–10 mg over 5 minutes

For other patients who are haemodynamically stable, treatment started within the first 2 weeks and continued for many months seems to reduce the reinfarction rate by about 25%, with a similar reduction in the occurrence of sudden deaths. This effect is most noticeable with agents without intrinsic sympathomimetic activity. Prime candidates are those patients with post-infarction angina and hypertension. Therapy should be continued for at least 18 months, and the agents at present recommended are metoprolol, timolol and propranolol.

BRETYLIUM TOSYLATE

Bretylium (Bretylate) is an adrenergic neurone-blocking agent that suppresses noradrenaline release. It has Class II antidysrhythmic properties and is useful in ventricular dysrhythmias, especially resistant ventricular fibrillation. It is not commonly used in the UK but is in the USA, where the choice of antidysrhythmic agents is limited.

Dose 5–10 mg/kg infused intravenously over 10–30 minutes. This may be repeated after 1–2 hours, to a total dose of 30 mg/kg.

Side-effects Postural hypotension is common, and dopamine support may be required if there are severe hypotensive episodes. Bretylium is excreted by the kidneys, and reduced doses are required in renal impairment.

BUMETANIDE

Bumetanide (Burinex) is a loop diuretic similar to frusemide. Following an intravenous injection, a diuresis starts within a few minutes, reaching a maximum within 15–30 minutes. Orally, the onset is usually after 30–60 minutes, and the diuresis continues for about 3–4 hours. One milligram is about equivalent to 40–60 mg of frusemide, but at high doses direct comparison of doses is not possible, and dosage requires titration. Bumetanide may increase urine output in patients with renal failure who are unresponsive to frusemide.

Dose 1–2 mg orally or intravenously, but doses over 5 mg are required in renal failure.

Side-effects Potassium depletion, myalgia and skin rashes.

CALCIUM CHLORIDE

Calcium ions can cause the asystolic heart to beat, as well as strengthening contractility. It is also useful to counteract the effect of hyperkalaemia. However, the routine administration of calcium salts during cardiopulmonary resuscitation is questionable. Calcium may cause coronary and cerebral vasospasm, as well as increasing ventricular irritability in patients taking digoxin. Small doses may be useful for cardiac arrest complicated by hypocalcaemia or hyperkalaemia or for patients on high doses of calcium-channel blocking agents (e.g. nifedipine, verapamil or nicardipine). Calcium may be of value in the treatment of electromechanical dissociation, especially if the QRS complex is widened.

Dose 2–4 mg/kg intravenously (2 ml 10% calcium chloride solution).

Side-effects Sudden death may occur if the patient is digitalised. Intramuscular or subcutaneous administration can cause tissue necrosis.

CALCIUM-CHANNEL BLOCKING AGENTS

Calcium-channel blocking agents are a heterogeneous group of therapeutic agents with a widening range of indications (Braunwald et al, 1985; Kenny, 1985). They are remarkably safe, considering the importance of transmembrane calcium flux in many biological systems. Calcium is needed in the formation of the cardiac action potential, the regulation of cardiac contractility and the contraction of arterial smooth muscle. By preventing calcium uptake by cells, these effects are reduced, resulting in an antidysrhythmic activity, a reduction in myocardial work and vasodilatation. The calcium-channel blocking agents are able to modify the transmembrane transport of calcium ions in various tissues, although their mechanism of action and pharmacological effects differ. Following the introduction of verapamil and nifedipine, there has been a proliferation of newer drugs and modified-release formulations, producing a lot of confusion over prescribing. Verapamil has marked effects on the cardiac conduction system, whereas nifedipine and nicardipine produce peripheral vasodilatation, as well as preventing coronary vasospasm. Diltiazem acts preferentially on coronary vessels, producing vasodilatation, with less effect on systemic vessels.

The calcium antagonists are used predominantly in the treatment of hypertension and angina and sometimes in the management of supraventricular dysrhythmias. All are of value in angina associated with coronary artery spasm. There is some evidence that sudden withdrawal of calcium-channel blockers may be associated with an exacerbation of angina.

The routine use of calcium antagonists as an alternative to beta-blockade after myocardial infarction does not improve survival (Lau et al, 1992), but diltiazem may reduce the risk of reinfarction in patients who present with non-Q wave infarction (Gibson et al, 1986). Verapamil may be of value in patients who are unable to tolerate beta-blockade and have good left ventricular function following myocardial infarction (DAVITT II, 1990).

Verapamil (Cordilox, Berkatens, Securon)

The most striking effect of verapamil is on AV nodal conduction, making it very useful for treatment of supraventricular tachycardias. Verapamil is a Class IV antidysrhythmic agent, which inhibits calcium influx through slow channels into the myocardial cells. Electrical activity in the SA and AV nodes is largely dependent on calcium ions, so verapamil is of major value in supraventricular tachycardias. As re-entry is responsible for 70% of cases of supraventricular tachycardias, verapamil is the drug of choice. Following an intravenous injection (5–10 mg), AV conduction is quickly reduced, and re-entry tachycardias at the AV node are terminated (Talano and Tommaso, 1982). Orally, it is not so effective, because much is metabolised by the liver. If given to a patient on beta-blockers, profound hypotension or bradycardias may be produced, so care is needed. Although it is useful with digoxin in controlling the ventricular rate in atrial fibrillation and atrial flutter, it is contraindicated in atrial fibrillation complicating the Wolff–Parkinson–White syndrome, as it gives rise to preferentially accessory conduction, which may result in ventricular fibrillation.

Dose The recommended dose is 5–10 mg intravenously over 2–3 minutes, which may be repeated after 30 minutes. Care is needed if the patient is taking other agents that act on the sinus and AV nodes (especially beta-blockers), to prevent heart block and heart failure developing. Oral therapy is 40–120 mg three times a day. Higher doses are required for the treatment of angina (40–120 mg three times daily) and hypertension (120–240 mg twice daily).

Nifedipine (Adalat)

Nifedipine reduces peripheral and coronary vascular resistance. It has a mild negative inotropic effect, which is usually offset by increasing sympathetic activity secondary to its vasodilator effect. The dose is 15–60 mg/day in divided doses, although a sustained release form is available (Adalat SR), which is of particular value in the treatment of hypertension (up to 320 mg/day).

Nicardipine (Cardene)

This agent is similar to nifedipine, although cardiodepression is not so marked. It is used in the treatment of angina and hypertension.

Dose   20–30 mg 8 hourly.

Diltiazem (Tildiem)

Diltiazem inhibits transmission in cardiac conducting tissue and gives rise to a mild resting bradycardia. It vasodilates coronary arteries and, to a lesser extent, peripheral arteries. Whilst used predominantly in the treatment of angina, it may also be used in higher doses for hypertension. Diltiazem and verapamil are both useful in the prophylaxis of recurrent supraventricular tachycardias. In addition, they are useful in controlling the ventricular rate in patients with atrial fibrillation, with or without digoxin.

Dose   60–320 mg daily, in divided doses.

Others

Amlodipine and felodipine are similar to nifedipine but do not reduce myocardial contractility.
   Lacidipine and isradipine are indicated for hypertension only.

Uses of the calcium-channel blocking agents

Angina

The calcium blocking agents have been used most extensively in the treatment of myocardial ischaemia. The main indication for these drugs is stable angina, and all are effective. They probably work by reducing myocardial work. Nifedipine used alone may produce a tachycardia, thus worsening stable angina, and is often better combined with a beta-blocker. The well-documented anti-anginal effects of beta-blockers may be augmented by the addition of a calcium-channel blocker. Verapamil usually slows the heart and is probably superior to nifedipine when used alone (Subramanian et al, 1982). However, the combination of verapamil and a beta-blocker may depress myocardial function and conduction, to produce heart block and heart failure (Winniford et al, 1985).
   Calcium-channel blockers are effective in coronary artery spasm and are useful in variant angina. Spasm also plays an important role in the genesis of crescendo

angina, and the calcium-channel blockers are effective, providing symptomatic relief and reducing the rate of myocardial infarction or the need for coronary arterial surgery. Diltiazem is probably the drug of choice in these cases.

Hypertension

Nifedipine and nicardipine are powerful peripheral vasodilators and do not have much effect on cardiac conduction. Nifedipine has emerged as a potent antihypertensive agent and is often prescribed as a first-line agent. It is also useful in hypertensive crises. Verapamil and diltiazem are also useful, but their place in the routine treatment of hypertension is unclear (Breckenridge, 1984). This specific peripheral vasodilatory effect makes them good agents for treating Raynaud's disease and perhaps in the prevention of migraine attacks.

Cardiac dysrhythmias

Intravenous verapamil is very effective in supraventricular tachycardia, with a success rate of 85% (Talano and Tommaso, 1982). It may be given as a prophylactic drug for paroxysmal supraventricular dysrhythmias and is also sometimes successful in ventricular tachycardia.

Diltiazem similarly impairs AV and sinus conduction and may also be useful in the management of supraventricular dysrhythmias.

Side-effects

The calcium-channel blocking agents are remarkably safe drugs. The most serious side-effects are those on cardiac conduction. Varying degrees of heart block and asystole can occur, especially in those with nodal disease or in patients taking beta-blockers. The drugs should not be given intravenously to those taking beta-blockers. Myocardial depression can also produce heart failure. Vasodilator effects (flushing, headache and dizziness) sometimes occur at the start of therapy, and these are most pronounced with nifedipine. Fluid retention is common, often resulting in ankle oedema. Verapamil can produce constipation and also reduces digoxin excretion. If these two drugs are given together, the dose of digoxin should be halved. Diltiazem appears to produce fewer side-effects than the other calcium blockers, as it has less effect on the heart than verapamil and less effect on the peripheral vessels than nifedipine.

As with beta-blockers, sudden withdrawal of calcium blockers may be associated with symptoms of myocardial ischaemia or even myocardial infarction.

CORTICOSTEROIDS

Very large doses of intravenous steroids cause vasodilatation in patients with shock and peripheral vasoconstriction. This enables fluids to be given and tissue perfusion to be re-established.

Dose Variable. Single doses of methylprednisolone (30 mg/kg) have been used, with vasodilatation occurring after 2–4 hours.

Side-effects Many and usual. Gastrointestinal haemorrhage and hypokalaemia are often a problem.

DIAZOXIDE

Diazoxide (Eudemine) is useful in lowering systemic vascular resistance and is most effective when given with a loop diuretic. It has a very rapid action intravenously and should thus be given with care.

Doses 300 mg in 20 ml as an intravenous bolus. Orally, 400–1000 mg in two or three daily doses.

Side-effects Hyperglycaemia is inevitable and often needs concomitant treatment with tolbutamide. Fluid retention may require diuretic therapy.

DIGOXIN

Digoxin (Lanoxin) increases the force of myocardial contraction and, via the vagus, exerts a slowing of conduction at the sinus and AV nodes. Therapeutic doses cause shortening of the QT interval and flattening (or inversion) of the T waves, with ST segment sag. False positive ST changes may develop during exercise stress testing.

Digoxin is rapidly and almost entirely absorbed, but the effects are not directly correlated with blood levels of the drug. This is because of variable protein binding, penetration and uptake by the myocardium and other factors. It is primarily metabolised by the kidneys within 2–3 days but may accumulate in renal impairment. In some patients, digoxin is inactivated by gut flora, necessitating large oral doses to achieve satisfactory blood levels. If these patients are given broad-spectrum antibiotics that affect the gut flora, digoxin toxicity may be precipitated.

The principal use of digoxin is for controlling the ventricular rate in atrial fibrillation, especially when it occurs with heart failure. Digoxin has an acute positive inotropic effect, although whether this is chronically maintained is debated (*Lancet*, 1985). It is of little value in cases of high-output failure, cor pulmonale and restrictive cardiomyopathy. Long-term use in congestive heart failure without rhythm disturbance is controversial, since many patients in sinus rhythm remain well after therapy with digoxin is discontinued. In patients with paroxysmal atrial fibrillation, digoxin may maintain sinus rhythm, although it is contraindicated in atrial fibrillation complicating the Wolff–Parkinson–White syndrome. Atrial flutter is converted to atrial fibrillation and sinus rhythm may then be reinstated on stopping the drug. In patients with thyrotoxicosis, very large doses, often supplemented with propranolol, may be required to slow the ventricular rate.

Ventricular ectopics and ventricular tachycardia have been treated with digoxin, although it must be ensured that the dysrhythmia is not actually caused by digoxin.

Digoxin following myocardial infarction

The role of digoxin in acute myocardial infarction is very controversial (*Lancet*, 1989). In patients with left ventricular failure following acute myocardial infarction, digoxin is effective, but concern surrounds the increased myocardial work caused by the positive inotropic effect of the drug, which may extend the area of myocardial necrosis. Beneficial haemodynamic effects are greatest in patients with moderate left ventricular failure, and the risk of extending myocardial damage is probably least in these patients. Post-infarction survival in patients with congestive heart failure and with multifocal ventricular ectopics may be improved by withholding or discontinuing digoxin.

Doses

Digoxin is very irritant to the tissues and should only be given orally or intravenously. A single intravenous dose of 1 mg by infusion produces an effect in about 10 minutes, with maximal effect at 1–2 hours. The half-life is 36–48 hours. By mouth, the effect is noted within 1 hour and persists for 2–3 days. However, some effect may still be present for a week. Digitalisation will take about 1 week if no loading dose is given (0.125–0.25 mg twice daily). The faster method is by giving 1.0–1.5 mg over 24 hours in divided doses. The usual amount of digoxin required to produce a therapeutic blood level (in a patient weighing 70 kg) is about 0.75–1.0 mg. Care is needed in the elderly and if there is coexisting hypokalaemia, hyponatraemia or hypocalcaemia.

Radioimmunoassay techniques are available for determining blood levels of digoxin, which should not be measured within 6 hours of the last oral dose. Therapeutic levels are quoted as 0.5–2.5 ng/ml, but it must be remembered that the diagnosis of digoxin toxicity is clinical and too much reliance should not be placed on laboratory results. For example, digoxin toxicity can occur at normal blood levels if there are concomitant electrolyte upsets, thyroid disease, renal impairment or hypoxia. Additionally, patients with levels greater than 2.5 ng/ml may display no signs of toxicity.

Digoxin toxicity

A major drawback to the treatment with digoxin is the narrow margin between therapeutic doses and toxicity. Hence, adverse drug actions are very common, with as many as 20% of patients on the drug manifesting toxicity at some time (Aronson, 1983). There are many factors that may result in toxicity, including electrolyte imbalance and deteriorating renal function, especially in the elderly (who are most likely to be on digoxin). The early symptoms of overdose are nausea, vomiting and diarrhoea. Headache and confusion, often with visual disturbances, are more serious. Classically, *xanthopsia* (yellow vision) is reported, but flickering dots, halos and scotomata can occur.

Digoxin toxicity can produce any rhythm disturbance, including ventricular fibrillation. The more common problems are ventricular ectopics (especially ventricular bigeminy), sinus bradycardia, heart block and paroxysmal atrial tachycardia with block. Atrial flutter and rapid atrial fibrillation have been described but are uncommon. The ECG usually shows other signs of toxicity (ST/T wave changes or increased PR interval). Ventricular tachycardia is usually precipitated by short runs of ventricular ectopics. Nodal tachycardias usually occur in patients previously in atrial fibrillation and should be suspected if the pulse rate becomes rapid and regular.

Treatment of toxicity

If stopping digoxin is inadequate, potassium chloride is very effective in the treatment of digoxin-induced tachydysrhythmias, particularly if there is hypokalaemia. ECG monitoring is desirable during parenteral administration of any potassium salt to observe for signs of hyperkalaemia. Potassium canrenoate (400 mg iv over 5 minutes) can be used for more urgent cases (de Guzman and Yeh, 1975). Propranolol (2 mg iv) is especially useful for supraventricular dysrhythmias, and phenytoin, amiodarone and lignocaine are effective in digitalis-induced ventricular dysrhythmias. Digibind (antidigoxin antibody fragments) should be used in all serious cases, and whilst electrical cardioversion may occasionally be required, pretreatment with lignocaine or phenytoin is recommended.

In the case of digoxin-related bradydysrhythmias, potassium supplements should be stopped, because they potentiate heart block. Symptomatic bradycardias may require intravenous atropine, isoprenaline or even temporary cardiac pacing.

DIPYRIDAMOLE

Dipyridamole (Persantin) is an antiplatelet agent that may potentiate the effect of aspirin. It is often used as an adjunct to oral anticoagulation in patients with prosthetic heart valves, to prevent emboli.

Dipyridamole may be used to increase coronary perfusion during nuclear scanning. Blood is diverted away from areas of poor perfusion, which makes scanning more accurate, but may precipitate angina.

Dose   300–600 mg/day in three to four divided doses.

Side-effects   May worsen coronary ischaemia. Interacts with adenosine to produce an enhanced effect.

DISOPYRAMIDE

Disopyramide (Rythmodan, Dirythmin) is a Class I antidysrhythmic agent, with electrophysiological properties similar to quinidine. It decreases automaticity in ectopic pacemaker cells and lengthens the effective refractory period in atrial and ventricular muscle. It thus has both ventricular and supraventricular activity.

Dose The dose is 2 mg/kg by very slow intravenous injection, to a maximum of 150 mg in the first hour. An infusion of 0.4 mg/kg per hour may then be employed, or oral therapy (400–800 mg in four doses). If the drug is going to work, it does so in the first 15–20 minutes. The usual therapeutic plasma levels are 2–4 µg/ml. Over half the drug is excreted unchanged in the urine, and dose reduction is required in patients with hepatic and renal impairment. The half-life is between 6 and 12 hours.

Side-effects Disopyramide has a marked negative inotropic effect, related to both serum levels and speed of administration. It should, therefore, be used cautiously in patients with heart failure. Sinus node depression also sometimes occurs, so care is needed in heart block. Anticholinergic activity may cause glaucoma, retention of urine and constipation.

DOBUTAMINE

Dobutamine (Dobutrex) is a synthetic adrenergic agent, modified from isoprenaline. It stimulates beta-adrenergic cardiac receptors and thereby directly increases the force of myocardial contraction, with only small increases in heart rates. Unlike with dopamine, there is little systemic vasoconstriction. This is because dopamine acts indirectly (by causing noradrenaline release), whereas dobutamine acts directly.

It is used short term in the treatment of cardiogenic shock and heart failure and is best administered when full cardiovascular monitoring techniques are available (including Swan–Ganz catheterisation). The left ventricular filling pressure falls and the cardiac output rises.

Dose It is supplied in ampoules containing 250 mg dobutamine. Following dilution, it is added to 250 or 500 ml of dextrose or saline, giving 1000 µg/ml or 500 µg/ml respectively. It is infused intravenously, and most patients respond to a dose of 2.5–10.0 µg/kg per minute. Some patients may need 40 µg/kg per minute. Dobutamine is often given in combination with low-dose dopamine, which is used to promote renal perfusion.

DOPAMINE

Dopamine (Intropin) is the natural precursor of noradrenaline and has similar alpha- and beta-stimulatory actions, particularly at beta-1 sites. Stroke volume is increased, with little effect on heart rate. It causes peripheral vasoconstriction, which raises blood pressure, but, unlike other sympathetic agents, produces selective renal and cerebral arterial vasodilatation. This is, therefore, of great use in renal hypoperfusion. At low doses, the renal effects are most marked, but as the dose increases, vasoconstriction and positive inotropic and chronotropic effects are more marked (see below). Dopamine is of major value in cardiogenic and other types of shock, and prolonged low-dose infusion is useful in heart failure.

It is given intravenously by continuous infusion, preferably by a central line. This is because of the dangers of extravasation; profound localised tissue ischaemia may result in gangrene. This can even result in the absence of extravasation when large doses are used for long periods. Should signs of tissue necrosis develop, the area should be infiltrated with phentolamine (10 mg in 10 ml saline).

Dose   Each ampule contains 800 mg dopamine, which is diluted in 500 ml of dextrose or saline, yielding 1600 µg/ml.

Calculating the rate of administration

Dopamine exerts it effect by action on different receptors (Table 15.2). The infusion is given by continuous metered infusion.

Administration of the required dose is calculated in drops per minute by the formula: Required dose (µg/kg/min) × Body weight (kg) × Total volume of infusion (ml) × Number of drops/ml dispensed by infusion pump, divided by Amount of dopamine added to infusion (mg) × 1000.

For example, for an infusion of 5 µg/kg/min in an 80 kg man given via a standard drip (20 drops/ml), the infusion rate would be:

$$\frac{5 \times 80 \times 520 \times 20}{800 \times 1000} = \frac{4\,160\,000}{800\,000}$$
$$= 5.2 \text{ drops/min}$$

Dopamine is contraindicated in patients with uncontrolled dysrhythmias and those taking monoamine-oxidase inhibitors. Hypovolaemia should always be corrected before its use, and therapy should be withdrawn slowly and not stopped abruptly.

Table 15.2   Effects of dopamine at different doses

Dose (µg/kg/min)	Effect
1–5	Dilates renal and mesenteric arterioles to produce increased renal blood flow and glomerular filtration rate and urine output
6–20	Direct inotropic effect on the heart, with dose-related increase in cardiac output and heart rate
>20	Direct alpha-action leads to peripheral vasoconstriction, which raises blood pressure. There are further inotropic and chronotropic effects on the heart

ENOXIMONE

Enoximone (Perfan) is a phosphodiesterase-inhibitor that inhibits the breakdown of myocardial cyclic AMP. The rate and force of myocardial contraction directly relates to the myocardial concentration of cyclic AMP, an effect that may be augmented by simultaneous administration of dopamine. Cyclic AMP also relaxes vascular smooth muscle, to effect vasodilatation. As a consequence, phosphodiesterase-inhibitors will improve cardiac output, and there is usually no change in blood pressure, heart rate or oxygen consumption.

There is no evidence that enoximone improves survival, but it may be used for the short-term, intravenous treatment of severe heart failure refractory to conventional treatment, providing the patient is monitored invasively.

Dose 90 µg/kg per minute is given over 30 minutes to load the patient. A continuous infusion of not more than 24 mg/kg should be given over 24 hours, in the range 5–20 µg/kg per minute.

Side-effects Dysrhythmias.

ESMOLOL HYDROCHLORIDE

Esmolol hydrochloride (Brevibloc) is a cardiospecific beta-blocker with a very short duration of action, which may be used in the treatment of supraventricular tachycardias, sinus tachycardia and hypertension, especially postoperatively.

Dose 50–200 µg/kg per minute by iv infusion.

FLECAINIDE

Flecainide (Tambocor) is a Class Ic agent, which has no effect on the duration of the action potential but slows conduction through the His–Purkinje system and prevents retrograde conduction through accessory pathways. It is useful in chronic ventricular dysrhythmias and in re-entry tachycardias, especially the Wolff–Parkinson–White syndrome.

Dose It is available for intravenous and oral use, and its long half-life allows a twice-daily dosage. Intravenously it should be given by slow injection or infusion (2 mg/kg). Oral maintenance is 100–200 mg twice daily.

Side-effects Proarrhythmic effects are described, particularly in those with acute myocardial ischaemia and in those with cardiac pacemakers. Flecainide is contraindicated in the treatment of dysrhythmias following acute myocardial infarction (CAST Investigators, 1989). Dizziness and blurred vision may occur, and the drug is negatively inotropic.

FRUSEMIDE

Frusemide (Lasix, Dryptal, Aluzine) is a powerful loop diuretic, similar to bumetanide. When given intravenously for left ventricular failure, the relief is almost immediate and occurs before a diuresis has taken place. This suggests that the prime value in acute heart failure is due to a vascular effect, by causing increased venous capacitance, and that the diuretic effect is secondary.

Dose The usual dose is 40–80 mg orally, intramuscularly or intravenously. Patients with refractory oedema or renal impairment may require very large doses (500–1000 mg).

Side-effects Transient or permanent deafness may result if frusemide is injected too rapidly, particularly in those with renal impairment. Large doses must be diluted, and intravenous infusion is then a preferable method of administration.

HEPARIN

Heparin is a naturally-occurring, high molecular weight mucopolysaccharide with marked anticoagulation properties. It is inactive orally and must, therefore, be given subcutaneously or intravenously. Intramuscular injection may produce large haematomas. It has been used prophylactically to prevent thromboembolism and in the treatment of deep vein thrombosis and pulmonary emboli (Goldberg et al, 1984).

It acts by combining with antithrombin III in the coagulation cascade, preventing the formation of factor Xa. It probably also reduces platelet stickiness. Unlike warfarin, it does not block prothrombin formation in the liver.

The activated partial thromboplastin time (APTT) is used as an index of efficacy and should be maintained at about twice normal. Thrombocytopenia often occurs, and platelet counts should be checked on alternate days.

Overdose, producing prolonged coagulation times, should be corrected by reducing the dose of stopping the drug altogether (the half-life is only 1.5 hours). More urgent cases can be treated with protamine sulphate (1 mg neutralises 100 U heparin within 5 minutes). However, since protamine is a weak anticoagulant itself, doses exceeding 50 mg should not be given.

Heparin regimens

- *Low dose* (prophylaxis): 5000 U twice daily, subcutaneously. APTTs are not required
- *Medium dose* (treatment of deep vein thrombosis or disseminated intravascular coagulation): 30 000–45 000 U daily by infusion or 4 hourly by intravenous injection. After 48 hours, the dose is reduced by about 50% and adjusted according to APTTs. Warfarin is usually started at the same time

● *High dose* (pulmonary embolism, systemic embolisation): a bolus loading dose of 5000–10 000 U should be given, followed by intravenous infusion, but there should be no reduction in dose at 48 hours as above. Warfarin is usually not started acutely.

Heparin following thrombolysis

Following publication of the ISIS-3 study results (1992), controversy exists regarding the efficacy of heparin in maintaining coronary patency after thrombolytic treatment for acute myocardial infarction. Whilst most physicians accept that heparin is not required following thrombolysis with streptokinase, it is usual in most centres to anticoagulate with intravenous heparin, to prevent recurrent thrombosis where clot-specific agents have been used. The concept of post-thrombotic vulnerability to reocclusion after TPA is supported by several studies, including TAMI-3 (Topol et al, 1989) and the European Co-operative study (de Bono et al, 1992). Our current practice is to use an intravenous heparin bolus of 5000 U followed by 1000 U/hr for 24 hours following thrombolysis with TPA. It is essential to ensure that the heparin is achieving therapeutic concentrations, by monitoring the APTT or heparin levels.

HIRUDIN

Hirudin and its derivatives are recently-developed intravenous anticoagulants, with specific and potent antithrombin effects.

They are more predictable than heparin in clinical use and are not associated with thrombocytopenia. They are more effective in inhibiting fibrin-bound thrombus and hold promise for preventing coronary reocclusion following successful thrombolysis.

HORMONE REPLACEMENT THERAPY

The effect of hormone replacement therapy (HRT) on cardiovascular risk is unclear (Findlay et al, 1994). There is good evidence that small doses of oestrogen given over several years following the menopause will reduce the incidence of stroke and myocardial infarction, but most recent trials (e.g. Khaw, 1992) have been based upon unopposed oestrogen, that is, oestrogen given without progesterone as in usual HRT. Although no large randomised, controlled trial has yet been carried out, current opinion is that hormone replacement therapy probably helps to prevent coronary heart disease. Decisions regarding HRT must be individualised, depending on the competing risks of coronary heart disease, osteoporosis, menopausal symptoms and endometrial and breast cancer.

HYDRALAZINE

Hydralazine (Apresoline) is an arteriolar vasodilator used in the treatment of aortic dissection, heart failure and hypertension. It increases heart rate and cardiac output by reducing afterload and also increases renal and cerebral perfusion. However, myocardial work and oxygen consumption are also increased, and angina may be precipitated.

Dose   The oral dose is 25–75 mg three or four times daily.

Side-effects   Due to vasodilatation, with postural hypotension, headache and flushing. Long-term therapy may cause a lupus syndrome, with positive LE cells (SLE).

INSULIN

Hyperglycaemia in the peri-infarction period is best treated with insulin, since oral hypoglycaemic agents may cause unwanted metabolic side-effects, particularly if there is renal and hepatic hypoperfusion. Soluble insulin of human origin (e.g. Humulin S) is probably the best choice (to prevent formation of insulin antibodies) and should, preferentially, be given by intravenous infusion. Hypoglycaemia should be avoided, as the induced catecholamine response may lead to tachydysrhythmias.

ISOPRENALINE

Isoprenaline is most often used to stabilise patients with profound bradycardia, heart block and hypotension, whilst awaiting pacemaker insertion.

Dose   4 mg in 500 ml 5% dextrose is infused at a rate that produces a suitable pulse rate and blood pressure.

Side-effects   Tremor, sweating and dysrhythmias.

LIGNOCAINE

In addition to its local anaesthetic properties, lignocaine is a Class I antidysrhythmic agent, which has been used for many years for the control of ventricular dysrhythmias complicating acute myocardial infarction. Its major action during cardiac arrest is to inhibit the initiation of re-entry dysrhythmias in the ischaemic myocardium, but its use makes defibrillation more difficult. Its routine use is, therefore, to be discouraged, although it may be considered after prolonged arrest.

Lignocaine by infusion may be of value following ventricular fibrillation to prevent recurrence, although the trend these days is to give smaller doses for shorter periods (up to 12 hours) than in the past. The incidence of side-effects is then very much reduced, without an apparent increase in further episodes of ventricular fibrillation.

Dose

- *Bolus therapy*: 0.5 mg/kg every 10 minutes
- *Infusion*: 1–4 mg/min (usually 25–50 µg/kg per minute)

Side-effects   Toxicity may result in hypotension, bradycardia, vomiting and fits. Reduced hepatic circulation may make lignocaine toxicity more likely, and no more than 3 mg/kg should be administered.

LIPID-LOWERING AGENTS

Drug therapy to lower plasma lipids should be used only after other risk factors have been addressed and following a careful trial of diet, employing the most rigorous diet achievable by the individual (Jowett and Galton, 1987). Appropriate drug therapy depends upon the particular lipid abnormality, and, in general, those with clinical vascular disease are treated more aggressively than those treated for primary prevention (Betteridge et al, 1993).

Initial drug therapy for those with hypercholesterolaemia is with bile acid sequestrant resins. The hydroxy-methyl-glutaryl co-enzyme-A (HMG-CoA) reductase-inhibitors ('statins') are being increasingly used and are extremely effective, particularly when used with low-dose bile sequestrants.

Those with mixed hyperlipidaemias are usually treated with fibric acid derivatives, especially if the triglyceride levels are markedly elevated.

Treatment of isolated hypertriglyceridaemia remains controversial. Nicotinic acid is sometimes very effective and is very popular in the USA, where it has been shown to be safe in long-term usage. Unfortunately, cutaneous flushing often limits its use. Acipimox is an analogue that may be more acceptable. Fish oils may be of benefit in reducing triglyceride levels as part of the basic diet, but have not proved useful pharmacologically.

1. *Anion exchange (bile sequestrant) resins* (e.g. cholestyramine, probucol): These bind bile acids, preventing reabsorption. Cholesterol is diverted into making more bile acids, so is progressively excreted.

Absorption of drugs, particularly digoxin and diuretics, is sometimes impaired. Anticoagulants may be enhanced or depressed.

2. *HMG-CoA inhibitors* (e.g. pravastatin, simvastatin): The HMG-CoA reductase-inhibitors ('statins') competitively inhibit the rate-limiting enzyme in cholesterol synthesis. They are very potent.

Side-effects are myositis and hepatic dysfunction.

3. *Fibrates* (e.g. bezafibrate, ciprofibrate, gemfibrozil, fenofibrate): These act on lipoprotein lipase and lower both cholesterol and triglycerides. They have the side-effect of myositis.

4. *Nicotinic acid group* (e.g. nicotinic acid, acipimox, nicofuranose): These inhibit triglyceride synthesis, but flushing limits their use.

5. *Fish oils*: The omega-3 marine triglycerides (Maxepa) may reduce triglyceride levels and have been advocated in the maintenance of bypass grafts and following coronary angioplasty.

MAGNESIUM

A number of trials (e.g. Teo and Yusuf, 1993) have seemed to show a reduction in mortality in patients treated with intravenous magnesium following acute myocardial infarction. Unfortunately, this has not been confirmed in the much bigger ISIS-4 (1995) study, and the routine use of magnesium cannot be recommended. However, it should be given in addition to potassium to hypokalaemic patients with serious dysrhythmias.

Dose 8 mmol of magnesium sulphate in 100 ml 5% dextrose over 15 minutes, followed by 72 mmol over 24 hours.

METOCLOPRAMIDE

Metoclopramide (Maxolon) is a centrally-acting anti-emetic agent, which also promotes gastric emptying. Oesophageal reflux is reduced, and small bowel transit time is increased.

Dose 10 mg orally, iv or im.

Side-effects Drowsiness, dizziness and dystonic movements of the head and neck.

MEXILETINE

Mexiletine (Mexitil) is very similar to lignocaine, but can be given orally, and sometimes works in lignocaine-resistant dysrhythmias. It is used in the treatment of ventricular dysrhythmias in coronary heart disease and following myocardial infarction.

Dose An intravenous loading dose of 100–250 mg is given over 5–10 minutes and is followed by a reducing infusion, starting at 2 mg/min for 1 hour, then 1 mg/min for 2 hours, down to 0.05 mg/min until no longer required or until oral therapy is instituted.

Oral loading is with 400 mg, followed by 200–250 mg three or four times daily. A slow-release preparation is available.

Side-effects These are related to blood levels, and a reduction in dose may be required for light-headedness, tremor and blurred vision. Gastrointestinal side-effects (nausea, vomiting and hiccoughs) sometimes limit its value.

MILRINONE

Milrinone (Primacor) is another phosphodiesterase-inhibitor, similar to enoximone (see above) and suitable for short-term inotropic support. Despite its beneficial haemodynamic actions, long-term therapy with oral milrinone increases mortality and morbidity in patients with severe heart failure (Packer et al, 1991).

Dose

- Loading: 50 µg/kg over 10 minutes
- Maintenance infusion: 0.375–0.750 µg/kg per minute (total daily dose should be less than 1.13 mg/kg)

Side-effects Dysrhythmias and hypotension.

MORICIZINE

Moricizine (Ethmozine) is a Class I antidysrhythmic agent for the treatment of ventricular dysrhythmias in patients with cardiac disease. However, in the CAST II study (1992), there was no benefit in mortality shown following myocardial infarction gained by suppression of ventricular ectopic activity with moricizine, and, acutely, the drug was associated with increased mortality. The drug should not be used early following acute myocardia infarction for asymptomatic dysrhythmias. No serious interaction occurs with digoxin, propranolol or heart failure medication.

Dose Initially, 600–900 mg daily in three divided doses, adjusted every 3 days to a maximum of 900 mg/day.

Side-effects Cardiodepression and proarrhythmia are less common than for flecainide, but gastrointestinal side-effects are common.

NALOXONE

Naloxone is a specific opiate antidote and is indicated if there is coma or respiratory failure following administration of diamorphine or morphine. It has a short intravenous half-life and needs repeated doses, depending upon the respiratory pattern.

Dose 0.8–2.0 mg, repeated every 2–3 minutes intravenously, or by infusion.

Side-effects Dysrhythmias.

NITRATES

Organic nitrates have been the mainstay in the treatment of angina pectoris for over 100 years and more recently have been used in the treatment of heart failure. The benefits arise from the combination of coronary and non-coronary actions, and different forms of coronary heart disease may respond differently. Nitrates relax vascular smooth muscle, mainly in the venous system, to increase capacitance and thus reduce preload to the heart. Arteriolar relaxation also occurs, with a fall in peripheral resistance (afterload). Although not a main action, coronary dilatation probably occurs, which may improve regional myocardial blood flow. These effects are most marked when the coronary arterial stenosis is due to spasm rather than a fixed lesion. Nitrates are, however, less effective than calcium antagonists in the treatment of coronary artery spasm and Prinzmetal angina (Conti, 1985). Sublingual glyceryl trinitrate (GTN) is accepted as the standard treatment for acute episodes of angina, and the longer-acting variants are used as prophylaxis against attacks. Tolerance may develop rapidly after the initiation of therapy but disappears quickly after discontinuing the drug (Cowan, 1986). Cross-tolerance with different preparations is also thought to occur. Tolerance appears to be a function of constant plasma levels of nitrates and is less likely to occur when nitrate levels fluctuate. Preparations designed to give 24-hour therapeutic plasma levels (e.g. transdermal nitrates) may, therefore, be associated with tolerance and should probably only be used at night in cases of nocturnal angina. Long-acting oral nitrates should, therefore, be given as intermittent therapy, two or three times daily, allowing a nocturnal nitrate-free period (Parker et al, 1987).

Uses

The most common indication for nitrate therapy is in the treatment and prophylaxis of angina. Recently, nitrates have been used in acute left ventricular failure, hypertension and the early phase of evolving acute myocardial infarction, with the hope of diminishing peri-infarction ischaemic zones and thus limiting the size of infarction (Conti, 1985; Johansson, 1986).

Choice

The haemodynamic effects of GTN are short lasting, and many different preparations have, therefore, been developed to prolong their effect and make them useful as prophylactic agents.

Sublingual GTN (0.3, 0.5 or 0.6 mg)

These tablets should be used as early as possible after the onset of angina or, prophylactically, before physical activity. If the pain persists, the tablets may be repeated at 5-minute intervals until relief is obtained. It must always be explained that the drug is neither addictive nor to be reserved only for emergencies. Headache and hypotension are common and may be avoided if the pill is swallowed or spat out as soon as relief is obtained. The tablets are deactivated by heat and light and must, therefore, be kept cool and in a dark bottle. The activity of the drug after opening lasts only 8 weeks, and old tablets should be discarded. Tablets are also deactivated if cotton-wool is placed in the bottle: the chemicals are absorbed by it.

Oral nitrates

There is an extensive 'first-pass' effect on nitrates when taken orally. That is, the amount of drug reaching systemic circulation is very much reduced because of metabolism by the liver (the first major organ encountered after drug absorption from the gut). As a result, as little as 10% of the drug may reach the circulation, although prolonged action can be achieved by using higher or more frequent doses. Isosorbide dinitrate (Isordil, Sorbitrate, Cedocard) is swallowed whole in doses of 10–60 mg 4–6 hourly. The onset of action is after about 30 minutes but sooner if the tablet is chewed. Isosorbide mononitrate (Ismo 20, Elantan) is thought not to be so extensively removed on first pass, which allows smaller doses to be given (20–40 mg 8 hourly).

Buccal nitrates

Sublingual GTN, Sorbichew and Nitrolingual sprays are rapidly-acting preparations that can bypass the hepatic circulation and may, consequently, have better effect. Suscard Buccal is a form of nitrate that has been impregnated into an inert polymer matrix, allowing slow diffusion of the drug across the buccal mucosa. The pill is tucked under the top lip without chewing, and a gel-like coating forms around the drug, allowing it to adhere to the buccal mucosa. Slow absorption can then take place as long as the pill remains intact (usually 3–5 hours).

Transdermal nitrates

The use of cutaneous nitrates has been known for 30 years, and GTN ointment and slow-release skin preparations that hold a reservoir of GTN are available. Cutaneous applications circumvent the first-pass metabolism of swallowed nitrates. Therapeutic blood levels are achieved within 1 hour and last for up to 24 hours. The patches are applied to any clean, dry, non-hairy part of the skin, although the extremities should be avoided. Absorption depends upon site and blood flow, and large amounts are sometimes required to produce therapeutic blood levels. Skin irritation and variable absorption limit their use, but there is a high placebo effect, especially if patches are applied over the heart. GTN ointment (Percutol) is messy to use and requires frequent application to produce a sustained effect. Each tube is provided with a measure, so that the required length of cream (1–2 inches) can be applied, under waxed paper, for 4–8 hours. Cutaneous prepacked patches containing 5 or 10 mg of GTN behind a special slow-release membrane (Transiderm-Nitro, Deponit 5) prevent the application from being rubbed or washed off and may last much longer. About 5 mg GTN is released in 24 hours.

Intravenous nitrates

Intravenous GTN (Tridil) and isosorbide dinitrate (Isoket) are useful in the management of unstable angina, prolonged infarction pain and left ventricular failure. The dose required for pain relief varies widely, and the infusion rate (1–10 mg/hr) must be titrated against pain and blood pressure.

Side-effects

The major side-effects of nitrates are due to vasodilatation, which may give rise to hypotension, tachycardia and headache. Alcohol will potentiate the effects. Side-effects will not be as prominent with continued use, if the patient can be persuaded to persevere. Beta-blockers given at the same time may help to slow the heart and relieve the headache. The nitrate ion reacts with haemoglobin to produce methaemoglobinaemia, but quantities are usually trivial.

Hypotension and reflex tachycardia during intravenous infusion can be treated by slowing or stopping the infusion, since the half-life of intravenous GTN is only 1–2 minutes.

NORADRENALINE

Noradrenaline stimulates cardiac beta-1 receptors to produce a positive inotropic effect and raise the blood pressure (especially the systolic blood pressure). Baroreceptor stimulation limits a simultaneous tachycardia. Alpha-adrenergic vasoconstriction takes place in vascular beds, except in the cerebral and coronary vessels, which dilate.

Noradrenaline may be useful in septic shock, although not following acute myocardial infarction. It augments coronary perfusion and raises the blood pressure, although peripheral vasoconstriction may increase cardiac afterload and myocardial work without increasing cardiac output. Noradrenaline may also constrict renal capillary beds, leading to renal hypoperfusion.

Dose 1–2 µg/min are infused centrally until the blood pressure rises.

Side-effects Renal hypoperfusion and increased myocardial work. If the drug is allowed to run in too fast, hypertensive crises may occur, leading to stroke and myocardial infarction.

PHENYTOIN

Although primarily used as an anticonvulsant, phenytoin (Epanutin) has Class Ib antidysrhythmic action and is of particular value in ventricular dysrhythmias, especially those that are digitalis induced. This is because it shortens prolonged QT intervals, increases AV nodal conduction and suppresses ventricular ectopic activity.

Dose An intravenous dose of 250 mg produces an effect in 5–20 minutes. Oral doses are 200–600 mg daily.

Side-effects Ventricular fibrillation, heart block and respiratory depression may result following intravenous administration. Oral therapy may be limited by ataxia, skin rashes and blood dyscrasias.

PROCAINAMIDE

Procainamide (Pronestyl) is derived from the local anaesthetic procaine and has Class I antidysrhythmic properties, similar to quinidine (see below). It is seldom an agent of first choice but is of value in the treatment of ventricular ectopics, ventricular tachycardia and paroxysmal atrial tachycardia.

Dose Oral treatment is preferred: 250 mg four times daily. The usual effective antidysrhythmic plasma concentration is 4–8 µg/ml.

Intravenous administration should be under ECG control, 100 mg being given over 5 minutes or by infusion.

Side-effects Toxicity is rare at plasma levels under 12 µg/ml. Gastrointestinal side-effects are common, and a lupus syndrome (SLE) has been described with long-term usage.

PROCHLORPERAZINE

Prochlorperazine (Stemetil) is a phenothiazine derivative often used in the treatment of nausea and vomiting. It may be associated with postural hypotension, and metoclopramide may, therefore, be a better choice in coronary care units.

Dose Can be given orally (5–10 mg), rectally (5 mg) or by deep intramuscular injection (12.5 mg). Intravenous injection is not recommended, as it is an irritant.

Side-effects Dry mouth, drowsiness and extrapyramidal signs.

PROPAFENONE

Propafenone (Arrhythmol) is a Class I antidysrhythmic agent, used in the treatment and prophylaxis of supraventricular and ventricular dysrhythmias.

Dose 150 mg three times daily, increasing to a maximum of 300 mg three times daily.

Side-effects Atropine-like side-effects, including dry mouth, constipation and blurred vision. It is contraindicated in severe bradycardia, uncontrolled heart failure and advanced chronic respiratory disease.

QUINIDINE

Quinidine (Kinidin) is the dextro-isomer of quinine and, in addition to antipyretic properties, has Class I antidysrhythmic properties, similar to procainamide. It also has anticholinergic activity, thus aiding AV conduction. It is not now commonly used, because it is unpleasant to take (nausea and vomiting) and can cause severe side-effects, such as ventricular fibrillation and heart block.

Dose   Orally, 500 mg twice daily, adjusted as required.

Side-effects   Gastrointestinal symptoms are common. Cardiodepression and heart block may occur, and the drug should be stopped if the QRS duration increases to longer than 0.14 second.

SODIUM BICARBONATE

Intravenous sodium bicarbonate has been widely used in the past for correcting the metabolic acidosis that follows cardiac arrest. However, there is little evidence that this therapy improves outcome, and its use is no longer recommended, because of the frequent occurrence of deleterious side-effects, including increasing carbon dioxide levels, hypernatraemia, inactivation of concurrently-administered catecholamines and tissue necrosis if accidentally given extravascularly.

Critically-ill patients in hospital may warrant early therapy with sodium bicarbonate, if there is developing hyperkalaemia or acidosis that might precede a cardiac arrest, but these occasions are now the exception rather than the rule.

SODIUM NITROPRUSSIDE

Sodium nitroprusside (Nipride) is a well-tolerated and potent parenteral vasodilator, which may be employed in hypertensive emergencies and severe left ventricular failure. It relaxes both arteriolar and venous smooth muscle. It acts rapidly (within 2 minutes) and should be given by controlled intravenous infusion. The drug is light sensitive. Solutions are normally red/brown in colour, and deterioration is marked by a colour change to blue.

Dose   The drug should be freshly prepared (in 5% dextrose) and used within 4 hours. The normal adult dose for heart failure is 10–15 µg/min, adjusted as required. Doses should normally not exceed 400 µg/min. The maximal dose is 700–800 mg in 24 hours, and the drug is best not given for periods exceeding 72 hours, because of the build-up of plasma cyanide. If therapy is needed for more than 3 days, cyanide and thiocyanate levels should be assayed.

Side-effects   Nausea, sweating, dizziness and twitching denote toxicity. These should be treated by stopping the drug and administering sodium thiosulphate if signs persist. Unexplained cyanosis may be due to formation of methaemoglobin-aemia. Large doses of hydroxocobalamin (vitamin B12, 1.5 mg/kg) may be used prophylactically to reduce plasma cyanide levels.

THROMBOLYTIC (FIBRINOLYTIC) AGENTS

Thrombolytic agents work by activating the body's natural fibrinolytic system. Streptokinase, Alteplase (TPA) and Anistreplase (APSAC) have all been shown to break up coronary thrombus and reduce mortality following myocardial infarction (Fibrinolytic Therapy Trialists' Collaborative Group, 1994). Streptokinase has to combine with plasminogen to form an activator complex, which acts on other circulating plasminogen to form plasmin, which, in turn, effects systemic fibrino-lysis. TPA, in contrast, is much more clot specific, since it binds directly to fibrin and does not activate circulating plasminogen (i.e. it is plasminogen independent). APSAC tends not to be used much these days. Pro-urokinase is effective in treat-ment of myocardial infarction but is not available currently in the UK. Urokinase is available for the treatment of pulmonary emboli. The use of fibrinolytic agents in coronary thrombosis is discussed in detail in Chapter 6.

The two major problems with thrombolysis in acute myocardial infarction that still need to be addressed are the reocclusion rates following thrombolysis and the risks of haemorrhage, particularly stroke. New protocols for drug administration are being tried (e.g. TIMI-9 and GUSTO II), as well as combination treatments and novel genetically-engineered agents. Antibody-targeted thrombolysis, using conjugates of antifibrin antibodies and a thrombolytic agent, have been tried, as have combinations of TPA and pro-urokinase. The role of antithrombotic agents such as hirudin (see above) is being explored.

TRANEXAMIC ACID

Tranexamic acid inhibits plasminogen activation and fibrinolysis. It is, therefore, of great value in severe haemorrhage complicating thrombolytic therapy. However, fresh frozen plasma should also be given.

Dose   0.5–1.0 g by slow iv injection 8 hourly.

Side-effects   Dizziness may follow rapid iv injection.

VERAPAMIL

See Calcium-channel blockers.

WARFARIN

Warfarin (Marevan) inhibits the action of vitamin K in the liver and thus inhibits synthesis of four plasma procoagulants (II, VII, IX and X). Its effect commences at about 12 hours and lasts for 2–5 days. Numerous dosage schedules have been described (e.g. 10 mg daily for 3 days and then adjusted to keep the prothrombin time at two to three times normal). Over-anticoagulation is treated by reducing the daily dose or stopping the drug altogether. If required, vitamin K1 (phytomenadione) may be given (10 mg over 2–3 minutes).

Many factors affect the potency of warfarin:

- *Increased potency*: heart failure, liver disease, fever, alcohol, aspirin, cimetidine, diuretics, antibiotics and oral hypoglycaemics
- *Decreased potency*: diabetes, hypothyroidism, hyperlipidaemia, sedatives, oral contraceptives, cholestyramine and antacids

The introduction of the World Health Organisation system for international standardisation of prothrombin times has allowed comparison of anticoagulant control regimens, based upon common systems of reporting, termed international normalised ratios (INRs) (see Table 15.3).

Anticoagulant therapy in acute myocardial infarction

Whilst the role of aspirin following acute myocardial infarction is clear (see above), the use of anticoagulants as an alternative method of secondary prevention is still debated (Hirsh, 1990). In contrast to aspirin, both heparin and warfarin will interrupt the coagulation cascade and could help to prevent infarct extension and coronary reocclusion, as well as preventing deep vein thrombosis and pulmonary emboli.

Patients, particularly those with large anterior infarcts involving the apex, are at risk of peripheral embolisation from left ventricular thrombus for up to 12 weeks following myocardial infarction. This complication may be minimised by routine anticoagulation with subcutaneous heparin (SCATI, 1989; Turpie et al, 1989). Patients at high risk should be fully anticoagulated with warfarin for 3 months to prevent thromboembolism and longer term to prevent infarction in patients with non-transmural infarction (Yedinak and Sproat, 1993). Concomitant low-dose aspirin should be considered for high-risk patients, despite the inherent dangers of

Table 15.3 Proposed therapeutic ranges of warfarin (after Poller, 1985)

INR	Condition
2–2.5	Prophylaxis
2–3	Treatment of deep vein thrombosis, pulmonary emboli and transient ischaemic attacks
3–4.5	Recurrent thromboembolic phenomena, arterial grafts, prosthetic valves, myocardial infarction and heart failure

bleeding. The current Veterans' Affairs Co-operative Study should help consideration of this aspect.

Those with atrial fibrillation, recurrent dysrhythmias, cardiac dilatation and
severe heart failure also should receive long-term anticoagulation.

References

Anti-platelet Trialists' Collaboration (1994) Overview I. Prevention of death, myocardial
infarction and stroke by prolonged anti-platelet therapy in various categories of patients.
Overview II. Maintenance of vascular graft or arterial patency by anti-platelet therapy.
British Medical Journal, **308:** 81–106, 159–168.

Aronson J K (1983) Digitalis toxicity. *Clinical Science*, **64:** 253–258.

Betteridge D J, Dodson P M, Durrington P N, Hughes E A, Laker M F, Nicholls D P,
Rees J A E, Seymour C A, Thompson G R, Winder A F, Wincour P H and Wray R
(1993) Management of hyperlipidaemia: guidelines of the British Hyperlipidaemia
Association. *Postgraduate Medical Journal*, **69:** 359–369.

Braunwald E, Muller J E and Stone P H (1985) Use of calcium channel blocking agents in the
management of ischaemic heart disease. *European Heart Journal*, **6:** 31–34.

Breckenridge A (1984) A third drug in hypertension. *British Medical Journal*, **289:** 859–860.

CASCADE Investigators (1993) Randomised anti-arrhythmic drug therapy in survivors of
cardiac arrest – the CASCADE study. *American Journal of Cardiology*, **72:** 280–287.

CAST Investigators (1989) Effect of encainide and flecainide on mortality in a randomised trial
of arrhythmia suppression after myocardial infarction (the Cardiac Arrhythmia
Suppression Trial). *New England Journal of Medicine*, **321:** 406–412.

CAST II Investigators (1992) Effect of the anti-arrhythmic agent Moricizine on survival after
myocardial infarction. *New England Journal of Medicine*, **327:** 227–233.

Conti C R (1985) Nitrate therapy in ischaemic heart disease. *European Heart Journal*, **6:** 3–11.

Cowan J C (1986) Nitrate tolerance. *International Journal of Cardiology*, **12:** 1–19.

DAVITT II (1990) Danish Study Group on verapamil in myocardial infarction. The effect of
verapamil on mortality and major events after acute myocardial infarction. *American
Journal of Cardiology*, **66:** 779–785.

de Bono D P, Simoons M L, Tijssen J, Arnold A E R, Betriu A, for the European Co-operative
Study Group Trial (1992) Effect of early intravenous heparin on coronary patency, infarct
size and bleeding complications after alteplase thrombolysis. *British Heart Journal*, **67:** 122–
128.

de Guzman N T and Yeh B K (1975) Potassium canrenoate in the treatment of long-term digoxin
induced arrhythmias in conscious dogs. *American Journal of Cardiology*, **35:** 413–420.

Fibrinolytic Therapy Trialists' Collaborative Group (1994) Indications for fibrinolytic therapy
is suspected acute myocardial infarction: collaborative overview of early and major
mortality from all randomised trials of more than 1000 patients. *Lancet*, **343:** 311–322.

Findlay I, Cunningham D and Dargie H J (1994) Coronary heart disease, the menopause and
hormone replacement therapy. *British Heart Journal*, **71:** 213–214.

Frishman W H (1981) Beta-adrenergic antagonists. New drugs and new indications. *New
England Journal of Medicine*, **305:** 500–506.

Gibson R S, Boden W E, Theroux P, Strauss H D and Pratt C M (1986) Diltiazem and reinfarction in patients with non-Q-wave myocardial infarction. *New England Journal of
Medicine*, **315:** 423–429.

Goldberg R J, Gore J M and Dalen J E (1984) The role of anticoagulant therapy in acute
myocardial infarction. *American Heart Journal*, **108:** 1387–1393.

Hirsh J (1990) Effectiveness of anti-coagulant therapy in reducing morbidity and mortality in
acute myocardial infarction. In *The Management of Acute Myocardial Ischaemia*,
Chamberlain D'A, Julian D G and Sleight P (eds), pp. 99–110. London: Chapman & Hall.

ISIS-2 Collaborative Group (1988) Randomised trial of intravenous streptokinase, oral
aspirin, both or neither amongst 17,187 cases of suspected acute myocardial infarction.
Lancet, **ii:** 349–360.

ISIS-3 (Third International Study of Infarct Survival) Collaborative Group (1992) A randomised comparison of streptokinase vs tissue plasminogen activator vs anistreplase and of aspirin plus heparin vs aspirin alone among 41,299 cases of suspected myocardial infarction. *Lancet*, **339:** 753–770.

ISIS-4 Collaborative Group (1995) A randomised factorial trial assessing early oral Captopril, oral mononitrate, and intravenous magnesium sulphate in 58,050 patients with suspected acute myocardial infarction. *Lancet*, **345:** 669–685.

Johansson B W (1986) Nitrate therapy today. *Acta Pharmacologica et Toxicologica*, **59**(supplement 6): 7–16.

Jowett N I and Galton D J (1987) The management of the hyperlipidaemias. In *Drugs for Heart Disease*, 2nd edn, Hamer J (ed.), p. 359. London: Chapman & Hall.

Katritsis D and Camm A J (1994) Anti-arrhythmic drug classifications and the clinician: a gambit in the land of chaos. *Clinical Cardiology*, **17:** 142–148.

Kenny J (1985) Calcium channel blocking drugs and the heart. *British Medical Journal*, **291:** 1150–1152.

Khaw K T (1992) Hormone replacement therapy. *British Medical Bulletin*, **48:** 249–476.

Lancet (1985) Needless digoxin. *Lancet*, **ii:** 1048.

Lancet (1986) Intravenous beta-blockade during acute myocardial infarction. *Lancet*, **ii:** 79–80.

Lancet (1989) Digoxin: new answers, new questions (Editorial). *Lancet*, **ii:** 79–80.

Lau J, Antman E M and Jimenez-Silva J (1992) Cumulative meta-analysis of therapeutic trials for myocardial infarction. *New England Journal of Medicine*, **327:** 248–254.

McGovern B, Garan H, Kelly E and Ruskin J N (1983) Adverse reactions during treatment with amiodarone hydrochloride. *British Medical Journal*, **287:** 175–180.

Packer M (1992) Patho-physiology of chronic heart failure and treatment of heart failure. *Lancet*, **340:** 88–95.

Packer M, Carver J R, Rodeheffer R J, Ivanhoe R J, DiBianco R, Zeldis S M, Hendrix G H, Bommer W J, Elkayam U and Kukin M L (1991) Effect of oral milrinone on mortality in severe chronic heart failure. The PROMISE Study Research Group. *New England Journal of Medicine*, **325:** 1468–1475.

Parker J O, Farrell B, Lahey K A and Moe G (1987) Effect of intervals between doses on the development of tolerance to isosorbide dinitrate. *New England Journal of Medicine*, **316:** 1440–1444.

Podrib P J, Lampert S, Graboys T B, Blatt C M and Lown B (1987) Aggravation of arrhythmia by anti-arrhythmic drugs. Incidence and predictors. *American Heart Journal*, **59:** 38E–43E.

Poller L (1985) Therapeutic ranges in anticoagulant administration. *British Medical Journal*, **290:** 1683–1686.

SCATI Study Group (1989) Randomised controlled trial of subcutaneous calcium heparin in acute myocardial infarction. *Lancet*, **ii:** 182–186.

Shah P K, Nalos P and Peter T (1987) Atropine resistant post-infarction complete AV block: possible role of adenosine and improvement with aminophylline. *American Heart Journal*, **113:** 194–195.

Sleight P (1986) Beta-adrenoreceptor blockade in the treatment of coronary heart disease. *European Heart Journal*, **7**(supplement C): 79–91.

Subramanian V B, Bowles M J, Khurmi M S, Davies A B and Raftery E B (1982) Randomized double blind comparison of verapamil and nifedipine in chronic stable angina. *American Journal of Cardiology*, **50:** 696–703.

St John Sutton M (1994) Should ACE inhibitors be used routinely after infarction? Perspectives from the SAVE trial. *British Heart Journal*, **71:** 115–118.

Talano J V and Tommaso C (1982) Slow channel calcium antagonists in the treatment of supraventricular tachycardia. *Progress in Cardiovascular Diseases*, **25:** 141–156.

Teo K K and Yusuf S (1993) Role of magnesium in reducing mortality in acute myocardial infarction. A review of the evidence. *Drugs*, **46:** 347–359.

Topol E J, George B S, Kereiakes D J and the TAMI group (1989) A randomised controlled trial of intravenous TPA and early intravenous heparin in acute myocardial infarction. *Circulation*, **79:** 281–286.

Turpie A G G, Robinson J G, Doyle D J, Muiji A S, Mishkel G J et al (1989) Comparison of high-dose with low-dose subcutaneous heparin in the prevention of left ventricular mural thrombosis in patients with acute anterior myocardial infarction. *New England Journal of Medicine*, **320:** 352–357.

Vaughan Williams E M (1984) A classification of antiarrhythmic actions reassessed after a decade of new drugs. *Journal of Clinical Pharmacology*, **24:** 129–147.

Vedin A and Wilhelmsson C (1985) Medical treatment of ischaemic heart disease – beta blockers. *European Heart Journal*, **6:** 13–27.

Winniford M D, Fulton K L, Corbett J R, Croft C H and Hillis L D (1985) Propranolol–verapamil versus propranolol–nifedipine in severe angina of effort: a randomised double blind crossover study. *American Journal of Cardiology*, **55:** 281–285.

Yedinak K C and Sproat T T (1993) Heparin and warfarin therapy after acute myocardial infarction. *Clinical Pharmacy*, **12:** 197–215.

Yusuf S, Peto R, Lewis J, Collins R and Sleight P (1985) Beta-blockade during and after myocardial infarction: an overview of the randomised trials. *Progress in Cardiovascular Diseases*, **27:** 335–371.

Appendix 1

Useful Addresses

ASH (Action for Smoking on Health)   109 Gloucester Place, London W1H 3PH.
Tel: 0171–935 3519

British Heart Foundation   14 Fitzhardinge Street, London W1H 4DH.
Tel: 0171–935 0185

British Holistic Medical Association   14 Harley House, Upper Harley Street,
London NW1 4PR.
Tel: 0171–935 7848

Chest, Heart & Stroke Association   CHSA House, 123–127 Whitecross Street,
London EC1Y 8JJ.
Tel: 0171–490 7999

Coronary Artery Disease Research Association (CORDA)   Tavistock House,
North Tavistock Square, London EC1Y 8JJ.
Tel: 0171–387 9779

Health Education Authority   Hamilton House, Mabledon Place, London WC1H
9TX.
Tel: 0171–383 3833

International Society for Humanism in Cardiology   43 Weymouth Street, London
W1N 3LD.
Tel: 0171–486 4191

National Forum for Coronary Heart Disease Prevention   Hamilton House,
Mabledon Place, London WC1H 9TX.
Tel: 0171–383 7638

Resuscitation Council UK   9 Fitzroy Square, London W1P 5AH.
Tel: 0171–388 4678

Appendix 2

Acronyms of the Major Cardiac Trials

Large multicentre cardiology trials have become increasingly common and of great clinical importance in recent years. The adopted design of these trials has been 'large and simple', so that 'definitive' answers can emerge, with practical implications for the management of coronary heart disease (Yusuf et al, 1984). Almost as important as trial design is the development of an acronym! Cardiologists now meet in huddles to discuss important research implications using this shorthand, and it is important to have a guide (Brown, 1992).

Below are some of the acronyms mentioned in this book, with a brief summary of the trial aim. A more extensive list of over 200 cardiological acronyms has been compiled by Cheng (1992).

ACME (1992): Angioplasty Compared to Medicine.
Comparison of angioplasty with medical therapy in the treatment of single-vessel coronary artery disease.

AIMS (1988): APSAC Intervention Mortality Study.
Investigation of the effect of intravenous APSAC on mortality after acute myocardial infarction.

AIRE (1993): Acute Infarction Ramipril Efficacy.
Effect of Ramipril on mortality and morbidity of survivors of acute myocardial infarction with clinical evidence of heart failure.

ASSET (1988): Anglo-Scandinavian Study of Early Thrombolysis.
Study of early administration of tissue plasminogen activator (TPA) in acute myocardial infarction.

BASIS (1990): Basel Anti-arrhythmic Study of Infarct Survival.
Effect of antiarrhythmic therapy on mortality in survivors of myocardial infarction with asymptomatic complex ventricular arrhythmias.

BHAT (1982): the Beta-blocker Heart Attack Trial.
A randomised trial of propranolol in patients with acute myocardial infarction.

BRESUS (1992): British Resuscitation Survey.
Survey of cardiopulmonary resuscitations in British hospitals.

CASS (1981): Coronary Artery Surgery Study.
Effect of bypass surgery on survival.

CAST: Cardiac Arrhythmia Suppression Trial.

- CAST I (1989): Effect of encainide and flecainide on mortality in arrhythmia suppression after myocardial infarction.

● CAST II (1992): Effect of moricizine on survival after myocardial infarction.

CONSENSUS: Co-operative North Scandinavian Enalapril Survival Study.
● CONSENSUS I (1987): Effect of enalapril on survival in severe congestive heart failure.
● CONSENSUS II (1992): Effect of early administration of enalapril on mortality in patients with acute myocardial infarction.

DAVIT: Danish Verapamil in Myocardial Infarction Trial.
● DAVIT I (1984): Effect of verapamil on mortality and major events given early in acute myocardial infarction.
● DAVIT II (1990). Effect of late administration of verapamil on mortality and major events after acute myocardial infarction.

EMIP (1988): European Myocardial Infarction Project.
Study investigating potential time saving with prehospital intervention in acute myocardial infarction.

EMIRAS (1993): Estudio Multicentrico Estreptoquinasa Rupublicas de America del Sur.
A study of late thrombolysis for acute myocardial infarction.

ESVEM (1993): Electro-physiologic Study Versus Electro-cardiographic Monitoring.
Comparison of Holter monitoring with electrophysiological testing to predict anti-dysrhythmic drug efficacy for ventricular dysrhythmias.

EXCEL (1990): Expanded Clinical Evaluation of Lovostatin.
Cholesterol-lowering trial.

FATS (1990): Familial Atherosclerosis Treatment Study.
Regression of atherosclerosis with hypolipidaemic therapy.

GISSI: Gruppo Italiano per lo Studio della Streptochinasi (Sopravvivenza) nell'Infarto miocardico.
● GISSI-1 (1986): The role of thrombolysis in acute myocardial infarction.
● GISSI-2 (1992): Survival of patients with acute myocardial infarction randomised between alteplase and streptokinase, with or without heparin.
● GISSI-3 (1994): Effects of lisinopril and nitrates in patients with acute myocardial infarction.

GREAT (1992): The Grampian Region Early Anistreplase Trial.
Feasibility, safety and efficacy of domiciliary thrombolysis by general practitioners.

GUSTO (1993): Global Utilisation of Streptokinase and Tissue plasminogen activator for Occluded coronary arteries.
A comparison of four thrombolytic strategies for acute myocardial infarction.

HART (1990): Heparin–Aspirin Reperfusion Trial.
A comparison of heparin and low-dose aspirin as an adjunct to thrombolysis with TPA.

HINT (1987): Holland Inter-university Nifedipine/metoprolol Trial.
Efficacy of nifedipine and metoprolol in the early treatment of unstable angina.

ISAM (1986): Intravenous Streptokinase in Acute Myocardial infarction.
Trial showing the efficacy of streptokinase.

ISIS: International Studies of Infarct Survival

- ISIS-1 (1988): Early mortality reduction produced by beta-blockade started early in acute myocardial infarction.
- ISIS-2 (1988): Randomised trial of intravenous streptokinase, oral aspirin, both or neither in suspected acute myocardial infarction.
- ISIS-3 (1992): Randomised comparison of streptokinase vs tissue plasminogen activator vs anistreplase and of aspirin plus heparin vs aspirin alone in suspected myocardial infarction.
- ISIS-4 (1994): Effects of oral mononitrate, of oral captopril and of intravenous magnesium in acute myocardial infarction.

LATE (1992): Late Assessment of Thrombolytic Efficacy.
The effect of alteplase given late after acute myocardial infarction.

LIMIT (1992): Leicester Intravenous Magnesium Intervention Trial.
Value of intravenous magnesium sulphate in suspected acute myocardial infarction.

MIAMI (1985): Metoprolol In Acute Myocardial Infarction.
The effect of beta-blockade following myocardial infarction.

MRFIT: Multiple Risk Factor Intervention Trial.
On-going trial assessing the impact of risk factor modification on coronary heart disease.

PAMI (1993): Primary Angioplasty in Myocardial Infarction.
Immediate angioplasty following thrombolysis for acute myocardial infarction.

POSCH (1990): Programme on Surgical Control of Hyperlipidaemias.
The effect of surgical interventions to reduce hypercholesterolaemia and coronary mortality.

PRIMI (1989): Pro-urokinase In Myocardial Infarction.
Trial of pro-urokinase versus streptokinase for thrombolysis.

PROMISE (1991): Prospective Randomised Milrinone Survival Evaluation.
Effect of oral milrinone on mortality in severe chronic heart failure.

RITA (1993): Randomised Intervention Trial of Angina.
A comparison of angioplasty versus coronary artery surgery.

SAVE (1992): Survival and Ventricular Enlargement.
Effect of captopril on mortality and morbidity in patients with left ventricular dysfunction after myocardial infarction.

SCATI (1989): Studio sulla Calciparina nell'Angina e nella Trombosi ventricolare nell'Infarto.

Trial of subcutaneous calcium heparin for the prevention of left ventricular thrombus following acute myocardial infarction.

SOLVD (1992): Studies Of Left Ventricular Dysfunction.

- Prevention arm: Effects of enalapril on mortality and the development of heart failure in asymptomatic patients with reduced left ventricular ejection fractions.
- Treatment arm: Effect of enalapril on survival of patients with mild to moderate heart failure.

SPRINT (1988): Secondary Prevention Re-infarction Israeli Nifedipine Trial.
The value of nifedipine in acute myocardial infarction.

STARS (1992): St Thomas' Atheroma Regression Study.
Effects on coronary artery disease of lipid-lowering diet or diet plus cholestyramine.

SWIFT (1991): Should We Intervene Following Thrombolysis?
The role of delayed elective intervention versus conservative management following thrombolysis.

TAMI Studies (from 1987): Thrombolysis and Angioplasty in Myocardial Infarction.
Trials of immediate and delayed angioplasty with different thrombolytic regimens.

TAPS (1992): TPA-APSAC Patency Study.
The effect of accelerated (front-loaded) TPA versus APSAC in an angiographic study.

TEAHAT (1990): Thrombolysis Early in Acute Heart Attack Trial.
A study of very early thrombolysis in suspected myocardial infarction.

THRIFT (1992): Thrombo-embolic Risk Factors Trial.
Risks of, and prophylaxis for, venous thromboembolism in hospital patients.

TIMI (from 1987): Thrombolysis in Myocardial Infarction studies.

- TIMI: Comparison of coronary and systemic routes of thrombolysis with TPA.
- TIMI-I: Comparison of TPA and streptokinase.
- TIMI-IIA and IIB: Comparison of angioplasty and conservative strategies after treatment with intravenous TPA in acute myocardial infarction.
- TIMI-IIIA and IIIB: TPA in unstable angina.
- TIMI-IV, V, VI, VII, VIII and IX are still to report.

NB: Angiographers now refer to the degree of obstruction of acutely occluded coronary arteries by the 'TIMI Grade of Occlusion'. Basically, TIMI-0 is a completely occluded vessel, and TIMI-3 is a completely patent vessel. TIMI-1 and TIMI-2 grades of occlusion are partially-opened vessels. The object of thrombolysis is to attain TIMI grade 3.

UNASEM (1992): Unstable Angina Study using Eminase.
Thrombolysis in patients with unstable angina.

V-HeFT I and II (1991): Veterans Heart Failure Trials.
Vasodilator therapy trials in congestive heart failure.

WARIS (1992): Warfarin Re-infarction Study.
Oral anticoagulation for secondary prevention after myocardial infarction.

References

Brown J D (1992) Acronymy. *Medical Journal of Australia,* **157:** 356.
Cheng T O (1992) Acronyms of major cardiologic trials. *American Journal of Cardiology,* **70:** 1512–1514.
Yusuf S, Collins R and Peto R (1984) Why do we need some large, simple randomised trials? *Statistics in Medicine,* **3:** 409–420.

Index

Page numbers in **bold** refer to figures; those in *italics* refer to tables.